Get Through

MRCP Part 2: 450 Best of Fives

Second Edition

To my mother and sister for all their support

Get Through

MRCP Part 2: 450 Best of Fives

Second Edition

Aruna Dias BSc MBBS MRCP (UK)
Specialist Registrar in Gastroenterology & Teaching Fellow,
Newham University Hospital, London and
Clinical Research Fellow,
Queen Mary School of Medicine and Dentistry
London

Editorial Advisor
Eric Beck FRCP (London, Glasgow and Edinburgh)

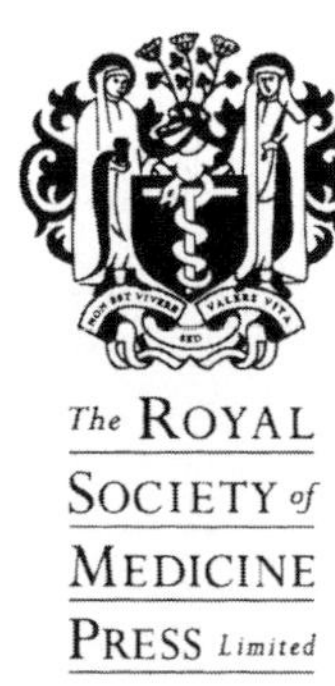

The ROYAL SOCIETY of MEDICINE PRESS Limited

First Edition 2004
Second Edition 2007

Published by the Royal Society of Medicine Press Ltd
1 Wimpole Street, London W1G OAE, UK
Tel: +44 (0) 207 7290 2921
Fax: +44 (0)20 7290 2929
E-mail: publishing@rsm.ac.uk
Website: www.rsmpress.co.uk

British Library Cataloguing in Publication Data
A catalogue record for this book is available from the British Library

ISBN: 978-1-85315-664-9

Distribution in Europe and Rest of the World:
Marston Book Services Ltd
PO Box 269
Abingdon
Oxon OX14 4YN, UK
Tel: +44 (0)1235 465500
Fax: +44 (0)1235 465555
Email: direct.order@marston.co.uk

Distribution in USA and Canada:
Royal Society of Medicine Press Ltd
C/o BookMasters Inc
30 Amberwood Parkway
Ashland, OH 44805, USA
Tel: +1 800 247 6553/ +1 800 266 5564
Fax: +1 410 281 6883
Email: order@bookmasters.com

Distribution in Australia and New Zealand:
Elsevier Australia
30–52 Smidmore Street
Marrickville NSW 2204, Australia
Tel: +61 2 9517 8999
Fax: +61 2 9517 2249
Email: service@elsevier.com.au

Phototypeset by tbc
Printed and bound by Krips b.v., Meppel, The Netherlands

Contents

Acknowledgements vii
Recommended reading ix
Reference values xi
List of abbreviations xv

Introduction 1
Paper 1: Questions 3
Paper 1: Answers 48
Paper 2: Questions 66
Paper 2: Answers 110
Paper 3: Questions 127
Paper 3: Answers 170
Paper 4: Questions 187
Paper 4: Answers 231
Paper 5: Questions 248
Paper 5: Answers 289
Paper 6: Questions 307
Paper 6: Answers 351

Plate Section 370

Index 401

Acknowledgements

I am deeply indebted to the many SHOs, registrars and consultants at William Harvey Hospital, Broomfield Hospital and Newham University Hospital for providing helpful suggestions and proof reading the text. In particular, I would like to thank: Dawn Bayford, Graham Bradley, Ronan Breen, Selina Brewerton, Stuart Coltart, Colley Crawford, Paul Dawkins, Abhishek Deo, Chulanie De Silva, Owen Epstein, Jane Fisher, Jeremy Fletcher, Sue Gelding, Keith Hattatowa, Kate Jones, Reena Joshi, Sam Khandhadia, Cho Cho Khin, Jeshen Lau, Linda Leung, James O'Beirne, Omi Parikh, Ilanga Samaratunga, Amanda Samarawickrama, Alcira Serrano-Gomez, John Sewell, Andrew Solomon, Arul Srinivasan, Chula Wijesurendra, and Yiannis Zoukos.

The imaging questions in this book would not have been possible without the help given to me by the following:

Dr Philip Gishen of Hammersmith Hospital for allowing me to use his extensive collection of radiological imaging; Mrs Bunny Kallipetis of King's College Hospital for helping to retrieve them; Cheryl Richardson at The Royal Marsden Foundation Trust; and Dr Paras Dalal of Lewisham University Hospital for reviewing all of the radiology questions with me.

Dr Mark Monaghan of King's College Hospital for providing the echocardiograms.

Mrs Pamela Walsh and Mrs Sue Walker of the Paula Carr Trust, William Harvey Hospital, for providing the ophthalmology pictures in the original edition of this book, and Dr Shamira Perera of Southampton University Hospital for providing the new ophthalmology pictures, questions and answers in this revised edition.

Dr Wendy Thurrell of William Harvey Hospital and Professor Paul Dhillon, Dr Florence Deroide and Dr Federica Grillo of the Royal Free Hospital for providing the histopathology imaging.

Dr James Nash of Public Health Laboratory Service, Ashford, Kent for providing the microbiology imaging.

Dr Catriona Irvine of William Harvey Hospital and Dr Hilary Dodds of Broomfield Hospital for providing the dermatology pictures.

Dr Wendy Mills, of Newham University Hospital for providing the blood films.

Dr Koolan Nagendran of Broomfield Hospital for providing the neurophysiology pictures.

Dr Del Turner, of Broomfield Hospital and the coronary care units of Broomfield Hospital and William Harvey Hospital for providing the ECGs.

I would also like to thank the following: Dr Una Coales, author of the sister Part I book, for introducing me to the idea of doing this book, Dr Eric Beck for laboriously checking every single question and giving expert guidance on both versions of this book; and Laura Compton and Peter Richardson of RSM Press for publishing this book and being very patient with me while I painstakingly completed this task.

Aruna Dias

Recommended reading

Adair OV (2001) *Cardiology Secrets*, 2nd edn. Philadelphia: Hanley & Belfus

Albert RK et al (2006) *Clinical Critical Care Medicine*. London: Mosby

Bacon BR et al (2005) *Comprehensive Clinical Hepatology*, 2nd edn. London: Mosby

Baker H (1989) *Clinical Dermatology*, 4th edn. London: Baillière Tindall

Beck ER et al (2003) *Tutorials in Differential Diagnosis*, 4th edn. Edinburgh: Churchill Livingstone

Bolognia JL et al (2003) *Dermatology*. London: Mosby

Feldman M et al (2006) *Sleisenger & Fordtran's Gastrointestinal and Liver Disease Pathophysiology/Diagnosis/Management*, 8th edn. Philadelphia: WB Saunders

Greenhalgh T (2006) *How to Read a Paper: the Basics of Evidence-Based Medicine*, 3rd edn. London: Blackwell

Hoffbrand AV, Petit JE (2006) *Essential Haematology*, 5th edn. Oxford: Blackwell

Hricik DE et al (2002) *Nephrology Secrets*, 2nd edn. Philadelphia: Hanley & Belfus

Kumar PJ, Clark M (2005) *Clinical Medicine*, 6th edn. Philadelphia: WB Saunders

McDermott MT (2004) *Endocrine Secrets*, 4th edn. Philadelphia: Hanley & Belfus

McNally PR (2005) *GI/Liver Secrets*, 3rd edn. Philadelphia: Hanley & Belfus

Milner AD & Hull (1998) *Hospital Paediatrics*, 3rd edn. Edinburgh: Churchill Livingstone

Provan D et al (2004) *Oxford Handbook of Clinical Haematology*, 2nd edn. Oxford: Oxford University Press

Ramrakha PS, Moore KP (2006) *Oxford Handbook of Acute Medicine*, 2nd revised edn. Oxford: Oxford University Press

Rolak LA (2005) *Neurology Secrets*, 4th edn. Philadelphia: Hanley & Belfus

West SG (2007) *Rheumatology Secrets*, 2nd edn. Philadelphia: Hanley & Belfus

Wood ME (2003) *Haematology/Oncology Secrets*, 3rd edn. Philadelphia: Hanley & Belfus

The following websites are highly recommended as knowledge sources:

www.emedicine.com
www.uptodate.com

Reference values

HAEMATOLOGY		
Hb	Male	13.0–18.0 g/dl
	Female	11.5–16.5 g/dl
MCH		28–32 pg
MCV		80–96 dl
MCHC		32–35 g/dl
WCC	Total	$4–11 \times 10^9$/L
	Neutrophils	$1.5–7 \times 10^9$/L
	Lymphocytes	$1.5–4 \times 10^9$/L
	Monocytes	$0–0.8 \times 10^9$/L
	Eosinophils	$0.04\text{-}\times 10^9$/L
	Basophils	$0–0.1 \times 10^9$/L
Platelets		$150–400 \times 10^9$/L
Reticulocyte count		0.5–2.5%
ESR	Male	0–20 mm/1st h
	Female	0–30 mm/1st h
CLOTTING		
APTT		30–40 s
Bleeding time		3–8 min
D-dimer		< 1 mg/L
Factor II, V, VII, VIII, IX, X, XI, XII		50–150 IU/dl
FDP		< 100 mg/L
Fibrinogen		1.8–5.4 g/L
INR		< 1.4
PT		11.5–15.5 s
Von Willebrand factor		45–150 IU/dl
BIOCHEMISTRY		
ALT		5–35 U/L
Albumin		37–49 g/L
Aldosterone		
Supine		135–400 pmol/L
Upright		330–830 pmol/L
ALP		45–105 U/L (over 14 years)
Ammonia (plasma)		12–55 mol/L
Amylase		60–180 U/L
Anion gap		12–16 mmol/L
AST		1–31 U/L
Bicarbonate		22–30 mmol/L

Bilirubin	
Total	1–22 mmol/L
Conjugated	0–3.4 mmol/L
C-reactive protein	< 10 mg/L
Caeruloplasmin	200–350 mg/L
Calcitonin	< 27 pmol/L
Calcium (corrected)	2.2–2.6 mmol/L
Chloride	95–107 mmol/L
Cholesterol	
Total	< 5.2 mmol/L
LDL	< 3.36 mmol/L
HDL	> 1.55 mmol/L
Cholecalciferol/25-vitamin D_3	60–105 nmol/L
25-OH-Cholecalciferol/1,25 vitamin D_3	45–90 nmol/L
Complement	
C_3	65–190 mg/dl
C_4	15–50 mg/dl
Copper	12–26 mol/L
Creatine kinase	
Male	25–195 U/L
Female	35–170 U/L
Creatinine	60–110 mmol/L
Ferritin	15–300 g/L
Folate	
Serum	2.0–11.0 g/L
Red cell	160–640 g/L
Gastrin	< 55 pmol/L
GGT	4–35 U/L
Globulin	23–35 g/L
Glucose (plasma)	
Fasting normal	3.0–6.0 mmol/L
Haemoglobin A_1C	3.8–6.4%
Haptoglobin	0.13–1.63 g/L
Immunoglobulin	
IgA	0.8–3.0 g/L
IgG	6.0–13.0 g/L
IgM	0.4–2.5 g/L
IgE	< 120 kU/L
Iron	12–30 mol/L
Lactate (plasma)	0.6–1.8 mmol/L
LDH	10–250 U/L
Magnesium	0.75–1.05 mmol/L
Osmolality (plasma)	278–305 mosmol/kg
PTH (plasma)	0.9–5.4 pmol/L
Phosphate	0.8–1.4 mmol/L
Potassium (K)	3.5–5.0 mmol/L
Prolactin (plasma)	< 360 mU/L

Protein	60–76 g/L
PTH-related peptide	< 1.8 pmol/L
Renin (plasma)	
Supine	1.1–2.7 pmol/ml/h
Upright	3.0–4.3 pmol/ml/h
Sodium (Na)	135–145 mmol/L
Thyroid binding globulin (plasma)	13–28 mg/L
TSH (plasma)	0.4–5 mU/L
Thyroxine	
Total T_4	58–174 nmol/L
Free T_4	10–25 pmol/L
Total T_3	1.07–3.18 nmol/L
Free T_3	5–10 pmol/L
TIBC	45–75 mol/L
Transferrin	2.0–4.0 g/L
Triglyceride	0.45–1.69 mmol/L
Troponin I	< 0.4 g/L
Troponin T	< 0.1 g/L
Urate	
Male	0.23–0.46 mmol/L
Female	0.19–0.36 mmol/L
Urea	2.5–7.5 mmol/L
Vitamin B_{12}	160–760 ng/L

BLOOD GASES

H^+	35–45 nmol/L
pH	7.35–7.45
$PaCO_2$	4.7–6.0 kPa
PaO_2	11.3–12.6 kPa
Base excess	± 2 mmol/L
Carboxyhaemoglobin	
Non-smoker	< 2%
Smoker	3–15%

CSF

Cell count	
Neutrophils	None
Lymphocytes	60–70%
Monocytes	30–50%
Protein	0.15–0.45 g/L
Glucose	3.3–4.4 mmol/L
Opening pressure	5–18 cmH_2O

URINE

5-HIAA	10–47 mol/24 h
Adrenaline	< 144 nmol/24 h
Albumin	< 30 mg/24 h

Calcium	2.5–7.5 mmol/24 h
Dopamine	< 3100 nmol/24 h
Glomerular filtration rate	70–140 ml/min
Noradrenaline	< 570 nmol/24 h
Osmolality	350–1000 mosmol/kg
Protein	< 0.2 g/24 h
VMA	5–35 mol/24 h

List of abbreviations

ACE	angiotensin-converting enzyme
ACTH	adrenocorticotrophic hormone
ADH	antidiuretic hormone
AF	atrial fibrillation
AFP	α-fetoprotein
ARDS	acute respiratory distress syndrome
ALP	alkaline phosphatase
ALT	alanine aminotransferase
ANA	antinuclear antibody
ANCA	antineutrophil cytoplasm antibody
APS	autoimmune polyglandular syndrome
APTT	activated partial thromboplastin time
ARR	absolute risk reduction
AST	aspartate transaminase
AV	atrioventricular
AZT	azidothymidine
CA	cancer antigen
CEA	carcinoembryonic antigen
CD	cluster designation
CJD	Creutzfeldt–Jakob disease
CK	creatine kinase
CMV	cytomegalovirus
COPD	chronic obstructive pulmonary disease
CRP	C-reactive protein
CSF	cerebrospinal fluid
CT	computed tomography
CVP	central venous pressure
DAT	direct antibody test
DDAVP	1-deamino-8-D-vasopressin
DEXA	dual-energy X-ray absorptiometry
DIP	distal interphalangeal
DKA	diabetic ketoacidosis
DLCO	carbon monoxide diffusion in the lung
ds-DNA	double-stranded DNA
ECG	electrocardiogram
EEG	electroencephalogram
ERCP	endoscopic retrograde cholangiopancreatography
ESR	erythrocyte sedimentation ratio
FBC	full blood count
FEV_1	forced expiratory volume in 1 second
FiO_2	fractional concentration of oxygen in inspired gas
FOB	faecal occult blood
FSGS	focal segmental glomerulosclerosis

FSH	follicle-stimulating hormone
FVC	forced vital capacity
G6PD	glucose-6-phosphate dehydrogenase
GBM	glomerular basement membrane
GCS	Glasgow coma scale
GGT	γ-glutamyltransferace
GI	gastrointestinal
GVHD	graft versus host disease
5-HIAA	5-hydroxyindoleacetic acid
HAART	highly active antiretroviral treatment
Hb	haemoglobin
HBcAg	hepatitis B core antigen
HBeAg	hepatitis B e antigen
HbsAg	hepatitis B surface antigen
HCG	human chorionic gonadotrophin
HCV	hepatitis C virus
HDL	high density lipoprotein
HIV	human immunodeficiency virus
HMA	homovanillic acid
HOCM	hypertrophic obstructive cardiomyopathy
HSMN	hereditary motor and sensory neuropathy
HSP	Henoch–Schönlein purpura
HSV	herpes simplex virus
Ig	immunoglobulin
INR	international normalised ratio
ITP	idiopathic thrombocytopenic purpura
JVP	jugular venous pressure
KCO	diffusion coefficient
LBBB	left bundle branch block
LDH	lactate dehydrogenase
LDL	low density lipoprotein
LFT	liver function test
LH	luteinising hormone
MCH	mean corpuscular haemoglobin
MCHC	mean corpuscular haemoglobin concentration
MCV	mean corpuscular volume
MEN	multiple endocrine neoplasia
MI	myocardial infarction
MRCP	magnetic resonance cholangiopancreatography
MRI	magnetic resonance imaging
MSU	midstream urine
NG	nasogastric
NNT	number needed to treat
NSAID	non-steroidal anti-inflammatory drug
OR	odds ratio
PAWP	pulmonary artery wedge pressure

PCO_2	partial pressure of carbon dioxide
PCR	polymerase chain reaction
PCV	polycythaemia rubra vera
PEF	peak expiratory flow
PEG	percutaneous endoscopic gastrostomy
PO_2	partial pressure of oxygen
PRV	polycythaemia rubra vera
PSA	prostate specific antigen
PT	prothrombin time
PTC	percutaneous transhepatic cholangiogram
PTH	parathyroid hormone
RBBB	right bundle branch block
RBC	red blood cell
RCT	randomised controlled trial
RNA	ribonucleic acid
RTA	renal tubular acidosis
SIADH	syndrome of inappropriate ADH secretion
SLE	systemic lupus erythematosus
T_3	tri-iodothyronine
T_4	thyroxine
TB	tuberculosis
TIBC	total iron binding capacity
TLC	total lung capacity
TPA	tissue plasminogen activator
TSH	thyroid-stimulating hormone
TT	thrombin time
U&E	urea and electrolytes
VIP	vasointestinal peptide
VMA	vanillylmandelic acid
VT/VF	ventricular tachycardia/fibrillation
WCC	white cell count
WPW	Wolff–Parkinson–White

Introduction

Medical training is going through a radical upheaval with the abolition of the old SHO grade and the introduction of the new ST grade. What has not changed is the need to pass the MRCP examination. The MRCP (UK) examination is an obstacle that, in the UK, has to be passed after a statutory minimum period of prescribed medical training and before completing specialist training. Finding the time to study -while dealing with on-call duties, shift patterns, ward work, not forgetting other aspects of social life, is not an easy task.

Although no book can guarantee you will have every answer at your fingertips, it can help you to make the best use of your knowledge by familiarising you with new formats illustrated by copious examples.

Both the Part 1 and Part 2 exams are wholly MCQ. Generally, a stem will have five completions each having some degree of correctness/plausibility and the task is to choose the SINGLE best answer (hence best of five [BOF]). A relatively new introduction to the exam involves completions extended to 10–15, and two or three answers have to be chosen. There is no negative marking and the pass rate is no longer predetermined as a fixed percentage of candidates (peer reference). Rather a predetermined standard is set by the examiners and all candidates achieving it will pass (criterion reference). Candidates are no longer competing against each other.

The details of criterion referencing/standard setting in Parts 1 and 2 have not been made public. In this book, as in the first edition, the degree of difficulty of each question is graded on a three-point scale, making a judgement on what proportion of candidates just passing the whole examination are likely to get that particular question right, viz:

*	25–50% 'just passing' candidates expected to get correct
**	50–75% 'just passing' candidates expected to get correct
***	75–100% 'just passing' candidates expected to get correct

Thus an easier paper will require a higher mark to pass, as shown in the accompanying table, where the notional pass marks in the six papers in the book range from 57% to 65%. (Note that 'blind' guessing gives up to a 1 in 5 or 20% chance of being correct!)

Criterion referencing of the six papers in the book (note that although there are 75 questions in each paper a few questions are extended, requiring two or three answers):

Paper	Difficulty of questions *	**	***	Pass mark	% mark
1	18	41	18	48/77	63
2	23	41	18	50/82	65
3	18	43	15	47/76	62
4	14	42	21	50/77	65
5	20	44	11	45/77	58
6	28	39	11	45/78	57

As the questions are now multiple choice a much wider syllabus is covered and questions can be asked from different angles. Examiners setting questions go to great lengths to avoid ambiguity in their wording. However, sometimes an answer may be so blindingly obvious that it would be difficult to find four plausible distracters; look out for the occasional format of: 'Every answer is true **EXCEPT** for ...' .

Generally, in answering the question, think of the answer you would give before looking at each distracter. If you find your answer among them you are probably right and need not waste valuable time weighing up the pros and cons of each distractor in turn. Incidentally, the order in which they appear is usually alphabetical so do not look for patterns of favoured responses in the ABCDE – they do not exist.

The vast majority of these questions are based on real patients and clinical scenarios. The key to passing is your ability to apply the largely theoretical knowledge you have acquired in passing Part 1 to the individual clinical problems posed in Part 2.

The core specialities are covered but there are also questions on intensive care medicine, oncology, transplantation and HIV and genitourinary medicine. Questions from the earlier edition have been revised so as to keep up to date with new developments in medicine. The answers section gives you detailed explanations not only for why one is the best but also why the others are less good, including key references for further reading.

In the interests of uncluttered reading you will find at the beginning a list of abbreviations used throughout the book and in everyday life. You will find a list of normal values with only a few given in the text. Increasingly there is standardisation of test methods but enzymes and hormone measurement references may still vary. The index will help to locate particular points.

It is crucial for you visit the MRCP website (www.mrcpuk.org) as this gives you the most up to date information about the content, organisation and regulations governing the examination.

We hope you will find this a useful and pleasurable form of programmed learning even if you do not always agree with everything written.

We wish you the best of luck in the exam.

Paper 1

Questions

1.1 A 60-year-old man with a history of congestive cardiac failure and mild asthma presented with worsening shortness of breath that was now occurring at rest. He could walk only 20 m on flat ground and could only manage six stairs before having to stop to catch his breath. He had no chest pain. He slept with three pillows at night. He stopped smoking over 30 years ago and did not drink alcohol. He was currently on furosemide 80 mg o.d., enalapril 20 mg o.d. and salbutamol inhalers.

On examination his pulse was 72 regular and his blood pressure was 155/90. His JVP was elevated +4 cm above the sternal angle. Heart sounds were normal and there were no murmurs. His chest was clear and his respiratory rate was 18 breaths/min. O_2 saturation on air was 94% and peak flow was 300 L/min.

Bloods	Hb	15.0	WCC	10.0
	Platelets	300	Na	130
	K	4.2	Urea	5.8
	Creatinine	100		
Echocardiogram	Mild tricuspid regurgitation			
	No evidence of pulmonary hypertension			
	Severe left ventricular systolic dysfunction			
	Ejection fraction 35%			

The most appropriate management for this patient would be:

A add digoxin
B add low dose atenolol
C add low dose spironolactone
D change furosemide to co-amilofruse
E increase furosemide to b.d.

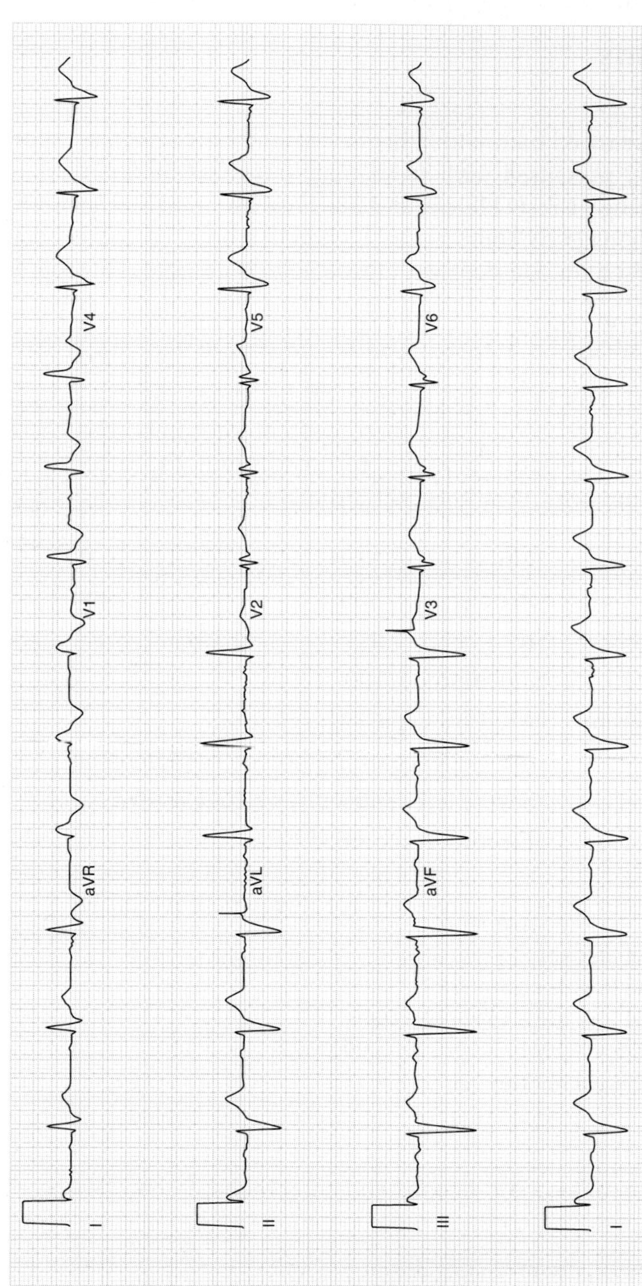
I
aVR
V1
V4
II
aVL
V2
V5
III
aVF
V3
V6
I

1.2 An 84-year-old woman was referred with dizziness.

ECG PR interval 0.20 s, QRS duration 0.16 s, QT interval 0.28 s

Her ECG shows:

- A left bundle branch block
- B right bundle branch block
- C right bundle branch block and left anterior fascicular block
- D right bundle branch block and left posterior fascicular block
- E trifascicular block

1.3 A 19-year-old woman was admitted with a salicylate overdose. She had taken 40 tablets 16 h ago. She complained of abdominal pain, vomiting, tinnitus and sweating. She was not on any other medication and had not drunk alcohol at the time of the overdose.

On examination she was hyperventilating. Her temperature was 38.0°C, pulse 98 regular and blood pressure 100/60. Her JVP was not elevated and heart sounds were normal. Her respiratory rate was 30 breaths/min and her chest was clear. She had diffuse abdominal tenderness. There was no focal neurological abnormality.

Bloods	Hb	13.8	WCC	10.0
	Platelets	180	INR	1.1
	Na	135	K	5.8
	Urea	19.8	Creatinine	240
	Protein	70	Albumin	39
	Bilirubin	14	ALT	55
	ALP	90	GGT	39
	Glucose	3.0		
Paracetamol	Not detected			
Salicylate	530 mg/L			
Arterial blood gases on air	pH	7.21	PCO_2	2.1
	PO_2	10.4	Bicarbonate	10.2
	Base excess	−15.4		

Of the following statements concerning her management the one which is correct is:

- A development of convulsions would be an indication for haemodialysis
- B forced alkaline diuresis is the treatment of choice
- C pyrexia would suggest underlying sepsis
- D immediate gastric lavage should be given
- E she should be treated with intravenous N-acetylcysteine

1.4 A 4-year-old boy presented with sudden onset fever and painful oral lesions. (Figure 1.4, page 370.)

The most likely organism to have caused this is:

A *Candida albicans*
B *Molluscum contagiosum*
C *Staphylococcus aureus*
D *Streptococcus pyogenes*
E *Varicella* zoster virus

1.5 A 55-year-old woman complained of pain in her legs and difficulty in walking over the past 2 months. She had a previous medical history of insulin dependent diabetes and had recently been diagnosed as having coeliac disease.

On examination her pulse was 72 regular and BP 154/90. Her chest was clear and abdominal examination was normal. She had no rash. Her lower limb muscles were tender and there was weakness of her quadriceps and hip girdle muscles but no wasting. There was normal tone, power, reflexes and sensation.

Bloods				
	Hb	12.2	MCV	101.3
	WCC	6.7	Platelets	325
	Na	144	K	4.5
	Urea	3.7	Creatinine	100
	Calcium	1.99	Phosphate	0.6
	ALP	140	Albumin	38
	Protein	70	Glucose	10.5
	HbA_{1c}	7.5%		

The most likely cause of her symptoms is:

A diabetic amyotrophy
B osteomalacia
C osteoporosis
D periodic paralysis
E peripheral neuropathy

1.6 It has been proposed that continued excessive alcohol intake is associated with the development of stomach carcinoma. You have been asked to design a study to investigate this possibility.

The most appropriate study design would be:

A case control study
B case reports
C cohort study
D cross-sectional study
E randomised controlled trial

1.7 A 55-year-old Caucasian woman with Crohn's disease presented with back pain. She had not had any falls. She had had numerous courses of prednisolone in the past but was not on hormone replacement therapy. A DEXA scan was performed and she has returned wanting to know the result.

DEXA scan of total hip	T score	–1.5
	Z score	–1.6

The interpretation of the DEXA scan result is:

A normal bone mass
B osteopaenia appropriate for her age
C osteopaenia inappropriate for her age
D osteoporosis appropriate for her age
E osteoporosis inappropriate for her age

1.8 A 13-year-old boy presented to Accident & Emergency with severe generalised bruising following a fall. Apart from a sore throat 1 week ago, he had no previous medical history.

On examination he was apyrexial. Physical examination was normal apart from bruising all over his body and limbs. There was no lymphadenopathy.

Bloods	Hb	12.9	MCV	78
	WCC	11.6	Platelets	15
	Neutrophils	5.8	Lymphocytes	5.1
	Monocytes	0.4		

The most likely diagnosis is:

A acute lymphoblastic leukaemia
B acute myeloid leukaemia
C aplastic anaemia
D idiopathic thrombocytopenic purpura
E Henoch-Schönlein purpura

1.9 A 16-year-old girl presented to Accident & Emergency with abdominal pain. She had had recurrent attacks in the past. The pain was generalised and was associated with nausea and shortness of breath. Until now the pain had resolved spontaneously but could last for hours. She had no bowel or urinary problems. She was not pregnant. Her mother used to suffer similar problems as a teenager.

On examination she was in pain. Her temperature was 37.0°C, pulse 120 regular and blood pressure 130/70. Her respiratory rate was 24 breaths/min and her chest was clear. There was generalized abdominal tenderness but bowel sounds were present. Rectal examination was normal.

Bloods	Hb	13.5	WCC	7.8
	Platelets	190	Na	140
	K	4.4	Urea	4.8
	Creatinine	80	Protein	74
	Albumin	42	Bilirubin	12
	ALT	25	ALP	85
	Amylase	50	Calcium	2.25
	PO_4	0.9	ESR	12
	CRP	10		
Urinalysis	No protein, glucose or white cells			
	HCG negative			
Chest X-ray	Normal			
CT abdomen	Some localized oedema in proximal jejunum			
Laparoscopy	No abnormalities detected			

The most likely diagnosis is:

A acute intermittent porphyria
B familial Mediterranean fever
C hereditary angioedema
D polyarteritis nodosa
E Wiskott–Aldrich syndrome

1.10 A 72-year-old man presented with a 1-week history of severe abdominal pain and diarrhoea with some blood mixed with stool. He opened his bowels up to eight times per day. He had a normal appetite but had lost some weight. Five days ago he had been discharged from hospital with an infective exacerbation of chronic obstructive pulmonary disease, where his treatment included steroids, nebulisers and antibiotics. He had no recent foreign travel.

On examination his temperature was 37.5°C, pulse 92 regular and blood pressure 123/88. His chest was clear. His abdomen was generally tender but there was no organomegaly. Flexible sigmoidoscopy was performed and biopsies taken. (Figure 1.10, page 370.)

The most likely diagnosis is:

A colorectal carcinoma
B Crohn's disease
C giardiasis
D melanosis coli
E pseudomembranous colitis

1.11 A 28-year-old man presented with a 7-day history of fever, watery diarrhoea and abdominal pain, and now had developed a dry cough. He had returned from South Africa 5 days ago where he had been on safari. He had no previous medical problems, was not on any medication and did not take malaria prophylaxis.

On examination he had a few cervical lymph nodes. His temperature was 39.0°C, pulse 95 regular and blood pressure 118/76. JVP was not elevated and heart sounds and chest were normal. His abdomen was soft and he had 2 cm non-tender hepatomegaly.

Bloods	Hb	12.9	WCC	2.7
	Neutrophils	1.3	Lymphocytes	1.0
	Eosinophils	0.1	Platelets	219
	Na	139	K	4.2
	Urea	3.8	Creatinine	78
	Protein	65	Albumin	35
	Bilirubin	13	ALT	25
	ALP	100	ESR	36
	CRP	43	INR	1.1
Malaria blood films	Negative			
Chest X-ray	Normal			

The most likely diagnosis is:

A amoebic dysentery
B blackwater fever
C dengue haemorrhagic fever
D typhoid
E yellow fever

1.12 A 24-year-old woman presented with a 6-week history of headache and blurred vision and this had affected her job. There was no significant previous medical history. She did not smoke and drank half a bottle of wine at the weekend. The headaches began at the back of her head and were associated with flashing lights and zigzag lines. There was no vomiting, falls or fits. Her appetite and weight were stable. There was no family history of migraine. Apart from the combined oral contraceptive pill she was not on any medication

On examination she was apyrexial, pulse 90 regular and blood pressure 142/84. Respiratory and neck examinations were normal. Examination of her cranial nerves and her peripheral nervous system was unremarkable. Fundoscopic examination was performed. (Figure 1.12, page 370.)

Bloods	Hb	13.8	WCC	5.8
	Platelets	190	ESR	8
	Na	141	K	4.6
	Urea	4.7	Creatinine	46
	CRP	13	PT	11.9
	APTT	30		
CT brain	Normal			

The most helpful investigation would be:

- A cerebral angiography
- B EEG
- C lumbar puncture
- D magnetic resonance venography
- E thrombophilia screen

1.13 A 35-year-old woman with insulin dependent diabetes mellitus was referred with recent onset blurred vision. Fundoscopy was performed. (Figure 1.13, page 371.)

The most likely cause of her worsening vision is:

- A branch retinal artery occlusion
- B branch retinal vein occlusion
- C diabetic maculopathy
- D traction retinal detachment
- E vitreous haemorrhage

1.14 A 65-year-old man had a colonoscopy to investigate the cause of his rectal bleeding. At the rectosigmoid junction a large ulcerated mass was found that extended halfway into the diameter of the lumen and bled readily on contact. A barium enema showed no other mass in his large intestine and abdominal ultrasound revealed no liver metastases.

He had a sigmoid colectomy. Histology of the mass revealed poorly differentiated adenocarcinoma with invasion through the serosa but no regional lymph node involvement.

Using the modified Dukes' classification system, this patient's tumour would be graded as:

A Dukes' A
B Dukes' B_1
C Dukes' B_2
D Dukes' C_1
E Dukes' C_2

1.15 A 44-year-old man presented with a 2-day history of painful, swollen left knee. It came on gradually and there was no history of trauma or joint pain. He did not have any other previous medical history. He was not on any medication.

On examination he was in pain. His temperature was 37.0°C, pulse 98 regular and blood pressure 130/88. Cardiovascular and respiratory examinations were normal. His left knee was swollen, erythematous and tender with an obvious effusion but normal range of movements. There was no rash, and tone, power, reflexes and sensation were normal.

Bloods	Hb 13.6		WCC	9.2
	Neutrophils 6.5		Platelets	348
	Na 138		K	4.3
	Urea 3.5		Creatinine	68
	ESR 24		CRP	49
Blood cultures	No growth			
Rheumatoid factor	Negative			
Left knee X-ray	Soft tissue swelling			
	No fracture			
Synovial fluid	Slightly turbid appearance			
	WCC 35 000			
	Neutrophils 60%			
	Protein 35			
	Crystals showing negative birefringence			

The most likely diagnosis is:

A bacterial septic arthritis
B gout
C osteoarthritis
D palindromic rheumatoid arthritis
E pseudogout

1.16 A 19-year-old student was admitted with headache, photophobia and malaise for 1 day. She had no previous medical history and was not on any medication.

On examination she had a decreased GCS of 9/15 with a temperature of 38.5°C, pulse 110 regular and blood pressure 90/55. JVP was not elevated and heart sounds were normal. Respiratory and abdominal examinations were normal. Cranial nerve examination was normal and pupils were equal and reactive with no papilloedema. Her arms were flexed and hands were clenched into fists. Her legs were extended and plantars were unresponsive. There was a non-blanching rash on her legs. (Figure 1.16, page 371.)

CT head Normal with no intracranial lesion seen

Concerning her management the statement which is correct is:

A in addition to antibiotics, treat with intravenous steroids
B perform a lumbar puncture if clotting and platelet count are normal
C treat with intravenous aciclovir and intravenous cefotaxime
D treatment with activated protein C is contraindicated
E unless this is meningococcal disease contact tracing is unnecessary

1.17 A 55-year-old man presented with collapse. His GCS at the time of presentation was 14/15.

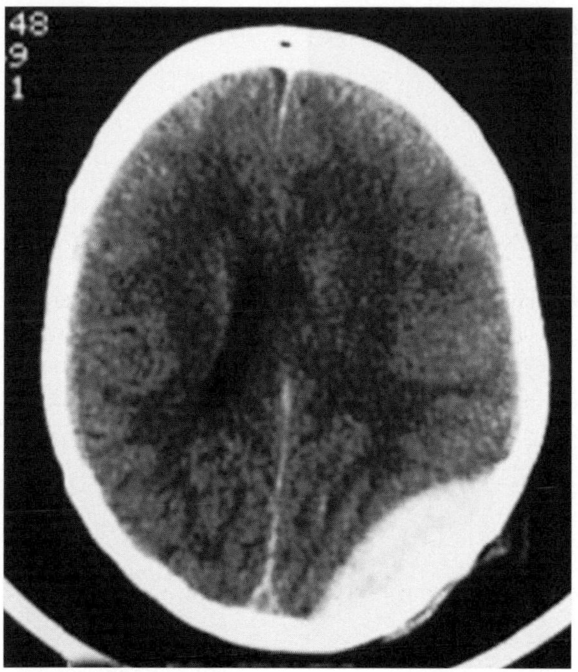

The CT scan shows:

- A cerebral abscess
- B extradural haematoma
- C intracerebral haemorrhage
- D subarachnoid haemorrhage
- E subdural haematoma

1.18 This is a barium Swallow in a 52-year-old woman presented with a 6-week history of progressive dysphagia and weight loss.

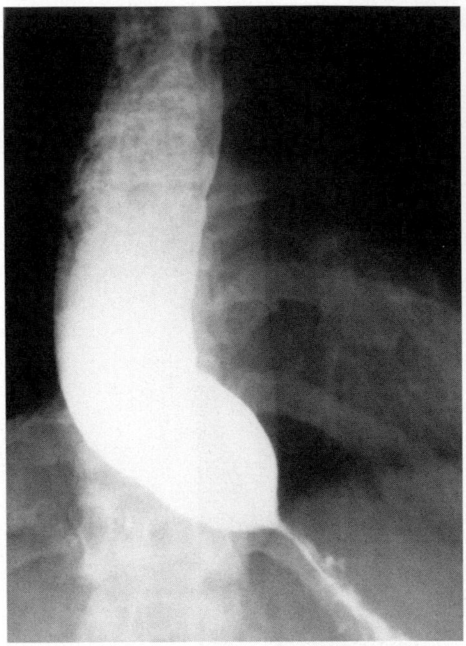

The most likely diagnosis is:

A achalasia
B benign stricture
C carcinoma of the oesophagus
D oesophageal candidiasis
E oesophageal varices

1.19 A 51-year-old woman was admitted with an anterior myocardial infarction (MI). She was treated with tissue plasminogen activator. She made an uneventful recovery.

Which **THREE** of the folowing medications/classes of medication have **NOT** been shown conclusively to improve prognosis post MI?

A angiotension converting enzyme (ACE) inhibitors
B aspirin
C atenolol
D calcium antagonists
E clopidogrel
F low molecular weight heparin
G N3 polyunsaturated fat fish oils
H nicorandil
I nitrates
J simvastatin

1.20 A 75-year-old man was referred for a pacemaker check because he complained of dizziness. He had no chest pain or shortness of breath. He had a previous history of myocardial infarction 10 years ago. He had a permanent pacemaker fitted 2 years ago for complete heart block. He was only on aspirin.

His pulse was 60 paced and blood pressure 116/58. His JVP was not elevated and both heart sounds were normal.

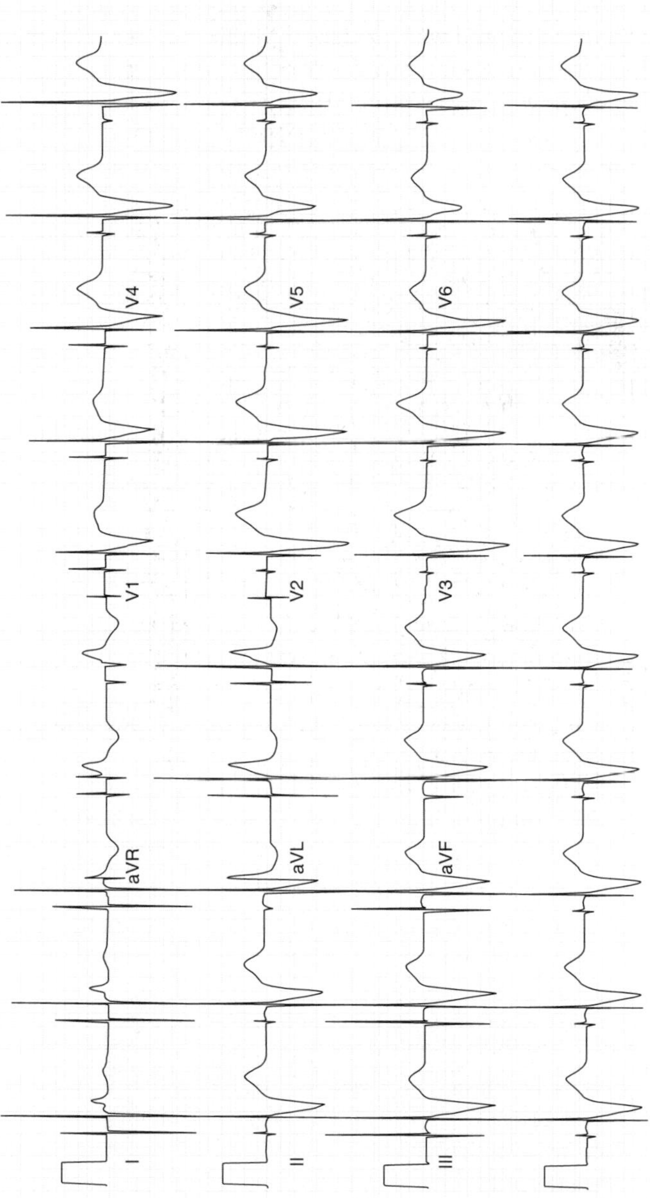

Of the following statements concerning this patient the one which is true is:

A anaemia can alter the rate of the pacemaker
B he is likely to have a VVI pacemaker
C his pacemaker is malfunctioning and that is the cause of his dizziness
D pyrexia can alter the rate of the pacemaker
E when he had his original pacemaker fitted he was likely to have been in atrial fibrillation

1.21 A 25-year-old man was brought in to the Accident & Emergency department after attempting suicide by inhalation of carbon monoxide. He had a headache and had vomited three times. He had no past medical problems and was not on any medication. He did not drink alcohol or smoke.

On examination he was drowsy and there was a red discoloration around his cheeks and some blueness of his lips. His pulse was 110 regular and blood pressure 100/74. His JVP was not elevated and heart sounds were normal. His respiratory rate was 24 breaths/min and his chest was clear. Abdominal examination was normal. There were no focal neurological abnormalities.

Arterial blood	pH	7.40	PCO_2	2.9
gases on air	PO_2	12.4	Bicarbonate	24
	Base excess	1.0		
	Carbon monoxide	30%		

The following statement concerning this patient is true:

A a high PCO_2 is associated with a worse prognosis
B carbon monoxide causes the oxygen-dissociation curve to shift to the right
C development of focal neurological signs is an indication for hyperbaric oxygen therapy
D intravenous doxapram would improve his condition
E pulse oximetery is an accurate measure of carboxyhaemoglobin (COHb)

1.22 A 29-year-old woman presented with a non-pruritic skin rash on her back, shoulders and arms. Ten days ago she had had a bout of tonsillitis. (Figure 1.22, page 371.)

The most likely diagnosis is:

A guttate psoriasis
B lichen planus
C pityriasis versicolor
D tinea corporis
E vitiligo

1.23 A 30-year-old woman who was 15 weeks pregnant developed sweating and tachycardia. She also complained of diplopia and a swelling in her neck.

On examination she had a temperature of 37.3°C, pulse 110 regular and blood pressure 140/65. She had a tender, smooth enlarged goitre and exophthalmos.

Bloods	TSH	< 0.1	Free T_4	45
	Free T_3	18		

The most appropriate treatment for this patient would be:

A atenolol
B prednisolone
C propylthiouracil
D iodine-131
E thyroidectomy

1.24 Two thousand patients with stroke were randomly allocated to treatment with either aspirin or placebo. At the end of 1 year five patients in the aspirin group had died compared to 15 of the placebo group.

The number needed to treat (NNT) to prevent one death is:

A 5
B 15
C 75
D 100
E 200

1.25 A 75-year-old woman was referred with black stools. It was late at night when she presented to Accident & Emergency. She had recently been started on diclofenac for osteoarthritis. There was no haematemesis but she had passed approximately 400 ml of dark motions today. She had no other medical problems and was not taking any other medication. She did not drink alcohol.

On examination she was apyrexial. Her pulse was 98 regular and blood pressure 120/70 with no postural drop. Abdominal examination revealed some epigastric tenderness but no guarding and bowel sounds were present. Rectal examination revealed fresh melaena.

Bloods	Hb	11.4	WCC	9.6
	Platelets	500	INR	1.2
	Na	139	K	4.5
	Urea	7.8	Creatinine	85
	Albumin	40	Protein	70
	Bilirubin	19	AST	26
	ALP	100	Amylase	95
Chest X-ray	No free gas under the diaphragm			
Abdominal X-ray	No evidence of obstruction			

Of the following, the next step in the immediate management of this patient would be:

- A immediate upper gastrointestinal endoscopy
- B intravenous terlipressin
- C intravenous omeprazole
- D intravenous propanolol
- E intravenous ranitidine

1.26 A 42-year-old woman was admitted with ascites, which had been increasing over the past 2 months. She also complained of progressive lethargy and that her skin bruised easily. Her urine was dark but stools were normal coloured. She did not drink alcohol, had no previous medical history and was not on any medication.

On examination she looked pale. She was apyrexial and there was no lymphadenopathy. Her pulse was 94 regular and blood pressure 110/75. Her abdomen was distended with generalized tenderness and there was 3 cm hepatomegaly.

Bloods	Hb	8.9	MCV	76.4
	WCC	2.9	Platelets	98
	Na	140	K	4.3
	Urea	5.9	Creatinine	90
	Protein	65	Albumin	32
	Bilirubin	18	ALT	65
	ALP	100	INR	1.1
Abdominal ultrasound	Hepatomegaly with enlarged caudate lobe			
	No flow in hepatic veins			
	Gross ascites			

The most helpful test to establish the diagnosis would be:

- A bone marrow aspirate and trephine
- B haemoglobin electrophoresis
- C Ham's test
- D osmotic fragility studies
- E Schumm's test

1.27 A 55-year-old man was referred with hepatomegaly and deranged liver function tests. He did not drink alcohol and had no risk factors for hepatitis. He had a previous medical history of rheumatoid arthritis, which affected his hands, elbows and knees. He was not on any medication. He had a normal appetite and stable weight.

On examination he was not jaundiced or pale. His pulse was 79 regular and blood pressure 140/89. Respiratory examination was normal. He had 6 cm hepatomegaly but no other signs of chronic liver disease.

Bloods	Hb 13.4		WCC	4.5
	Platelets	110	INR	1.4
	Na	132	K	4.8
	Urea	3.9	Creatinine	80
	Albumin	33	Protein	70
	Bilirubin	30	ALT	85
	ALP	105	GGT	39
	Glucose	5.4		
Hepatitis A, B, C serology	Negative			
Liver biopsy (H&E)	(Figure 1.27, page 372.)			

The most likely diagnosis is:

- A α_1-antitrypsin deficiency
- B amyloidosis
- D haemochromatosis
- D hepatocellular carcinoma
- E Wilson's disease

1.28 A 45-year-old man known to have contracted HIV was referred for HAART (highly active antiretroviral treatment). In the past year he had developed lobar pneumonia due to *Streptococcus pneumoniae*. He had no other medical problems but continued to inject heroin. He was hepatitis B and C negative. He had a normal appetite and his weight was stable.

Apart from oral candidiasis, no abnormalities were found on physical examination.

Bloods	Hb	12.4	WCC	3.9
	Platelets	150		
CD_4	450			
Viral load	26 000			

Of the following statements concerning this patient's management the one that is correct is:

- A zidovudine (AZT) should be avoided in anaemic patients
- B start on HAART
- C treat with long-term septrin
- D standard HAART treatment consists of two drugs
- E viral load is the most important determinant of when to start HAART

1.29 A 47-year-old man presented with inability to walk. His problem started yesterday with weakness but now he could not stand. He had not opened his bowels yet. He was able to use his arms normally and there were no problems with his eyes or swallowing but he had some shortness of breath on exertion. Two weeks ago he had had salmonella gastroenteritis. There was no previous medical history and he was not on any medication.

On examination he was anxious. His pulse was 120 regular and blood pressure 130/94. Respiratory examination was normal. There was no palpable bladder but normal anal tone. There was no muscle wasting or fasciculation. In the lower limbs tone was decreased, power was 0/5 and reflexes were absent. There was decreased sensation in the distal lower limbs. Upper limbs and cranial nerve examination were normal.

Bloods	Hb	12.8	WCC	7.4
	Platelets	223	ESR	36
	Glucose	5.6		
CSF	Glucose	3.6	Protein	1.7 g/L
	WCC	5		

Poor prognosis would be associated with the presence or development of:

- A *Escherichia coli* infection
- B loss of reflexes and sensory involvement
- C low peak expiratory flow rate (PEFR)
- D low vital capacity
- E *Salmonella typhi* infection

1.30 A 45-year-old woman was admitted with decreased level of consciousness. No history was available.

Arterial blood gases on air	pH	7.25	PCO_2	3.5
	PO_2	7.9	Bicarbonate	15.6
	Base excess	–7.6		

These blood gases show:

A metabolic acidosis and type I respiratory failure
B metabolic acidosis and type II respiratory failure
C metabolic alkalosis and type II respiratory failure
D mixed respiratory and metabolic acidosis and type II respiratory failure
E respiratory acidosis and metabolic alkalosis and type I respiratory failure

1.31 A 65-year-old woman was referred because of tiredness, shoulder and hip stiffness and pain, waking her at night persistently for 3 months. Paracetamol gave little relief. She was an insulin dependent diabetic with good control. She had no headache, visual problems, joint swellings or skin rashes.

On examination she was not in pain. Her pulse was 78 regular and blood pressure 143/88. She had normal tone, power, reflexes and sensation in her limbs. There was normal range of movements and no tenderness was elicited anywhere.

Bloods	Hb	14.4	WCC	6.8
	Platelets	369	ESR	88
	Na	145	K	4.1
	Urea	5.7	Creatinine	100
	Protein	72	Albumin	41
	Bilirubin	8	ALT	20
	ALP	130	GGT	65
	Creatine kinase	80	Glucose	7.8
	$HbA1_c$	6.9	TSH	1.4
	Free T_4	16		

The most likely diagnosis is:

A diabetic amyotrophy
B fibromyalgia
C giant cell arteritis
D polymyalgia rheumatica
E polymyositis

1.32 A 30-year-old woman presented with vaginal discharge and an unpleasant odour post-coitus. She was 18 weeks pregnant with her second pregnancy. The first pregnancy went to term and resulted in a healthy boy being delivered.

On speculum examination she produced a thin, watery, homogeneous discharge, pH 7.72. (Figure 1.32, page 372)

Microscopy No inflammatory cells, no lactobacilli

The most likely diagnosis is:

A Bacterial vaginosis
B *Candida* sp
C *Chlamydia* sp
D *Gonorrhoea* sp
E *Trichomonas* sp

1.33 A 23-year-old man presented to Accident & Emergency short of breath.

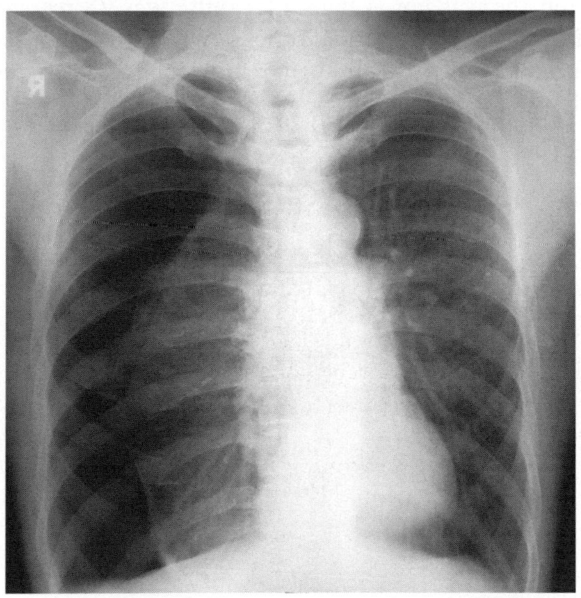

Of the following statements the one that is **FALSE** is:

A an inspiratory click may be heard on the affected side
B histiocytosis X could be the underlying cause of his chest problem
C needle thoracocentesis in the second left intercostal space at the midclavicular line should be undertaken
D pleuradhesis should be considered if this problem recurs
E the condition is more prevalent in young, thin men

1.34 A 65-year-old woman presented with early satiety and weight loss.

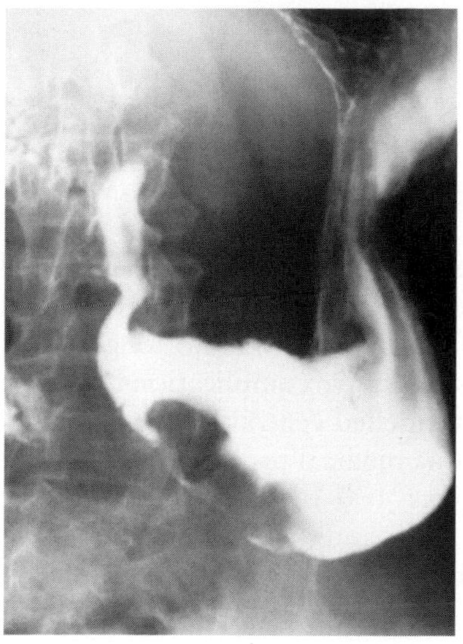

The risk factor that is **NOT** associated with her condition is:

A achlorhydria
B alcohol
C blood group O
D *Helicobacter pylori* infection
E smoking

1.35 A 45-year-old woman was admitted with weakness, headaches and palpitations. Her symptoms had been getting worse over the past month. She had no previous medical history. She did not smoke or drink alcohol.

On examination her pulse was 90 regular and blood pressure was 190/105. Her JVP was not elevated and heart sounds and chest examination were normal. Abdominal examination was normal.

Bloods	Na	140	K	2.8
	Urea	5.0	Creatinine	110
	Glucose	6.5	Magnesium	0.65
Arterial blood gases on air	pH	7.51	PCO_2	4.5
	PO_2	11.4	Bicarbonate	35
	Base excess	7.5		

The **LEAST** likely diagnosis in this patient is:

A Conn's syndrome
B Cushing's syndrome
C Liddle's syndrome
D liquorice ingestion
E phaeochromocytoma

1.36 A 55-year-old woman on the intensive care unit had been admitted after an emergency operation for bowel perforation. Now, 6 days later, she developed worsening shortness of breath. She was no longer being mechanically ventilated. Due to postoperative complications she was given total parenteral nutrition via a tunnelled central line, which had since been removed. She had no previous medical problems.

On examination her pulse was 100 regular and blood pressure 120/84. Her JVP was elevated + 4 cm and there was a pansystolic murmur. There were crackles at both lung bases.

Echocardiogram:

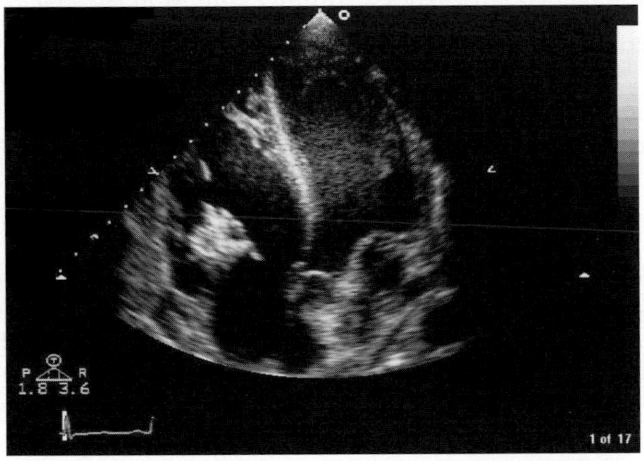

The most likely diagnosis is:

A atrial septal defect
B infective endocarditis
C intracardiac thrombus
D myxoma
E ventricular aneurysm

1.37 A 30-year-old woman complained of itching on her hands and forearms for 2 weeks. (Figure 1.37, page 372.)

The most appropriate treatment for this patient is:

- A oral chlorpheniramine
- B oral prednisolone
- C topical clotrimazole
- D topical hydrocortisone
- E topical malathion

1.38 A 56-year-old man was admitted to Accident & Emergency with general lethargy, abdominal discomfort and weight loss. He had been feeling unwell over the last 3 weeks.

Bloods	Calcium	3.22	Phosphate	1.2
	Albumin	35	ALP	120
	PTH	1.0		
	PTH related peptide	increased		

These findings are most consistent with:

- A adenocarcinoma of the kidney
- B medullary carcinoma of the thyroid
- C oat cell carcinoma of the lung
- D primary hyperparathyroidism
- E tertiary hyperparathyroidism

1.39 It has been proposed that serum CA19-9 could be used to screen for pancreatic carcinoma. A trial in 600 patients was carried out; of these 195 cases developed carcinoma. The CA19-9 detected 70 cases and 30 false positives.

The negative predictive value of CA19-9 as a screening test is:

- A 70/100
- B 70/195
- C 375/500
- D 375/405
- E 445/600

1.40 A 55-year-old man presented with a distended abdomen that had been getting progressively larger over the past 4 weeks and now caused difficulty with breathing. He admitted to having drunk 1 L of spirits a day for over 10 years.

On examination he was alert and orientated and apyrexial. His pulse was 70 regular and blood pressure 130/80. His chest was clear. His abdomen was tender with shifting dullness.

Bloods				
	Hb	10.5	WCC	4.8
	Platelets	130	INR	1.0
	Na	130	K	4.3
	Urea	4.5	Creatinine	70
	Albumin	28	Bilirubin	35
	Protein	58	ALT	45
	ALP	120		

The next step in this patient's management would be:

- A fluid restrict and institute a salt-free diet
- B intravenous furosemide
- C oral spironolactone
- D paracentesis with albumin cover
- E transjugular intrahepatic portosystemic stent shunt

1.41 A 58-year-old woman was referred because of burning sensation and weakness in her legs progressing over some months. She had no previous medical problems and was not on any medication.

On examination her back and legs showed no deformity. There was bilateral lower limb weakness. Tone was increased and the knee jerks were brisk. The ankle jerks were absent and plantar responses were extensor. There was decreased light touch, vibration sense and proprioception. Heel–shin coordination was normal. She walked with a stamping gait and Romberg's test was positive.

The most likely diagnosis is:

- A Friedreich's ataxia
- B motor neurone disease
- C multiple sclerosis
- D subacute combined degeneration of the cord
- E tabes dorsalis

1.42 A 15-year-old girl was admitted with difficulty in breathing. She had had a number of admissions in the past 2 years with the same problem, which had responded to antibiotics. She had a chronic cough, which produced thick yellow sputum. She had no other medical problems. Her current medication included salbutamol nebulisers, aminophylline and oral prednisolone when her breathing got very bad. She did not smoke or drink alcohol. She did not keep any pets and she lived in the middle of town.

On examination her temperature was 37.6°C, pulse 98 regular, blood pressure 100/68 and respiratory rate 22 breaths/min. She had bilateral wheeze plus crackles in the right lower zone of her chest. Abdominal examination was normal.

Bloods	Hb	12.9	WCC	11.0
	Neutrophils	6.3	Lymphocytes	3.5
	Eosinophils	1.2	Platelets	250
	Na	146	K	4.3
	Urea	3.8	Creatinine	67
	Protein	76	Albumin	40
	Bilirubin	10	ALT	24
	ALP	400		
Chest X-ray	Patchy shadowing in the right middle and lower lobe Basal atelectasis on right			

The feature that would be **LEAST** likely to be consistent with her condition is:

A elevated serum IgE
B proximal bronchiectasis on imaging
C restrictive pattern lung function tests
D serum precipitins to *Aspergillus* antigen
E sputum eosinophilia

1.43 A 48-year-old man was referred with a 3-month history of worsening pain in both legs. The pain came on at rest and kept him awake at night. His symptoms were worse in cold weather. He had tried changing shoes with little effect. He could walk about 25 m before he had to stop and rest. He had no previous medical history or family history of note. He was not on any medication. He smoked 30 cigarettes a day for over 30 years.

His pulse was 90 regular and blood pressure 140/88. His JVP was not elevated and heart sounds were normal. Respiratory and abdominal examinations were normal. There were no palpable pulses below the femoral arteries. He had normal lower limb tone, power and reflexes and sensation to light touch and pinprick. His legs appeared normal but he felt pain on elevating them 30° from the horizontal. He had normal range of movements in all joints.

Bloods	Hb	13.7	WCC	6.9
	Platelets	500	INR	1.0
	Na	139	K	4.6
	Urea	7.8	Creatinine	115
	Protein	70	Albumin	40
	Bilirubin	14	ALT	20
	ALP	60	ESR	20
	CRP	10	Glucose	4.4
Rheumatoid factor	Negative			
Antinuclear antibody	Negative			
ECG	Normal sinus rhythm			

The most likely diagnosis is:

A microscopic polyangiitis
B peripheral neuropathy
C polyarteritis nodosa
D sciatica
E thromboangiitis obliterans

1.44 A 40-year-old man who suffered from pruritus ani had developed a rash over the past 4 months. It was confined to the areas shown. He had been treated with topical betnovate with no improvement. (Figure 1.44, page 373.)

The most likely diagnosis is:

A Crohn's disease
B eczema
C guttate psoriasis
D pityriasis versicolor
E ringworm

1.45 A 36-year-old woman presented with a 2-day history of worsening dry cough and shortness of breath.

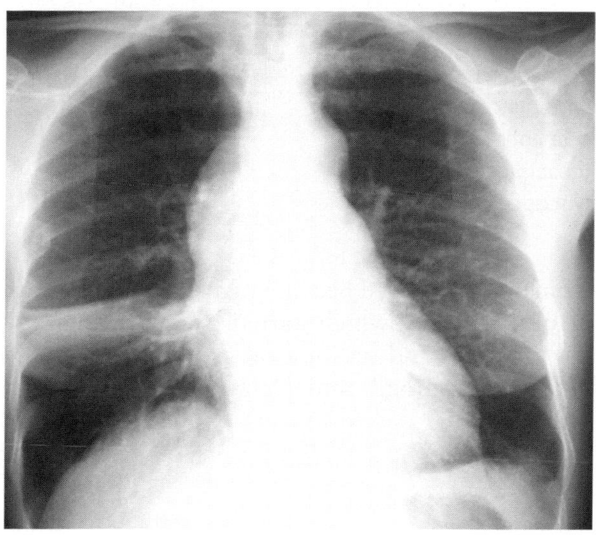

The most significant abnormality is in the:

A left lower lobe
B left upper lobe
C right lower lobe
D right middle lobe
E right upper lobe

1.46 A 78-year-old man was admitted having collapsed at home. He was sitting at the kitchen table eating his dinner when he suddenly collapsed. He remained unresponsive for about 2 min. There was no jerking of his limbs or tongue biting but he was incontinent of urine. After regaining consciousness his skin became flushed temporarily. He could not recall any warning, headache or nausea. He was not on any medication and had no previous medical history. His wife mentioned that this was the third time in 3 weeks this had happened without any warning. He did not drink alcohol or smoke.

On examination, he was well. His temperature was 36.7°C, pulse 42 regular and blood pressure 123/79. His JVP was not elevated and both heart sounds were normal. There were no murmurs, extra sounds or carotid artery bruits. Respiratory examination was normal. Central nervous system examination revealed no abnormality. He had normal tone, power, reflexes and sensation in all limbs. Cerebellar function was intact.

ECG Sinus bradycardia with rate of 42/min
No ischaemic changes

The most likely diagnosis is:

A orthostatic syncope
B Stokes–Adams syncope
C temporal lobe epilepsy
D transient ischaemic attack
E vasovagal syncope

1.47 A 53-year-old woman was referred because of a 3-month history of blisters occurring all over her body, which started off in her mouth. She had no other medical problems and was not on any medication. The skin surrounding the lesions was fragile and if pressed appeared to come off. (Figure 1.47, page 373.)

The most likely diagnosis is:

A bullous pemphigoid
B dermatitis herpetiformis
C epidermolysis bullosa
D pemphigus vulgaris
E scalded skin syndrome

1.48 A 19-year-old woman was referred with a 3-month history of excessive thirst and polyuria. She had no previous medical history but earlier in the year she was involved in a car accident in which she suffered minor injuries.

On examination she looked well and no abnormalities could be found. A water deprivation test was arranged.

Time after starting (h)	Plasma osmolality (mosmol/kg)	Urine osmolality (mosmol/kg)
0	295	110
2	300	115
4	306	122
6	310	127
DDAVP 2 μg given intramuscularly		
8	307	320
$Plasma_{ADH}$ post water deprivation test	Undetectable	

The most likely diagnosis in this patient is:

A complete central diabetes insipidus
B complete nephrogenic diabetes insipidus
C partial central diabetes insipidus
D partial nephrogenic diabetes insipidus
E primary polydipsia

1.49 A 57-year-old man was referred with a 7-month history of diarrhoea, opening his bowels four times a days with loose stools. There was no blood or mucus. There was no associated abdominal pain, nausea or vomiting. A year ago he was diagnosed with asthma and this had been difficult to control. He smoked 10 cigarettes a day and drank 2 units of alcohol in the evening.

On examination, he looked plethoric. He was apyrexial, pulse 100 regular and blood pressure 150/95. He had bilateral wheeze and palpable hepatomegaly. Rectal examination was normal.

Bloods	Hb	13.5	WCC	5.8
	Platelets	360	Na	140
	K	4.5	Urea	3.7
	Creatinine	90	Albumin	35
	Protein	72	Bilirubin	15
	ALT	35	ALP	130
	Chloride	75	Bicarbonate	24

The test that would give the definitive diagnosis is:

A serum gastrin
B serum vasointestinal peptide (VIP)
C stool laxative screen
D urinary 5-hydroxyindol acetic acid (5-HIAA)
E urinary vanillylmandelic acid (VMA)

1.50 A 65-year-old woman presented with back, hip and knee pain of 2 years' duration. She was currently taking diclofenac and paracetamol for her symptoms. She had not had any falls in the past. She had smoked 20 cigarettes a day for over 40 years and drank 2 units of alcohol a day.

On examination she was rather obese. She had tenderness and bony swelling of her distal and proximal interphalangeal joints. There was similar swelling and tenderness but no active inflammation of her knees and hips.

Of the following statements about this patient's condition it is true that:

A alcohol is not a predisposing factor
B early menopause is a predisposing factor
C her symptoms are likely to improve with exercising the joints
D previous trauma is not a predisposing factor
E steroids should be tried if current treatment is ineffective

1.51 A 69-year-old woman was referred because of painful hands. There had been tenderness and swelling in her hands and fingers for 4 months.

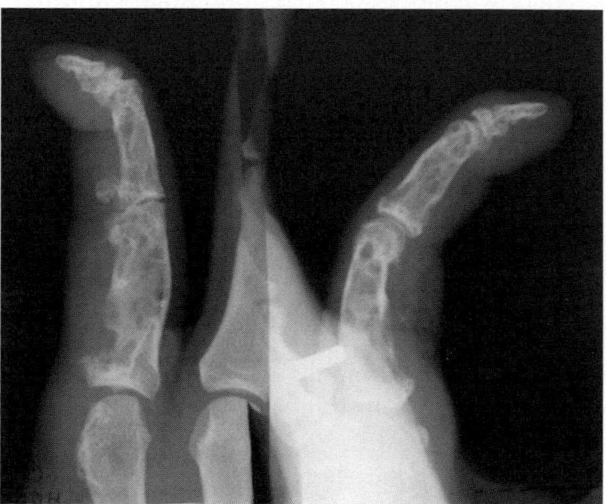

The most likely diagnosis is:

A gout
B hyperparathyroidism
C Paget's disease of bone
D rheumatoid arthritis
E sarcoidosis

1.52 A 3-year-old girl presented with her parents. They were concerned about bleeding from the lesion on her back. (Figure 1.52, page 374.)

Of the following statements concerning the girl's condition the one which is true is that:

A females are more likely to develop these lesions than males
B majority of the lesions are not present at birth
C approximately 5% of these lesions will undergo sarcomatous transformation
D she should undergo laser treatment as her lesion has not resolved
E the lesion is full of serous fluid

1.53 A 30-year-old woman was found to have an adrenal mass on CT abdomen. The surgeons wanted to resect the mass as it appeared to be localized purely to the adrenal gland. The anaesthetist has asked you to control her blood pressure preoperatively. Prior to admission she was treated with bendroflumethiazide.

Her pulse was 95 and her blood pressure 180/90. Cardiovascular, respiratory and thyroid examinations were normal.

Bloods	Na	138	K	4.3
	Urea	4.9	Creatinine	100
	Glucose	7.5	Bicarbonate	25
24-h urinary VMA	60			
ECG	Sinus tachycardia Left ventricular hypertrophy			
Chest X-ray	No evidence of failure			

The most appropriate antihypertensive for this patient would be:

A methyldopa
B nifedipine
C phenoxybenzamine
D propanolol
E spironolactone

1.54 A 45-year-old woman presented with a 3-month history of abdominal pain and loose stools, worse after eating meals. Four months ago she had had an uncomplicated laparoscopic cholecystectomy. Her appetite was normal with no weight loss. She had no other medical history and was not on any medication. She did not drink alcohol.

On examination she was apyrexial and was not jaundiced. Her pulse was 72 regular and blood pressure 130/75. There was mild upper abdominal tenderness and rectal examination was normal.

Bloods	Bilirubin	15	Albumin	35
	ALT	26	ALP	90
	GGT	50	Amylase	45
	CRP	5	Calcium	2.22
Abdominal ultrasound	Cholecystectomy noted, no gallstones seen No abnormalities of liver, pancreas, spleen, kidneys			

The most appropriate treatment would be:

A aluminium hydroxide
B cholestyramine
C gluten-free diet
D mebeverine
E prednisolone

1.55 A 19-year-old man was referred because of failure to develop secondary sexual characteristics. He had a cleft palate and was colour blind. He was not on any medication. He was adopted and knew nothing of his family history.

On examination there was no gynaecomastia. He had small, soft testes and normal but small male external genitalia.

Bloods	Testosterone	4	(normal 10–29 nmol/L)
	FSH	0.5	(normal 1–7 U/L)
	LH	0.5	(normal 1–6 U/L)
	Prolactin	100	
	TSH	2	
	Free T_4 26		
MRI pituitary	Normal		

This patient's most likely karyotype is:

A 45,XO
B 46,XO
C 46,XY
D 47,XXY
E 47,XYY

1.56 A 50-year-old woman was admitted because of recurrent upper abdominal pain. The pain was worse after eating and could last up to 24 h. It radiated to the back and there were no relieving factors. She had no previous medical history. She did not drink or smoke.

On examination she was not jaundiced or dehydrated. Her temperature was 37.6°C, pulse 95 regular and blood pressure 130/85. There was diffuse upper abdominal tenderness, no organomegaly and rectal examination was normal.

Bloods	Hb	13.9	WCC	12.5
	Platelets	300	INR	1.1
	Na	141	K	4.9
	Urea	4.5	Creatinine	75
	Bilirubin	18	Protein	65
	Albumin	38	ALT	250
	ALP	145	GGT	90
	Amylase	100		
Chest X-ray	Normal			
Abdominal X-ray	Normal			

The most likely diagnosis is:

- A acute appendicitis
- B acute pancreatitis
- C biliary colic
- D diverticulitis
- E peptic ulcer

1.57 A 32-year-old woman presented with a 2-month history of progressive weakness, fatigue and decreased appetite. She also complained of vague abdominal discomfort and nausea. She had three young children at home and felt depressed a lot of the time. Last year Graves' disease was diagnosed, from which she was making a slow recovery. Her mother suffered from type 1 diabetes.

On examination she still had some exophthalmos and a small goitre. Her skin was tanned but there was no jaundice or lymphadenopathy. Her pulse was 90 and her blood pressure was 100/65. Clinically she was euthyroid. Abdominal examination revealed generalised tenderness but no organomegaly or guarding.

Bloods	Hb	12.1	WCC	7.8
	Platelets	250	Na	132
	K	5.9	Urea	6.7
	Creatinine	69	Protein	70
	Albumin	39	Bilirubin	15
	ALT	26	ALP	110
	Calcium	2.34	TSH	2.3
	Free T_4	35	Glucose	3.2

The most likely diagnosis is:

A autoimmune polyglandular syndrome (APS) I
B APS 2
C multiple endocrine neoplasia (MEN) I syndrome
D MEN 2A syndrome
E MEN 2B syndrome

1.58 A 65-year-old homeless man was brought in looking dishevelled and smelling of alcohol. He was alert and coherent but felt tired.

On examination he had poor oral hygiene with gingivitis and bleeding gums. Cranial nerves were normal as was his gait. The rest of his physical examination was normal.

Bloods	Hb	11.5	WCC	5.7
	Platelets	150	MCV	77.5

The vitamin deficiency he is likely to have is:

A vitamin B_1
B vitamin B_2
C vitamin B_6
D vitamin B_{12}
E vitamin C

1.59 A 66-year-old woman was admitted with an anterior myocardial infarction for which she received thrombolysis. The next day she became very short of breath but had no chest pain or palpitations. Her medication included aspirin, simvastatin and atenolol.

Her temperature was 37.0°C, pulse 80 regular and blood pressure 75/40. Her JVP was elevated +8 cm and heart sounds were difficult to hear. There was dullness at both lung bases and the respiratory rate was 24 breaths/min.

ECG Normal sinus rhythm
Q waves and T wave inversion in V_{1-6}

Echocardiogram

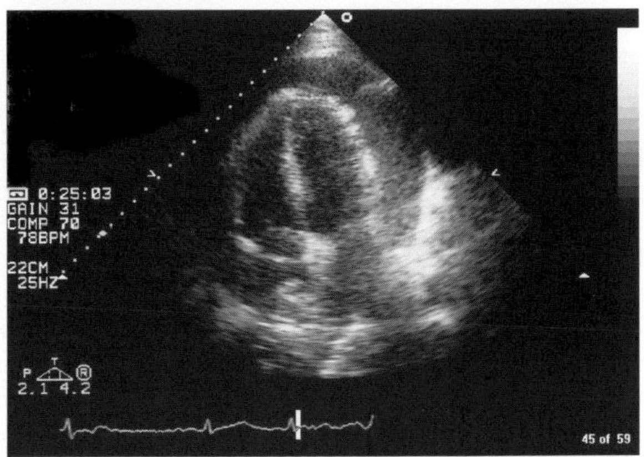

The most likely explanation for her deterioration is:

- A acute mitral regurgitation
- B dissection of thoracic aorta
- C pericardial effusion
- D right ventricular infarction
- E rupture of interventricular septum

1.60 A 30-year-old man presented with lethargy and malaise 2 days after starting chemotherapy for non-Hodgkin's lymphoma. He had mild abdominal discomfort but had not passed much urine despite drinking plenty.

On examination his temperature was 37.0°C, pulse 95 regular and blood pressure 140/78. His JVP was not elevated and heart sounds and chest were normal. His abdomen was soft and not tender with hepatosplenomegaly but no palpable bladder. Rectal examination was normal. Despite being catheterised he had only passed 200 ml of urine over the preceding 8 h.

Bloods	Hb	13.5	WCC	0.2
	Platelets	345	Na	130
	K	6.1	Urea	38.5
	Creatinine	450	Protein	65
	Albumin	35	Bilirubin	10
	ALT	35	ALP	130
	Calcium	2.0	Phosphate	2.0

Urinalysis Red cells 2+, granular casts

The prophylactic medication this patient should have received is:

A allopurinol
B furosemide
C gentamicin
D methotrexate
E methylprednisolone

1.61 A 22-year-old woman was referred to the clinic with persistent abdominal pain. This had been going on for a number of years. She was convinced that she had an allergy to eggs as she developed severe abdominal pain, vomiting and bloating about 5–6 h after eating any meal containing them; she now avoided eating eggs. Her previous medical history included asthma and hayfever, for which she regularly took inhaled salbutamol. She did not smoke or drink alcohol. Previously she had had a skin prick test done privately during which she had developed a skin wheal when pricked for eggs.

Physical examination was normal.

Of the following statements concerning this patient's diagnosis it is true that:

A eggs are not often a source of food allergy
B food allergies improve with age
C her history is consistent with IgE-mediated allergy to eggs
D skin prick tests have a high sensitivity and specificity for testing for food allergies
E skin prick tests should be done when not taking antihistamines

1.62 A 34-year-old man underwent a liver transplant for cryptogenic cirrhosis. Fourteen days postoperatively he was discharged from hospital. He was seen in the transplant clinic the following week complaining of abdominal pain and was noted to have worsening of liver function tests. He maintained that he was taking his immunosuppressive medication regularly and at the correct dose.

He had a temperature of 37.6°C, pulse 88 and blood pressure 135/75. His abdomen was soft with mild tenderness around the operation scar but there was no wound dehiscence.

Bloods	Hb	10.8	WCC	8.9
	Platelets	160	INR	1.4
	Na	138	K	4.2
	Urea	4.5	Creatinine	65
	Albumin	32	Bilirubin	38
	ALT	150	ALP	140

Liver ultrasound Normal

Percutaneous liver biopsy (the arrows 1–3 refer to different abnormalities, as described in the answer) (Figure 1.62, page 374.)

The complication that has occurred is:

A acute cellular rejection
B graft versus host disease
C ischaemic hepatitis
D recurrence of original disease
E sepsis

1.63 A 64-year-old man was admitted to the coronary care unit with an acute ST elevation myocardial infarction (STEMI). He was treated with thrombolysis, given aspirin and started on a statin. He appeared to have had a good response to treatment with resolution of his chest pain and ST elevation on the ECG. Twelve hours later he became clammy and short of breath with no chest pain. He was apyrexial with cool peripheries. His pulse was 105 regular and blood pressure had dropped from 120/80 to 85/50. His JVP was elevated to +6 cm and heart sounds were normal. There were bilateral basal crackles. He was put on high flow oxygen.

ECG Rate 115 sinus rhythm
Q waves in I, aVL, V_{4-6}

Chest X-ray Bilateral basal shadowing

Arterial blood gases on 15 L/min O_2	pH	7.21	PCO_2	3.4
	PO_2	45.5	HCO_3	15.4
	Base excess	–9.3	Lactate	5.3

Of the following statements concerning this patient's management the one that is correct is :

A glycoprotein IIb/IIIa inhibitors will worsen outcome
B inotropic support with dobutamine needs to be given
C a fluid challenge with 500 ml gelofusin over 1 h should be given
D an intra-aortic balloon pump should be considered
E verapamil is the drug of choice to control the tachycardia

1.64 A 20-year-old man was reviewed in the chest clinic 4 weeks after discharge from hospital following his second acute asthma attack of the year. Currently he was well but still got wheezy throughout the week. He was only taking salbutamol inhaler when he needed it, which was about twice a day on average. He had not been very compliant with medication in the past. He was now started on 800 μg of inhaled beclamethasone/day.

On examination he was apyrexial and he was not in distress. His chest was clear and respiratory rate was 18 breaths/min. His PEF was 250 L/min.

If the beclamethasone regimen does not relieve his symptoms, the **NEXT** step in his management would be:

A increase dose of beclamethasone to 1600 μg/day
B ipratropium bromide
C montelukast
D salmeterol
E theophylline

1.65 A 50-year-old woman was admitted with a stroke that caused left-sided facial and limb weakness. She had an unsafe swallow and so was kept nil by mouth. She had a previous medical history of congestive cardiac failure with peripheral oedema that was being treated with furosemide. Despite her admission sodium being 123, the furosemide was continued, now intravenously. She was given intravenous dextrose until a NG tube was inserted 5 days after admission. The next day she had a generalized seizure that lasted 5 min and stopped spontaneously.

On examination she was apyrexial, pulse was 78 regular and blood pressure was 130/78. JVP was +4 and heart sounds were clear and chest examination normal. There was still some residual weakness in the left upper and lower limbs. She had bilateral extensor plantars reflexes.

Bloods	Hb	12.4	WCC	6.6
	Platelets	248	INR	1.0
	Na	108	K	3.5
	Urea	6.5	Creatinine	80
	Glucose	5.0	TSH	4.3
	T_4	15.4		
Urinalysis	Na	24	Osmolality	80
Chest X-ray	Normal			
Urinalysis	No blood, glucose, protein			

Of the following statements concerning this patient's management it is correct that:

- A over rapid correction of sodium will result in cerebral oedema
- B she should be treated with demeclocycline
- C she should be treated with standard dextrose–saline
- D diuretics should be stopped and she should be fluid restricted
- E plasma sodium should not be raised by >12 mmol/L in the first 24 h

1.66 A 32-year-old man with chronic renal failure being treated with peritoneal dialysis presented to Accident &Emergency with a 1-day history of abdominal pain and cloudy effluent from his dialysis catheter. He had been established on dialysis for about 12 months and performed four exchanges per day at home and had had no problems hitherto.

On examination his temperature was 37.3°C, pulse was 78 regular and blood pressure was 138/92. Heart sounds and chest examination were normal. He had mild central abdominal pain around the catheter site but no crusting, erythema or swelling.

Catheter fluid	White cells	144/mm^3	Neutrophils	70%

Of the following statements concerning this patient it is true that:

- A antibiotics should be given for at least 2 weeks
- B blood cultures usually yield a positive result
- C fungi account for 50% of infections
- D he should be treated with intravenous vancomycin
- E the dialysis catheter should be removed

1.67 A 62-year-old man was referred by his GP because of progressive lower limb weakness and paraesthesia. He had also lost 6 kg in weight over the past 2 months and recently had developed haemoptysis. He had no previous medical history and used to work as an office manager. He had smoked 20 cigarettes a day for 40 years and drank at least 4 units of alcohol a day.

On examination he was apyrexial. Pulse was 72 regular and blood pressure 130/85. Cardiovascular, respiratory and abdominal examinations were normal. He had wasting of the quadriceps bilaterally. Tone was normal but there was loss of knee and ankle reflexes and plantar reflexes were absent. There was decreased sensation to pin prick and light touch up to the ankle bilaterally. The rest of the neurological examination was normal.

Bloods	Hb	13.4	WCC	8.5
	Platelets	62	MCV	113.6
	Na	130	K	3.9
	Urea	4.8	Creatinine	78
	Protein	70	Albumin	38
	Bilirubin	12	ALP	125
	ALT	58	GGT	90

Chest X-ray Opacity at left hilum

This patient's symptoms are most likely due to:

A alcoholic neuropathy
B carcinomatous neuropathy
C polymyalgia rheumatica
D polymyositis
E subacute combined degeneration of the cord

1.68 A 25-year-old man presented to Accident & Emergency with a 2-day history of shortness of breath, cough and haemoptysis. Five days ago he had returned from Vietnam where he had come into contact with poultry. He was previously fit and well and had no past lung problems. He did not smoke.

On examination his temperature was 38.2°C, pulse was 100 regular and blood pressure was 98/60. His JVP was not elevated and heart sounds were normal. There were crackles at both lungs and respiratory rate was 28 breaths/min. Abdominal and neurological examinations were normal.

Bloods	Hb	9.5	WCC	2.8
	Platelets	100	Lymphocytes	1.0
	Na	130	K	4.0
	Urea	7.9	Creatinine	90
	Albumin	30	Bilirubin	18
	ALT	130	ALP	135

Chest X-ray Bilateral patchy infiltrates

Arterial blood gases on 10 L/min O_2	pH	7.29	PCO_2	5.0
	PO_2	7.8	HCO_3	15
	Base excess	–8		

The patient was intubated and ventilated and nursed in a side room in ITU.

This patient should be treated with:

A amantadine
B immunoglobulin
C interferon-α
D oseltamivir
E ribavirin

1.69 A 20-year-old male student presented to the clinic with painful ulcers on the penis for the past 2 days with associated dysuria. He was heterosexual with multiple sexual partners.

On examination, temperature was 37.5°C. There were multiple, shallow, tender ulcers with associated tender inguinal lymphadenopathy.

The test that will establish the diagnosis is:

A dark ground microscopy of swabs from ulcer for *Treponema pallidum*
B HIV test
C skin scrapings for mycology
D syphilis serology
E viral culture swab for HSV

1.70 A 42-year-old woman was referred with a painful nodule on her elbow; there was no joint pain. She also had noticed purple skin lesions on her legs. Over the past 6 months she complained of paraesthesia in her legs. She had a previous medical history of asthma that was diagnosed 4 years ago and was difficult to control with $\beta 2$ agonists and inhaled steroids.

On examination she had multiple, non-pruritic purpuric lesions on both legs, and decreased sensation to light touch and pin prick in a stocking distribution up to mid-calf level in both legs. On the back of her left elbow was a tender, ulcerated nodule with surrounding erythema.

The complication **NOT** recognised as being associated with this condition is:

A bloody diarrhoea
B cerebral haemorrhage
C congestive cardiac failure
D glomerulonephritis
E lung carcinoma

1.71 A 36-year-old man was seen in the clinic complaining of profuse watery diarrhoea for the last week, opening his bowels up to five times per day. He had mild abdominal pain but no nausea or vomiting. He had a normal appetite and no weight loss. He had had a matched unrelated stem cell transplant for acute myeloid leukaemia 3 months ago and was on ciclosporin. Since then he had noticed an itchy rash all over his body.

On examination he was apyrexial. There was no jaundice, pallor or lymphadenopathy. Abdominal examination revealed mild generalised tenderness; rectal examination was normal. Flexible sigmoidoscopy revealed a few aphthous ulcers in the rectum and rectal biopsy was taken (the arrows 1–3 refer to different abnormalities, as described in the answer). (Figure 1.71, page 374.)

Bloods				
	Hb	13.0	WCC	5.4
	Platelets	229	ESR	24
	CRP	25	Albumin	35
	Bilirubin	22	ALT	60
	ALP	154		

Of the following statements concerning this patient's diagnosis and management it is true that:

A treatment should be with methotrexate in the first instance
B hepatic involvement is rare
C his diarrhoea is due to *Clostridium difficile* toxin
D steroids are likely to worsen symptoms
E risk of developing this condition would have been decreased if donor and recipient had been matched for gender

1.72 A 46-year-old woman was referred by her GP with persistent central abdominal pain for 5 months. Her appetite was normal and she had not lost weight or had night sweats. There was no history of foreign travel. She had no previous medical problems or family history of note. She smoked 10 cigarettes a day but did not drink alcohol.

Physical examination was normal.

CT abdomen	Para-aortic lymphadenopathy
CT guided lymph node biopsy	Poorly differentiated carcinoma Immunohistochemistry was inconclusive.
CT chest and pelvis	Normal
Upper gastrointestinal endoscopy	Normal
Colonoscopy	Normal
Mammogram	Normal
Barium follow through	Normal
FBC, U&E and LFTs	Normal
CA125, CA153, AFP	Normal

Chemotherapy treatment was suggested.

Of the following features the one that **BEST** suggests this patient's condition is likely to respond to chemotherapy is:

A age under 70 years
B elevated CEA
C female sex
D poorly differentiated adenocarcinoma on histology
E retroperitoneal lymphadenopathy

1.73 A 19-year-old female known asthmatic was admitted to Accident & Emergency. Despite treatment with nebulised salbutamol and ipratropium, intravenous steroids, magnesium and oxygen, her condition deteriorated and she became more drowsy and breathless.

Her respiratory rate was 33 breaths/min and she was using accessory muscles of respiration.

Arterial blood gases on 15 L/min O_2	pH	7.28	PCO_2	7.0
	PO_2	8.6	HCO_3	30
	Base excess	+2		

She was admitted to ITU for observation and possible ventilation; her breathing became more laboured and her breath sounds became quieter.

Of the following forms of ventilation the **ONE** that should be considered for this patient is:

- A continuous positive airways pressure ventilation (CPAP)
- B non-invasive positive pressure ventilation (NIPPV)
- C pressure control ventilation
- D pressure support ventilation
- E volume control ventilation

1.74 A 74-year-old man was brought to Accident & Emergency after slipping over in the street and falling on his chest.

Physical examination was normal. A chest X-ray was done and comparison with a previous chest X-ray taken 5 years ago showed no difference.

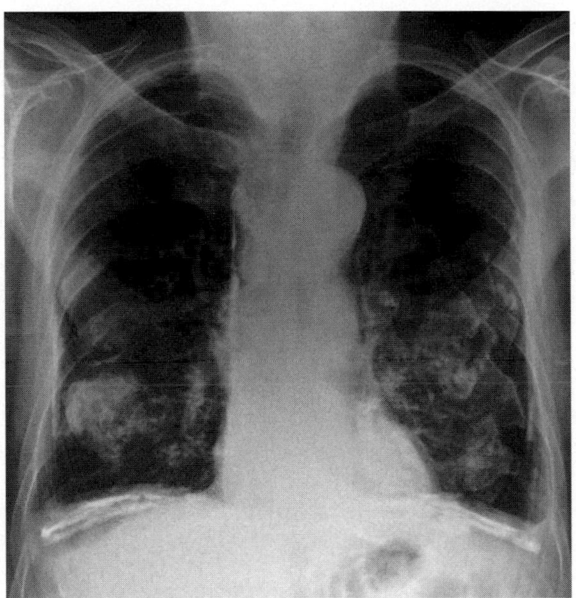

The chest X-ray findings are **MOST** consistent with:

- A asbestos exposure
- B bronchiectasis
- C mesothelioma
- D previous thoracic surgery
- E progressive massive fibrosis

1.75 A 70-year-old man complained of back pain. A MRI spine was performed.

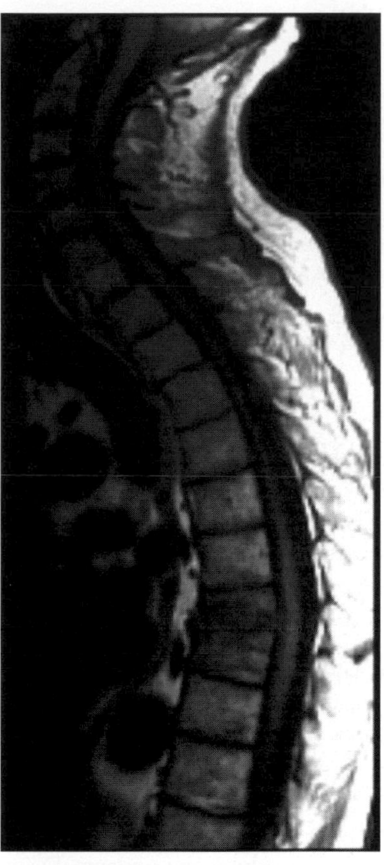

The correct diagnosis is:

A bone tumour metastasis
B discitis
C normal
D spinal cord compression
E syringomyelia

Paper 1

Answers

1.1 **C**** This is a patient with severe congestive cardiac failure that is getting worse. His condition would be classified as New York Health Association Grade IV failure as dyspnoea is occurring at rest. He needs intensification of his medication. The best treatment would be to add low dose spironolactone. The evidence for this comes from the RALES study.

Pitt B, Zannad F, Remme WJ, et al. (1999) The effect of spironolactone on morbidity and mortality in patients with severe heart failure. Randomized Aldactone Evaluation Study Investigators. *N Engl J Med* 341: 709–17.

1.2 **E*** The ECG shows right bundle branch block (RBBB) with a QRS complex > 0.12 s and second R wave in V_2. Left anterior fascicular block is shown by the presence of left axis deviation and an initial R wave in II, III and aVF. With left posterior fascicular block there is RBBB and right axis deviation. This is trifascicular block because there is also a prolonged PR interval.

1.3 **A**** Indications for haemodialysis in salicylate overdoses include: plasma salicylate concentrations > 700 mg/L; renal failure; pulmonary oedema; convulsions and central nervous system effects not resolved by correction of acidosis; and worsening metabolic acidosis. Delayed gastric lavage could be contemplated for up to 12 h, as it is possible that not all the pills will have been absorbed. Forced alkaline diuresis should not be used since it does not enhance salicylate excretion and may cause pulmonary oedema. Drug overdoses that can be treated with haemodialysis can be remembered using the mnemonic BLAST: Barbiturates, Lithium, Alcohol (including methanol and ethylene glycol), Salicylates and Theophylline.

1.4 **E*** This boy presents with primary varicella gingivostomatitis. Erosions, blisters and superficial ulcers can develop, with the clinical picture usually settling within 7–14 days. Systemic aciclovir is used for severe herpetic and varicella stomatitis.

1.5 **B***** A middle-aged woman with a malabsorptive disease complains of muscle pains and difficulty in walking. She has osteomalacia shown by low serum calcium and phosphate and high ALP. Diabetic amyotrophy presents with painful wasting of the thigh muscles with loss of knee reflexes. Here there is weakness but no wasting of the quadriceps. With osteoporosis there is no biochemical derangement. Periodic paralysis is associated with hyperthyroidism and hyperkalaemia.

1.6 **C**** The study design needs to allow comment to be made on prognosis. Cohort studies involve choosing a group of patients and following them up over a period of time to see if they develop the disease or not. A case control study could be employed but does not allow causality to be proved and so is not the most appropriate study design in this situation. If mass drop out of subjects were an issue, for practical purposes a case control study could be employed.

1.7 **B*** This woman is at risk of osteoporosis because she has had frequent courses of steroids. The T score compares the patient's bone mass with that of a normal young adult gender- and ethnicity-matched population. Using the World Health Organization scoring system, −1.0 means that the patient has a bone mass that is 1 standard deviation below that of the young reference population. The T score indicates whether or not a patient has osteoporosis. A T score of −1.0 or above is normal; between −1.0 and −2.5 means osteopaenia and below −2.5 means osteoporosis. The Z score compares the patient's bone mass with that of an age-, gender- and ethnicity-matched reference population. The Z score gives an indication of whether or not the bone mass is appropriate for the patient's age. A Z score below −2.0 suggests that there may be a secondary cause for the bone loss such as malabsorption, vitamin D deficiency or use of certain drugs like steroids.

1.8 **D***** A young teenager presents with bruising. He is recovering from a viral illness and his full blood count shows thrombocytopaenia and a mild lymphocytosis. The bruising is due to the low platelet count. In acute leukaemia a much higher white cell count would be expected and the blood film would show blasts. Henoch–Schönlein purpura (HSP) is a vasculitis that is associated with abnormal platelets but there is no significant drop in the platelet count. HSP, like idiopathic thrombocytopaenic purpura, can occur following a viral infection. There is no evidence of bone marrow failure as the haemoglobin is normal, making aplastic anaemia unlikely.

1.9 **C*** A patient presents with chronic recurrent abdominal pain that often resolves spontaneously and is normal at laparoscopy. Her mother had similar problems, suggesting an inherited component. This condition would be consistent with hereditary angioedema. Patients may present with abdominal pain due to visceral oedema, severe bronchospasm or facial angioedema, which does not respond to antihistamines. There are low/deficient levels of C1 esterase inhibitor as well as low C2 and C4. Acute treatment is with C1 esterase inhibitor or fresh frozen plasma. Long-term treatment is with danazol or α-aminocaproic acid, an inhibitor of plasmin. Acute intermittent porphyria could present similarly to this but some disturbance in the blood results would be expected, such as hyponatraemia, which would imply syndrome of inappropriate ADH secretion. Wiskott–Aldrich syndrome is an X-linked T and B cell disorder associated with eczema, thrombocytopaenia and lymphopaenia.

1.10 **E*** The history is of a patient with COPD treated with antibiotics who now presents with diarrhoea. The other options are possible but the histology shows the characteristic 'volcano' lesion of pseudomembranous colitis.

1.11 **D**** This patient has pyrexia, cough, altered bowel habit and abdominal pain without jaundice, which are all characteristic of typhoid. Rose spots tend not to develop until the second week of the illness. None of the other options is associated with cough or sore throat. Dengue and yellow fever are viral haemorrhagic fevers and so jaundice and evidence of bleeding would be expected with them. Malaria must always be excluded in a patient with pyrexia who has been abroad. Malaria is associated with a low/normal neutrophil count but to develop blackwater fever a low platelet count suggestive of haemolysis would be expected. Amoebic dysentery is usually associated with an increased neutrophil count.

1.12 **D*** In a young woman with chronic headaches, blurred vision, papilloedema and taking the contraceptive pill the most likely diagnosis is benign intracranial hypertension (BIH). CT brain shows no evidence of intracranial lesion, which would have to be excluded in a patient with papilloedema. Lumbar puncture with an opening pressure of 40 cm H_2O or more can confirm BIH. The aim would be to aspirate CSF not only for analysis but also to reduce the intracranial pressure. Treatments include acetazolamide and even repeat lumbar puncture to reduce the intracranial pressure. Blindness may occur through compression of the optic nerve and so visual field testing is necessary. Magnetic resonance venography is the correct answer because a differential diagnosis for BIH is sagittal vein thrombosis, which may not be detected by CT brain and could give a raised opening pressure as well.

1.13 **C**** This patient has diabetic maculopathy. There is a circinate of hard exudates in the macular area close to the centre. This implies there may be leakage of fluid affecting the centre of the macula. The patient may require laser treatment.

1.14 **C*** Using the modified Dukes' classification: Dukes' A colorectal carcinoma is limited to the mucosa; B_1 extends into the muscularis propria; B_2 extends into the serosa; C_1 has 1–4 regional lymph nodes involved; C_2 has >4 regional lymph nodes involved; and D involves distant metastases.

1.15 **B**** This middle-aged man presents with an acute monoarthritis. The main differential diagnoses are sepsis or crystal deposition disease, given the speed of onset. An acute hot, swollen, erythematous joint should be assumed to be infected until proven otherwise but there is nothing to suggest that this patient has a bacterial septic arthritis. He has crystals that show negative birefringence to polarized light and would look needle shaped. Pseudogout crystals are rhomboid shaped and show positive birefringence. Serum urate may be normal in up to 30% of patients during an acute attack.

1.16 **A**** This patient has bacterial meningitis until proven otherwise. The most likely organisms are *Neisseria meningitidis* or *Streptococcus pneumoniae*. Diagnostic tests that need to be undertaken include blood cultures, nasal and throat swabs for *N. meningitidis* carriage, serology for *N. meningitidis* and CSF for Gram stain. The normal CT head does not rule out raised intracranial pressure – this patient has a decreased GCS and decorticate posturing (arms flexed towards the chest and hands turning into clenched fists with extended legs), which is a contraindication to performing a lumbar puncture. High dose intravenous antibiotics should not be delayed but there is evidence that giving intravenous dexamethasone at initial presentation is associated with a better outcome. Activated protein C is an endogenous protein that has anti-inflammatory and fibrinolytic actions and is licensed for use in patients with severe sepsis and multiorgan failure. Contact tracing for all bacterial meningitis types is essential to ensure that close contacts are given antibiotic prophylaxis. There is nothing to suggest she has encephalitis and so she does not require treatment with aciclovir.

de Gans J, van de Beek D (2002) Dexamethasone in adults with bacterial meningitis. *N Engl J Med* **347**: 1549–56.

1.17 **B**** The CT scan shows a left posterior extradural haematoma most probably due to trauma to the middle meningeal artery. There is a potential space between the dura and the skull vault and any haematoma forming here will be convex in shape toward the brain and skull vault; hence the 'bulging' appearance. (see also **5.16**)

1.18 **A***** This barium swallow shows the characteristic 'bird's beak' appearance of a dilated proximal oesophagus tapering distally at the gastro-oesophageal junction.

1.19 D, H, I** While all the drugs help in the management of unstable angina, there is no conclusive evidence that they improve prognosis or reduce the risk of death post myocardial infarction. Other drugs that do not improve prognosis include magnesium, digoxin and antiarrhythmics such as flecainide or propafenone.

Aspirin: ISIS-2 (Second International Study of Infarct Survival). (1988) Collaborative Group Randomised trial of intravenous streptokinase, oral aspirin, both, or neither among 17,187 cases of suspected acute myocardial infarction: ISIS-2. *Lancet* **2**: 349–60.

Clopidogrel: CAPRIE Steering Committee (1966) A randomised, blinded, trial of clopidogrel versus aspirin in patients at risk of ischaemic events (CAPRIE). *Lancet* **348**: 1329–39.

Low molecular weight heparin: Antman EM, McCabe CH, Gurfinkel EP, et al. (1999) Enoxaparin prevents death and cardiac ischemic events in unstable angina/non-Q-wave myocardial infarction. Results of the Thrombolysis in Myocardial Infarction (TIMI) 11B Trial. *Circulation* **100**: 1593–1601.

Atenolol: First International Study of Infarct Survival Collaborative Group (1986) Randomised trial of intravenous atenolol among 16 027 cases of suspected acute myocardial infarction: ISIS-1. *Lancet* 2: 57–66.

ACE inhibitors: Yusuf S, Sleight P, Pogue J, et al. (2000) Effects of an angiotensin-converting-enzyme inhibitor, ramipril, on cardiovascular events in high-risk patients. The Heart Outcomes Prevention Evaluation Study Investigators. *N Engl J Med* **342**: 145–53.

Simvastatin: Scandinavian Simvastatin Survival Study Group (4S) (1994) Randomised trial of cholesterol lowering in 4444 patients with coronary artery disease. *Lancet* **344**: 1383–89.

n3 Polyunsaturated fat fish oils: GISSI-Prevenzione Investigators. (1999) Dietary supplementation with n-3 polyunsaturated fatty acids and vitamin E after myocardial infarction: results of the GISSI-Prevenzione trial. *Lancet* **354**: 447–55.

1.20 D* All permanent pacemakers are given a code describing their function. The first letter identifies the chamber/chambers being paced: A for atrium, V for ventricle and D for both. The second letter indicates the chamber/chambers whose activity is being sensed: A for atrium, V for ventricle and D for both. The third letter denotes the response to sensed information: I means that pacemaker output is inhibited by a sensed event; T means that stimulation is triggered by a sensed event; and D means that ventricular sensed events inhibit pacemaker output, whereas atrial sensed events trigger ventricular stimulation. VVI pacemakers are preferred for patients with complete heart block who are in atrial fibrillation because there are no P waves to trigger a ventricular impulse. As VVI pacemakers have only a single lead they would produce a pacing spike just before the QRS complex if they were working properly; this patient has two spikes before the QRS complex, suggesting he has a DDD pacemaker that is working well and therefore is not responsible for his symptoms. Pyrexia can alter the rate of a pacemaker but not anaemia. More advanced pacemakers can respond to body temperature.

1.21 C* Carbon monoxide exerts its toxic effects by binding to haemoglobin, preventing oxygen carriage, causing a left shift of the oxyhaemoglobin dissociation curve so that haemoglobin is less likely to give up oxygen, and by interfering with cytochrome oxidases. Pulse oximeters over-read because they cannot distinguish HbCO from HbO_2. Indications for hyperbaric oxygen therapy include pregnancy, coma, failure to respond to conventional therapy, development of neurological sequelae, and HbCO >40%. PCO_2 is not a determinant of prognosis.

1.22 A** This patient has droplet sized psoriasis papules on her back and extensor surfaces of her elbows, which have developed after a streptococcal infection. Psoriatic lesions are not necessarily associated with pruritus or silvery scales. Pityriasis versicolor is a superficial, non-inflammatory skin infection caused by the yeast, *Malassezia furfur*; it is characterized by sharply demarcated coffee-brown slightly scaling macules that may coalesce to form irregular forms. Lichen planus consists of small, violaceous flat-topped papules with a lacy white pattern on their surface called Wickham's striae.

1.23 C*** This pregnant woman has developed thyrotoxicosis. She needs treatment with propylthiouracil. Atenolol should be used with caution in pregnancy and would certainly not control her underlying thyroid disease.

1.24 D** NNT (number needed to treat) is the number of patients who would need to be treated with aspirin to prevent one death at the end of 1 year. It is the reciprocal of 1/ARR (absolute risk reduction).

Relative risk of death in aspirin group = 5/1000 = 0.005
Relative risk of death in placebo group = 15/1000 = 0.015
ARR = 0.015–0.005 = 0.01
NNT = 1/0.01 = 100

1.25 C*** All patients with haematemesis require endoscopy but only rarely would this need to occur immediately; in any case, patients need to be stabilised first. There is no evidence that H_2 blockers like ranitidine help; however, there is plenty of evidence that a proton pump inhibitor like omeprazole or pantoprazole may be beneficial. A possible reason for this is that haemostasis is more likely if the environment is as neutral as possible and this is more likely to be achieved with a proton pump inhibitor. There is evidence that a proton pump inhibitor is of benefit even if it is given orally. Terlipressin is the treatment of choice for oesophageal variceal bleed. As there is nothing in the history to suggest varices, management should be aimed at assuming this is an ulcer bleed.

1.26 **C*** This patient has paroxysmal nocturnal haemoglobinuria (PNH), which is a red cell abnormality characterised by the presence of a clone of red cells with an abnormal sensitivity to membrane lysis by complement. Patients may present with aplastic anaemia, myelodysplastic syndromes and acute myeloid leukaemia or with evidence of thombosis like Budd–Chiari syndrome (as in this case), deep vein thrombosis and cerebral vein thrombosis. In Ham's test, complement in the patient's serum is activated by acidification. CD59 could also be used to detect PNH.

1.27 **B*** The slide shows liver with very small, attenuated hepatocytes that stain pink. The paler pink material in between represents the amyloid. Amyloidosis would also stain with Congo red. With haemochromatosis, the hepatocytes would look normal in size but there would be periportal punctate deposits of haemosiderin pigment which stain with Perl's stain. The hepatocytes would look normal in Wilson's disease but the stain used then is rhodanine. There is not the fibrosis of cirrhosis, and hepatocellular carcinoma is associated with large hepatocytes with big nucleoli.

1.28 **A*** *HAART* should be delayed until the CD_4 count is <350 or the patient is symptomatic. The viral load does not influence the timing of starting HAART in non-pregnant adults but does influence the type of treatment regimen. Standard HAART consists of three drugs: two nucleosides + one non-nucleoside or two nucleosides + one protease inhibitor or three nucleosides. The danger of starting HAART too early is that viral resistance may develop and so treatment options will be limited with more advanced disease. Long-term septrin is given for *Pneumocystis juroveci* (formerly *carinii*) pneumonia. AZT can cause bone marrow suppression and so should be avoided in patients who are anaemic.

1.29 **D**** He has Guillain–Barré syndrome. Such patients can deteriorate quickly and may require intensive care admission, especially if there is respiratory compromise. Factors associated with severe disease include: *Campylobacter jejeuni* infection; hypoxia; autonomic neuropathy including arrhythmias, orthostatic hypotension, hypertension; bulbar involvement; age >40 years; worsening vital capacity (not peak flow); and rapid onset of symptoms.

1.30 **A**** Arterial blood gases are very easy to interpret if they are approached in a logical fashion. First, decide whether the condition is compensated or not compensated. Second, look at the PCO_2 and see if this is high; if so, there is a respiratory acidosis. Third, assess the bicarbonate to see if this is low, as this would be consistent with a metabolic acidosis. Finally, look at the base excess; the more negative the value, the greater the metabolic acidosis. The PO_2 is not strictly part of the acid–base equation and only gives an indication of hypoxia (PO_2 <8.0 kPa). Low PO_2 and low PCO_2 indicates type I respiratory failure, and low PO_2 and poisoning normal/high PCO_2 indicates type II respiratory failure. Using the above approach, this patient has an uncompensated metabolic acidosis with type I respiratory failure. This would be consistent with a salicylate overdose or ethylene glycol poisoning.

1.31 D*** Polymyalgia rheumatica is a large blood vessel vasculitis characterised by pain and stiffness in the shoulder and pelvic girdle muscles. While patients may complain of weakness, none is often found on clinical examination. It is associated with patients over 50 years of age and patients usually have high ESRs as well as mildly deranged liver function tests. One-third of patients may subsequently develop giant cell (temporal) arteritis. Fibromyalgia is associated with normal blood results and tender points on examination. Polymyositis would result in objective weakness and raised creatine kinase. Amyotrophy is more common in poorly controlled diabetics and would have associated muscle wasting.

1.32 A* Bacterial vaginosis is typically caused by *Gardnerella vaginalis*, *Bacteroides* sp, *Mobiluncus* sp and *Mycoplasma hominis*. It has a propensity to affect pregnant women and the type of discharge is characteristic in this patient. It is important to treat as it may cause premature delivery. *Trichomonas* produces a green, frothy discharge with itching. Chlamydia can produce a watery discharge but tends to affect younger women and results in inflammatory cells being seen. In gonorrhorea, female patients are usually asymptomatic, with no discharge unless they develop pelvic inflammatory disease, and microscopy may reveal lactobacilli. Candidal infections are associated with a thick, creamy discharge and itching.

1.33 C*** This patient has a large pneumothorax on the right. If he were in distress and had signs of a tension pneumothorax, needle thoracocentesis should be performed as soon as possible but on the side of the pneumothorax. There are a number of causes of secondary pneumothoraces but any condition that can cause cysts on the lung may rupture to produce a pneumothorax. Pleuradhesis should be considered if the patient develops a second pneumothorax on the same side. Hamman's sign is an inspiratory click sometimes heard in a patient with a small pneumothoraces.

1.34 C** The barium meal shows a mass in the stomach consistent with gastric carcinoma. Patients with blood group A have an increased risk of gastric carcinoma. *H. pylori* can cause chronic atrophic gastritis and in some patients there is decreased secretion of gastric acid leading to achlorhydria. It is for this reason that symptomatic patients who have *H. pylori* should have eradication treatment.

1.35 E** This middle-aged woman presents with hypokalaemia, metabolic alkalosis, hypertension and hypomagnesaemia. Most patients with Conn's syndrome do not present with any clinical features except hypertension and hypokalaemia. However, Cushing's syndrome due to an oat-cell tumour may not present with cushingoid features due to the advanced nature of their underlying disease. Liddle's syndrome is a renal tubular defect where there is increased sodium absorption and excessive potassium excretion but with no involvement of the renin–aldosterone system.

1.36 B** The echocardiogram shows a bright irregular mass on the tricuspid valve. This patient has infective endocarditis, probably introduced by the central venous catheter. Myxoma is a tumour that usually arises from the body or wall of the heart. Thrombus would have a darker echogenicity. The ventricle and interatrial septum are normal.

1.37 E** This patient has scabies and the photograph shows the characteristic burrow. The diagnosis is confirmed by identifying the mite microscopically. Treatment is with 0.5% malathion aqueous liquid or 5% permethrin cream. The patient is bathed in the ointment for 24 h but the itching may take 2–3 weeks to resolve.

1.38 A** This patient has hypercalcaemia of malignancy as evidenced by the normal PTH and the elevated PTH related peptide. PTH related peptide has a similar homology to PTH and causes bone resorption and inhibition of renal calcium excretion. It is produced by squamous carcinomas involving the lung, head, neck and oesophagus, and adenocarcinomas of the kidney, bladder, pancreas, breast and ovary.

1.39 C** The negative predictive value is the probability that a patient who tests negative really does not have the condition.

	Pancreatic cancer +	**Pancreatic cancer –**	
CA 19-9 +	70 (a)	30 (b)	100
CA 19-9 –	125 (c)	375 (d)	500
	195	405	600

Negative predictive value = d/d + c = 375/500 = 0.75

1.40 D** A patient with presu med alcoholic liver disease presents with tense ascites. The most appropriate treatment is to relieve his ascites with therapeutic paracentesis. If he had mild ascites, the plan would be to start oral spironolactone. Fluid restriction is useful if patients are hyponatraemic but it must first be established that they are passing urine adequately, otherwise such actions may cause renal failure. A salt-free diet will not help in the acute situation. The aim should be to drain as much fluid as possible with albumin cover.

1.41 **D**** Subacute combined degeneration of the cord is a consequence of vitamin B_{12} deficiency and results in degeneration of the dorsal columns and corticospinal/pyramidal tracts (causing the extensor plantars) along with demyelination of peripheral nerves (causing the absent ankle jerks). If the burning sensation in the spine and limbs occurs with neck flexion it is a referred to as Lhermitte's sign; it indicates that the cervical spinal cord and sensor tracts are diseased. It may occur in other conditions such as multiple sclerosis, cervical myelopathy, cervical cord tumours and syringomyelia.

1.42 **C*** The underlying condition in this child is likely to be cystic fibrosis with allergic bronchopulmonary aspergillosis (ABPA). This is an allergic reaction to *Aspergillus fumigatus* that often presents in asthmatics as an eosinophilic pneumonia. It is thought to be a type of hypersensitivity reaction but unlike other forms of aspergillus infection, this type is not invasive. There is no pathognomic test for ABPA but presence of all the criteria mentioned in the question would make the diagnosis very likely. ABPA would give an obstructive not restrictive lung function abnormality.

1.43 **E**** Thromboangitis obliterans or Buerger's disease is an inflammatory, obliterative, non-atheromatous vascular disease that affects small and medium-sized blood vessels. Patients are usually middle-aged men who smoke. The diagnosis can be confirmed by arteriography. The history is not suggestive of sciatic nerve damage, which would be associated with normal peripheral pulses and usually be unilateral.

1.44 **E***** This patient has sharply defined red, scaling, pruritic lesions with centrifugal spreading. If this were eczema it ought to respond to topical steroids, but as this is a fungal infection steroids allow the infection to spread.

1.45 **D***** The chest X-ray shows right middle lobe collapse. There is a raised right hemidiaphragm and shadowing of the right lower zone obscuring part of the right heart border. An inhaled foreign body, mucus plug, neoplasm or any cause of consolidation could cause this.

1.46 **B***** Stokes–Adams syncope is usually due to transient asystole or ventricular tachyarrhythmia. Patients typically develop sudden loss of consciousness, with no warning, that improves spontaneously. There is no jerking of limbs, tongue biting or headache, although incontinence does occur occasionally.

Vasovagal syncope typically occurs in the upright position and is usually preceded by vagally mediated symptoms such as nausea, yawning, sweating or apprehension. Orthostatic syncope is due to hypovolaemia or excessive venous pooling; it tends to occur when adopting the upright position after prolonged bed rest. Apart from the loss of consciousness there is no focal neurological lesion for this to be classed as a transient ischaemic attack.

1.47 D** This patient has blisters all over her body, which have burst to leave red, denuded areas. The bullae also involve mucous membranes, which are characteristic of pemphigus vulgaris; this is very rare in pemphigoid. If the skin next to the vesicles is pressed, the epidermal layers can be removed, and this is referred to as Nikolsky's sign and indicates that the keratinocytes within the epidermal tissue have been disturbed by acantholysis. Unlike pemphigoid, there are intercellular deposits of IgG and complement within the epidermis. Pemphigus vulgaris is lethal if left untreated.

1.48 A** Diabetes insipidus (DI) is characterised by a low urine osmolalilty that fails to concentrate with water deprivation. The fact that there is significant concentration of the urine after injection of desmopressin (DDAVP) is consistent with central or hypothalamic DI. This is complete central DI because there is an undetectable level of ADH circulating in the blood even after water deprivation. A plasma osmolality >295–300 mosmol/kg should be an adequate response for the release of ADH. With partial central DI, the kidneys still retain some concentrating ability; the urine osmolality would be expected to be higher than in complete central DI, the expected increase in urine osmolality would be less after DDAVP injection, and there would be reduced but detectable levels of ADH in the blood post deprivation test. The normal levels of $\text{plasma}_{\text{ADH}}$ post deprivation test would be 3–5 pg/ml.

1.49 D*** A patient with bronchospasm, flushing and chronic diarrhoea is most likely to have carcinoid syndrome. The definitive test is a 24-h urine collection for 5-HIAA.

1.50 A*** This patient has generalised osteoarthritis. Unlike inflammatory arthritides, pain and stiffness of joints is worse with activity, although non-weight bearing exercises like swimming can help. There is no role for oral or parenteral steroids. Predisposing factors for osteoarthritis include advanced age, previous joint trauma, certain occupations (e.g. machine tool operators), abnormal joint mechanics and smoking. Alcohol and early menopause are associated with osteoporosis.

1.51 **E**** The X-ray shows bone medullary lucency and expansion of the phalanx. There is also some soft tissue swelling. These findings would be consistent with sarcoidosis affecting the hands. (see also **4.30**).

1.52 **B**** This young girl has a strawberry naevus, which is a benign haemangioma and full of blood, so it could potentially haemorrhage. The tumour is not present at birth but usually appears within the first month of life. Most tumours start to involute during the first year and many have fully resolved by age 5–7. There is no sex predominance. This lesion would be too large to treat with laser and should be treated conservatively; otherwise surgery and steroids would be the treatment options of choice.

1.53 **C**** This patient is likely to have a phaeochromocytoma (see also **5.53**) Prior to the operation her blood pressure would need to be controlled. She needs α-adrenergic blockade **first** and then β-blockade, otherwise there will be unopposed α-adrenergic stimulation.

1.54 **B**** This patient has had a cholecystectomy and her symptoms are worse after eating. The history is suggestive of bile salt malabsorption. She would respond best to a bile acid sequestrant like cholestyramine. This could be investigated by a SeHCAT scan.

1.55 **C**** This patient has hypogonadotrophic hypogonadism or Kallman's syndrome, as there is also colour blindness and midline facial defects. These patients may also have anosmia. It can be inherited as an X-linked dominant condition. The basic defect is deficiency of gonadatrophin-releasing hormone from the hypothalamus. (see also **4.51**).

1.56 **C**** The history is very suggestive of biliary colic. Peptic ulcer disease is not always associated with eating but is more of a continuous disease rather than episodes of severe abdominal pain.

1.57 **B*** This patient has symptoms of adrenal insufficiency. The hyperkalaemia and hypoglycaemia are consistent with this diagnosis. The previous medical history of autoimmune thyroid disease and family history of diabetes suggests that this patient has an autoimmune polyglandular syndrome (APS). APS type 2 is associated with adrenal insufficiency, autoimmune thyroid disease and diabetes type 1. Patients may also suffer from gonadal failure or other autoimmune conditions like coeliac disease, vitiligo, pernicious anaemia, alopecia, Sjögren's syndrome and rheumatoid arthritis.

1.58 **E**** This patient has signs of scurvy (vitamin C deficiency). Lack of vitamin C is associated with mild iron deficiency anaemia. Wernicke–Korsakoff's syndrome due to thiamine deficiency tends to present with ataxia, ophthalmoplegia, nystagmus, global confusional state and polyneuropathy.

1.59 **C**** The four-chamber echo shows a dark layer surrounding the heart suggestive of a large pericardial effusion.

1.60 **A***** This patient has developed 'tumour lysis syndrome' which is a form of uric acid nephropathy. It is characterised by acute renal failure post chemotherapy with urine showing red cells and granular casts. In lymphoproliferative and myeloproliferative disorders there is increased cell turnover; after starting chemotherapy, massive cell necrosis occurs, leading to increased uric acid production. The uric acid crystals can become deposited in the renal tubules, causing obstruction and acute renal failure. The aim is to prevent the condition from happening by making sure patients are well hydrated and by giving prophylactic allopurinol to block xanthine oxidase to prevent hyperuricaemia. Once acute renal failure develops, patients may need dialysis.

1.61 **E***** This patient has evidence of atopy as she has a history of asthma, hayfever and IgE response to eggs. The history on the other hand is not consistent with IgE-mediated allergy because such patients typically develop multiorgan symptoms and signs (i.e. urticaria, angioedema, rhinoconjunctivitis, gastrointestinal anaphylaxis and general anaphylaxis) within a few minutes to 2 h post-ingestion. Such patients will avoid the allergen for fear of a fatal reaction and this fear does not diminish with time. Skin prick testing may have a high sensitivity for various allergens but a poor specificity, particularly when testing for food allergens. The test should be performed with the patient off antihistamines. If this is not possible, then immunoassay for food-specific IgE can be done. Eggs, milk, nuts, shellfish and fruit are the most common types of food allergy.

1.62 **A*** The diagnosis of acute cellular rejection is made on liver biopsy and certain features must be present: (1) mixed cellular infiltrate – lymphocytes, neutrophils, plasma cells and eosinophils; (2) endothelitis – characterised by activated lymphocytes and monocytes adhering to the vascular endothelium (here they are surrounding and infiltrating the blood vessel with endothelial cell drop off); (3) bile duct damage – inflammation and irregularity of the interlobular bile ducts with infiltration by lymphocytes and monocytes. Sepsis is characterised by large bile plugs. Graft versus host disease is very rare so soon after transplantation and is seen more often with stem cell transplantation (see **1.71**). Ischaemia is associated with centrilobular collapse (not seen here) and abnormal liver ultrasound.

1.63 D* This patient has developed cardiogenic shock complicating an acute anterior MI. It is defined as a state of inadequate tissue perfusion due to cardiac dysfunction. It is characterised by systemic hypotension, signs of systemic hypoperfusion and respiratory distress secondary to pulmonary congestion. Glycoprotein IIb/IIIa inhibitors have been shown to be beneficial in the treatment of non-STEMI, and increased survival rate in those who developed cardiogenic shock. Whilst the same result has not been conclusively shown in STEMI patients who have developed cardiogenic shock, there is no evidence it makes the condition worse. Negatively inotropic agents, i.e. β-blockers and calcium channel antagonists like verapamil, should be avoided, especially as the patient has pulmonary oedema. Tachyarrhythmias should be treated with amiodarone. Inotropic support will be necessary in this patient but dobutamine's vasodilator effect could worsen the hypotension; dopamine or noradrenaline (norepinephrine) should be used in the first instance. Despite the metabolic acidosis, bicarbonate should not be given as it can lead to fluid overload, hypernatraemia and post-recovery metabolic alkalosis. The acidosis will often respond to mechanical ventilation and hyperventilation. The balloon of the intra-aortic balloon pump is inserted into the femoral artery to lie in the distal descending thoracic aorta. It inflates and deflates in coordination with the cardiac cycle, increasing diastolic aortic pressure, improving coronary perfusion and reducing left ventricular afterload. It should be used in patients with evidence of tissue hypoperfusion that is unresponsive to vasopressors.

1.64 D*** This patient with poorly controlled asthma should be on inhaled steroids (200–800 μg of beclomethasone/day) because he has had exacerbations of asthma in the last 2 years, is regularly using inhaled β_2 agonists and is still getting regular symptoms. The next step if he remains symptomatic is to introduce a long acting β_2-agonist (LABA), such as salmeterol or formoterol. If LABAs in conjunction with inhaled steroids do not result in adequate control, then the LABA could be stopped. There are a number of further options, including increasing the inhaled steroid dose up to 2000 μg/day; leucotriene receptor antagonists (such as montelukast or zifirlukast); oral theophylline; or an oral β_2 agonist (salbutamol or bambuterol). Oral steroids should only be tried after these options have been shown not to be effective.

BTS/SIGN. British guideline on the management of asthma. April 2004.

1.65 E** The cause for this patient's hyponatraemia is the continued use of diuretics and intravenous dextrose. She appears to be euvolaemic, and have normal thyroid and renal function and low urinary sodium and osmolality, which do not support a diagnosis of SIADH. In an asymptomatic patient, fluid restriction may be the most sensible plan to prevent further hyponatraemia. With acute hyponatraemia the decreased plasma osmolality creates a gradient which favours the transport of water into the cells, leading to cerebral oedema. If this process occurs more chronically, then the brain can adapt by losing sodium and other organic solutes into the cerebrospinal fluid, reducing the amount of oedema and keeping the brain volume close to normal. Patients may be asymptomatic despite a plasma sodium concentration of 115–120 but below this level they can become confused, lethargic and dizzy, and have muscle cramps and sometimes seizures and coma. Unfortunately the brain is not so efficient at dealing with rapid increases in sodium concentration and this can lead to an osmotic demyelination – central pontine myelinolyis. The sodium should not be corrected by more than 10–12 mEq/L within the first 24 h. As this patient has symptomatic hyponatraemia treatment requires more than just fluid restriction. Dextrose saline (0.18% NaCl) has even less sodium than normal isotonic saline (0.9%). She will need slow administration of hypertonic saline (3% NaCl). The amount of sodium required is determined by calculating the sodium deficit:

Sodium deficit = total body weight x (desired Na – actual Na)

1.66 A* A patient with purulent effluent should be assumed to have peritonitis regardless of whether there is pyrexia or not. The white cell count is >100 cells/mm^3 and polymorphs are >50%, which is consistent with infection. Most infections are due to Gram-positive cocci, such as *Staphylococcus aureus*, but *Pseudomonas aeruginosa* is another common organism and empirical treatment should cover both these organisms. Treatment depends on local protocols but usually involves antibiotics being given intraperitoneally with the dose depending on the patient's weight. Antibiotics are given for at least 2 weeks. Fungal infections account for about 20% of infections. Fungi, *Pseudomonas*, multiple organisms and bowel perforation are all indications for removal of the catheter; otherwise it can be left in position. Blood cultures frequently do not grow the organism and patients may have so-called 'sterile peritonitis'.

International Society of Peritoneal Dialysis (ISPD) (2005) Peritoneal dialysis-related infections recommendations: 2005 update. *Peritoneal Dialysis Int* **25**: 107–31.

1.67 A*** This patient may well have a lung neoplasm, as suggested by the weight loss, haemoptysis and abnormal chest X-ray, but this cannot explain the macrocytosis, thrombocytopaenia and elevated GGT. Subacute combined degeneration of the cord due to vitamin B12 deficiency is not associated with thrombocytopaenia and loss of vibration sense is a common deficit. Polymyalgia and polymyositis would not cause those abnormalities of the blood results or the sensory disturbance. The low platelet count and macrocytosis with mild elevation of the LFTs is alcohol induced.

1.68 D** This patient has a severe pneumonia, pyrexia and evidence of coming into contact with wildfowl or poultry, and has recently returned from Vietnam. Avian influenza H5N1 is the most likely diagnosis. Influenza viruses are classified depending on their core protein (A, B or C), their species of origin and surface glycoprotein subtype: haemagglutinin (HA) and neuraminidase (NA). It is usually spread by aerosol contact from animal to human but there are reports of human to human spread. Patients can also present with watery diarrhoea, pancytopaenia and elevated aminotransferases. Diagnosis can be confirmed by viral culture and PCR detection of H5N1 viral RNA, but this has to be done at a specialist centre. There is a high mortality. Patients should be barrier-nursed in a single room with negative pressure. The neuraminidase inhibitors oseltamivir and zanamivir have been shown to be effective but specialist advice should be sought first. There is no vaccine currently available.

The Writing Committee of the World Health Organization (WHO). (2005) Consultation on Human Influenza A/H5 *N Engl J Med* **353**: 1374–85. http://www.hpa.org.uk/infections/topics-az/influenza/avian/case-definition.htm#introduction

1.69 E** There are a number of causes of genital ulceration: sexually transmitted infections, i.e. HSV, primary and secondary syphilis, chancroid, LGV and granuloma inguinale; trauma; Behçet's disease; erythema multiforme; pyoderma gangrenosum; fixed drug eruptions; inflammatory bowel disease; lichen planus; lichen sclerosis; and neoplasms, i.e. basal cell carcinoma, squamous cell carcinoma and melanoma. HSV is associated with multiple, painful shallow ulcers with associated tender regional lymphadenopathy. There are two main types of HSV infection: type 1 mainly affects the mouth and type 2 mainly affects the genitalia, but both viruses can affect either area. Patients can present with constitutional symptoms like fever, malaise and myalgia. The test of choice is viral cell culture with a sensitivity of >90% in a fresh sample. Treatment is with aciclovir. Syphilis presents with a single, non-tender ulcer. HIV seroconversion does not usually cause genital ulceration; this is more associated with pharyngitis, lymphadenopathy and rash. Candida usually causes balanitis in men.

1.70 E*** In a patient with asthma and evidence of vasculitis (nodules, skin changes and peripheral neuropathy), Churg–Strauss syndrome is the most likely diagnosis. Whilst lung involvement is not a universal finding, the disease usually starts with atopy, rhinitis and asthma before developing esoinophilia and vasculitis. A number of complications can occur – respiratory system: asthma, pulmonary infiltrates, nodules usually without cavitation, diffuse interstitial disease and pulmonary haemorrhage; nervous system: mononeuritis multiplex, polyneuropathy and cerebral infarction and haemorrhage; cardiovascular system: acute leading to constrictive pericarditis, congestive cardiac failure and myocardial infarction; gastrointestinal system: abdominal pain, bloody diarrhoea secondary to eosinophilic gastroenteritis and colitis, and vasculitic infarcts leading to gastrointestinal haemorrhage; joints: arthritis and arthralgia, although these are not common; and renal system: hypertension, glomerulonephritis, proteinuria and haematuria, but, unlike in Wegener's granulomatosis, renal failure is not common.

1.71 E* In a patient who has had a stem cell transplant and now presents with diarrhoea, skin rash and deranged liver function tests, graft versus host disease (GVHD) needs to be excluded. The rectal biopsy shows all the characteristic features: (1) lack of crypts, (2) apoptotic bodies which are not usually seen, and (3) inflammation. The diagnosis can be made on clinical grounds. The skin rash is typically pruritic and maculopapular, and affects the upper and lower limbs and neck but may spread across the whole body to form bullous lesions with toxic epidermal necrolysis. Hepatic involvement is relatively common and usually presents with raised bilirubin and ALP. Other organs that can be involved include the upper and lower gastrointestinal tract, and haemopoietic system, resulting in thrombocytopaenia and recurrent infections. There is still a significant mortality associated with GVHD. Risk factors for developing GVHD include HLA and gender disparity along with increasing age of the recipient. Most patients are not given immunosuppressive treatment post-stem cell transplantation, but if GVHD does develop then first-line treatment in a patient already on ciclosporin is methylprednisolone. Methotrexate, tacrolimus, mycophenolate and antithymocyte globulin are indicated in patients who fail, or cannot tolerate, initial treatment.

1.72 E* This patient has a malignancy of unknown primary origin. There is evidence that some patients do respond to platinum-based chemotherapeutic agents. Favourable features are a young age (<50 years old), histology showing a poorly differentiated carcinoma (as opposed to adenocarcinoma), no more than three metastatic sites, normal CEA and tumour confined to the retroperitoneal and peripheral lymph nodes.

Van der Gaast A, Verweig J, Henzen-Logmans SC, Rodenburg CJ, Stoger G (1990) Carcinoma of unknown primary: identification of a treatable subset? *Ann Oncol* **1**: 119–22

1.73 C** This patient has life-threatening asthma and appears to be on the verge of respiratory arrest. In this situation she needs elective intubation and ventilation. Her bronchospasm will generate high airways pressure and low lung compliance. Her agitation will require her to be paralysed before she can be ventilated. In pressure support ventilation each patient's breath is amplified by positive pressure supplied by the ventilator. The patient has control over the respiratory rate, inspiratory time and inspiratory flow rate. For this type of ventilation the patient needs to generate a spontaneous breath which cannot happen if neuromuscular blockade is induced. It is used to wean patients off the ventilator. Volume control is used in anaesthesia to give a set tidal volume. If used in this patient it could generate high airways pressure and thus a high risk of barotrauma and tension pneumothorax. One way of avoiding this is by paralysing the patient and allowing hypercapnia and hypoventilation, provided there is adequate oxygenation. This can be achieved by synchronised intermittent mechanical ventilation/pressure control ventilation.

1.74 A*** If this were his first presentation to hospital, then it would be reasonable to query a lung neoplasm in the right base. However the changes are chronic and a patient diagnosed with mesothelioma would not survive 5 years. The holly-shaped opacities and pleural plaques are consistent with previous asbestos exposure. Progressive massive fibrosis can occur after exposure to coal or silica and presents with multiple pulmonary nodules usually located in the upper lobes.

1.75 B** The scan shows destruction of the disc between T6 and T7; this is due to an infection such as *Staphylococcus aureus, Pseudomonas* spp, haemolytic streptococci and tuberculosis. Metastatic bone disease causes damage that is centred on the bone but does not usually involve the intervertebral disc. There is no cord compression.

Paper 2

Questions

2.1 A 44-year-old man was admitted to the coronary care unit with an anterior myocardial infarction. This was his first myocardial infarction. He was treated with thrombolysis and his chest pain settled. He was a non-insulin dependent diabetic. He had no retinopathy, neuropathy or nephropathy. He was a non-smoker. Current treatment was gliclazide 80 mg b.d. For the first 2 days he was put onto an intravenous infusion of insulin. Now his blood glucose stick measurements were between 10 and 15.

He was now apyrexial, pulse 70 regular and blood pressure 140/80.

Bloods	Glucose	10.9	HbA_{1c}	8.5
	Na	140	K	4.5
	Urea	6.7	Creatinine	90

The best way to manage his diabetes would be to:

A add metformin to gliclazide
B convert to metformin
C convert to subcutaneous insulin
D increase dose of gliclazide
E leave him on the current dose of gliclazide

2.2 A 70-year-old man was admitted with an acute coronary syndrome but did not receive thrombolysis. The next day he complained of chest pain and, as the doctor approached the patient to assess him, he collapsed suddenly. He had no pulse and was not breathing. The cardiac monitor next to his bed revealed the following trace.

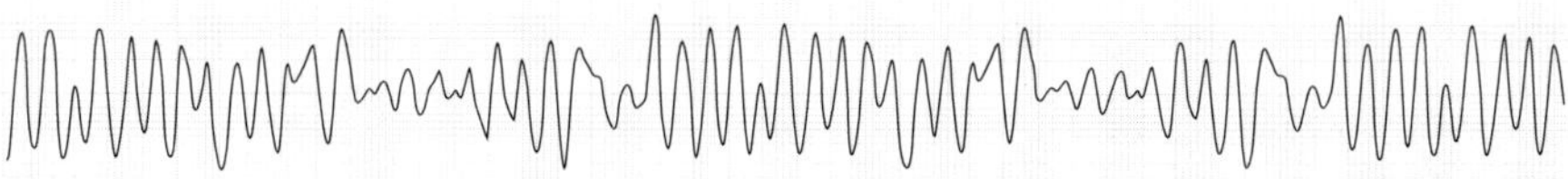

The next step in the immediate management of this patient would be:

A adrenaline 1 mg intravenously
B defibrillate 360 J (monophasic)
C lignocaine 100 mg intravenously
D precordial thump
E start cardiopulmonary chest compressions

2.3 A 42-year-old woman was brought in having collapsed at home. Her husband thought she had taken an overdose a few hours ago but did not know of what. She had a previous medical history of hypertension and depression. She did not drink alcohol.

On examination she was drowsy but could respond to commands. Her temperature was 38.2°C, pulse 120 regular and blood pressure 100/55. Her JVP was not elevated and heart sounds were normal. Respiratory and abdominal examinations were normal, although she had a palpable bladder. Her pupils were dilated but there were no other cranial nerve abnormalities; power, tone and reflexes were normal.

Bloods	Hb	14.0	WCC	7.9
	Platelets	239	INR	1.0
	Na	140	K	3.9
	Urea	4.6	Creatinine	88
	Protein	70	Albumin	40
	Bilirubin	9	ALT	25
	ALP	76	GGT	29
	Glucose	5.2		
Chest X-ray	Normal			
ECG	Sinus tachycardia			
Arterial blood gases on air	pH	7.39	PCO_2	4.1
	PO_2	10.8	Bicarb onate	23
	Base excess	−1.0		

The most likely drug overdose she has taken is:

A amitriptylline
B atenolol
C lithium
D paracetamol
E salicylate

Paper two questions

2.4 A 25-year-old woman returned from Kenya complaining of some itching in her right shin. She had spent most of her time on the beach or on safari. She had no other symptoms. (Figure 2.4, page 375.)

The most likely organism to cause this is:

A *Ancylostoma braziliense*
B *Ascaris lumbricoides*
C *Borrelia burgdorferi*
D *Treponema pertenue*
E *Trichophyton mentagrophytes*

2.5 A 70-year-old woman was brought in drowsy and confused. Her daughter said that she had been off her food and had vomited several times that day.

She had decreased skin turgor and a furred tongue. Her temperature was 38.2°C, pulse 105 regular and BP 100/55. Her JVP was not elevated and heart sounds were normal. Her chest was clear. There was vague lower abdominal tenderness. She was unable to walk independently.

Bloods	Hb	12.5	WCC	13.4
	Platelets	200	Na	152
	K	4.0	Urea	19.0
	Creatinine	184	Glucose	42
Blood gases	pH	7.34	PCO_2	4.6
on air	PO_2	10.5	Bicarbonate	28
Urine osmolality	300 mOsm/kg			
Urinalysis	Protein 2+, glucose 3+, ketones 1+			

The most likely diagnosis is:

A Addison's disease
B Cushing's syndrome
C diabetes insipidus
D diabetic ketoacidosis
E hyperosmolar non-ketotic state

2.6 In patients with hepatic encephalopathy there is increased serum ammonia. It has been suggested that measuring serum ammonia might be a useful screening tool for detecting encephalopathy. You have been asked to design a study to investigate this possibility.

The most appropriate study design would be:

- A case control study
- B case reports
- C cohort study
- D cross-sectional study
- E randomised controlled trial

2.7 A 53-year-old man was admitted with central abdominal pain and vomiting. He had had abdominal pain for 5 months but this had worsened over the past week. The pain radiated to the back and was exacerbated by eating. He denied any haematemesis or melaena but did complain of watery diarrhoea. He had lost 12 kg in that time period with associated poor appetite. He had a previous medical history of acute pancreatitis and had recently been diagnosed with diabetes for which he took insulin. He had drunk 50 units of alcohol a week for more than 30 years and smoked 20 cigarettes a day.

On examination he looked thin. He was apyrexial. His pulse was 88 regular and blood pressure 116/68. Cardiovascular and respiratory examinations were normal. He had diffuse abdominal tenderness but there was no guarding or organomegaly; bowel sounds were present.

Bloods	Hb	11.6	MCV	100.4
	WCC	8.8	Platelets	200
	Na	133	K	4.2
	Urea	5.7	Creatinine	58
	Albumin	37	Protein	63
	Bilirubin	18	ALT	65
	ALP	140	GGT	70
	Amylase	140	Glucose	8.6
	CRP	40		
Chest X-ray	No abnormality seen			

Of the following complications the one **LEAST** likely to be associated with this patient's condition is:

- A ascites
- B duodenal obstruction
- C protein losing enteropathy
- D pseudoaneurysm
- E splenic vein thrombosis

2.8 A 60-year-old man presented with sudden loss of vision in his left eye. Over the past 3 months he had noticed increased lethargy and loss of weight. He had no previous medical history.

On examination his temperature was 37.0°C, pulse 88 regular and blood pressure 145/90. Cardiovascular and respiratory examinations were normal. Abdominal examination revealed palpable splenomegaly. Cranial nerve examination was normal, ophthalmoscopy: (Figure 2.8, page 375.)

Bloods	Hb	8.0	MCV	98
	WCC	8.7	Neutrophils	5.0
	Lymphocytes	3.0	Monocytes	0.2
	Platelets	450	ESR	140
	Protein	84	Albumin	38
Immunoglobulins	IgG	1.9	IgA	1.2
	IgM	39.7		
Skeletal survey	No lytic lesions			

The most likely diagnosis is:

A chronic myeloid leukaemia
B monoclonal gammopathy of undetermined significance
C multiple myeloma
D myelofibrosis
E Waldenstöm's macroglbulinaemia

2.9 A 35-year-old HIV-positive man presented with shortness of breath and cough productive of green sputum. He was not on any treatment and had no other medical problems.

CD_4 count	95
Viral load	118 500

His current condition is **LEAST** likely to be due to:

A Cytomegalovirus
B *Haemophilus influenzae*
C *Histoplasma capsulatum*
D *Mycobacterium avium intracellulare*
E *Nocardia asteroides*

2.10 A 42-year-old Nigerian woman was referred with left-sided abdominal pain associated with change in bowel habit over the past 4 months. She opened her bowels 3–5 times per day associated with some mucus and blood. Her appetite had decreased and she had lost some weight. She was diagnosed with HIV last year but was not on any treatment. She had arrived from her native Nigeria 3 months ago.

Flexible sigmoidoscopy was performed and biopsies taken. (Figure 2.10, page 376.)

The most likely diagnosis is:

A cytomegalovirus colitis
B giardiasis
C irritable bowel syndrome
D Kaposi's sarcoma
E tuberculous colitis

2.11 A 38-year-old man presented with a 10-day history of fever and myalgia and a 3-day history of abdominal pain and watery diarrhoea. He had returned from the Gambia 2 weeks ago. He had no previous medical problems and apart from mefloquine malaria prophylaxis was not on any medication.

On examination he was not jaundiced. His temperature was 38.4°C, pulse 100 regular and blood pressure 110/80. His JVP was not elevated and heart sounds were normal. There was dullness at the right lung base. He had 4 cm tender hepatomegaly but no splenomegaly. There was no ascites and rectal examination was normal.

Bloods	Hb	12.5	WCC	11.5
	Neutrophils	8.7	Lymphocytes	1.3
	Eosinophils	0.2	Platelets	286
	Na	140	K	4.2
	Urea	4.3	Creatinine	86
	Protein	68	Albumin	35
	Bilirubin	12	ALT	30
	ALP	120	CRP	150
Malaria films	Negative			
Chest X-ray	Elevated right hemidiaphragm			

The most likely diagnosis is:

A amoebic liver abscess
B hepatitis A
C hydatid cyst
D schistosomiasis
E typhoid

2.12 A 60-year-old man developed right-sided weakness affecting his face and upper limb 8 h previously at breakfast. His speech became slurred and his right arm became weak, with some recovery of power in his arm when seen by the GP. There was no headache, loss of consciousness or fits. Three years ago while having an operation he was noted to have atrial fibrillation but was not on any medication. There was no other significant previous medical history. He did not smoke but drank 2 units of alcohol a night.

On examination he was fully conscious and alert. His temperature was 36.5°C, pulse 95 irregular and blood pressure 135/70. There were no murmurs or carotid bruits. There was a slight right facial droop and expressive dysphasia. His gag reflex was intact and he was able to swallow. Fundoscopy was normal. He had normal tone, power, reflexes and sensation in all limbs with flexor plantar responses.

Bloods	Hb	14.5	WCC	6.7
	Platelets	345	Na	140
	K	4.7	Urea	4.6
	Creatinine	78	PT	11.4
	ESR	6	Glucose	5.5

The most appropriate immediate treatment for this patient would be:

A aspirin 300 mg
B dipyridamole 75 mg
C no treatment until CT head is performed
D thrombolysis with tissue plasminogen activator
E warfarin

2.13 A 44-year-old woman was referred with vomiting. As part of the examination, fundoscopy was performed.(Figure 2.13, page 376.)

The fundoscopic appearance is most likely due to:

A central retinal vein occlusion
B choroidal metastases
C choroidoretinitis
D photocoagulation scars
E retinitis pigmentosa

2.14 A 50-year-old man who was a heavy smoker presented with shortness of breath and productive cough.

Arterial blood gases on air	pH	7.21	PCO_2	9.8
	PO_2	7.7	Bicarbonate	34.5
	Base excess	6.3		

These blood gases show:

- A mixed respiratory and metabolic acidosis with type I respiratory failure
- B mixed respiratory and metabolic acidosis with type II respiratory failure
- C respiratory acidosis but not in respiratory failure
- D respiratory acidosis with type I respiratory failure
- E respiratory acidosis with type II respiratory failure

2.15 A 55-year-old woman was referred with a 4-month history of back and shoulder pain. There was no history of trauma. Her symptoms mainly affected the neck, back and shoulder muscles with some shoulder joint pain. She had some morning stiffness, but normal appetite and no loss of weight. There was a previous medical history of migraine and severe tiredness. She did not smoke or drink alcohol. She took paracetamol self-medication.

On examination, she looked well. Her pulse was 74 regular and blood pressure 132/78. There was a full range of movements of all joints, although some muscle tenderness over the spine and shoulders. Power, tone, reflexes and sensation were normal.

Bloods	Hb	14.3	WCC	7.4
	Platelets	332	Na	138
	K	4.9	Urea	5.2
	Creatinine	83	Protein	70
	Albumin	40	Bilirubin	11
	ALT	18	ALP	68
	GGT	30	Creatinine kinase	75
	ESR	12	CRP	4
	TSH	2.5	Free T4	20
Rheumatoid factor	Negative			

The most likely diagnosis is:

- A cervical radiculopathy
- B fibromyalgia
- C osteoarthritis
- D polymyalgia rheumatica
- E polymyositis

2.16 A 45-year-old woman was referred with skin bruising. This is the appearance of her eyes; (Figure 2.16, page 377.)

The **LEAST** likely diagnosis is:

A Behçet's syndrome
B Ehlers-Danlos syndrome
C Marfan's syndrome
D osteogenesis imperfecta
E pseudoxanthoma elasticum

2.17 A 28-year-old woman was referred because of a 5-month history of progressive shortness of breath and pain in her hands and feet.

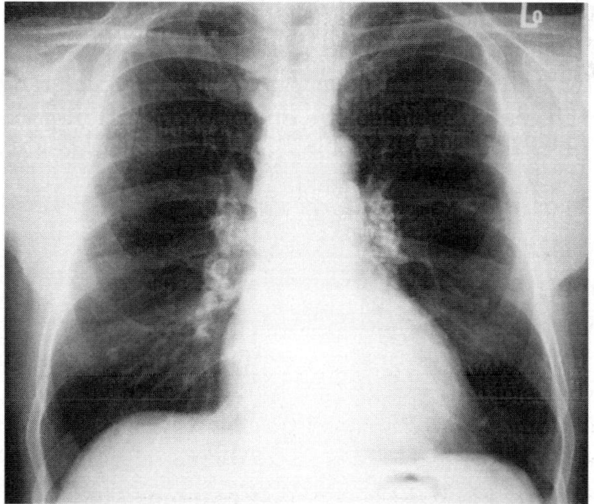

The most likely diagnosis is:

A histoplasmosis
B Hodgkin's lymphoma
C sarcoidosis
D systemic lupus erythematosus
E tuberculosis

2.18 A 21-year-old man presented with a 2-month history of back stiffness.

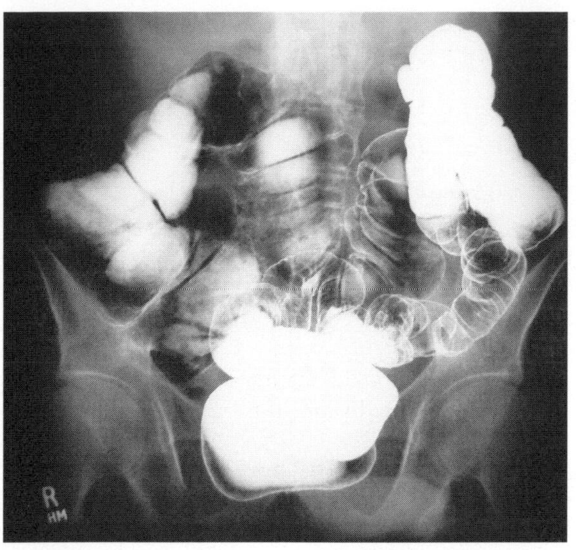

Of the following the one which is NOT associated with this patient's rheumatological condition is:

A amyloidosis
B atrioventricular conduction block
C Crohn's disease
D pulmonary fibrosis
E scleritis

2.19 A 15-year-old girl was referred for cardiac catheterisation because of progressive shortness of breath.

	Pressure (systolic/diastolic [mmHg])	Normal value (systolic/diastolic [mmHg])	O_2 saturation (%)
Right atrium	8	0–8	75
Right ventricle	32/11	15–30/0–8	76
Pulmonary artery	43/14	15–30/0–8	85
Left atrium (mean)	12	1–10	96
Left ventricle	132/12	100–140/3–12	97
Aorta	135/70	100–140/60–90	97

The most likely diagnosis is:

A atrial septal defect
B coarctation of the aorta
C Fallot's tetralogy
D patent ductus arteriosus
E ventricular septal defect

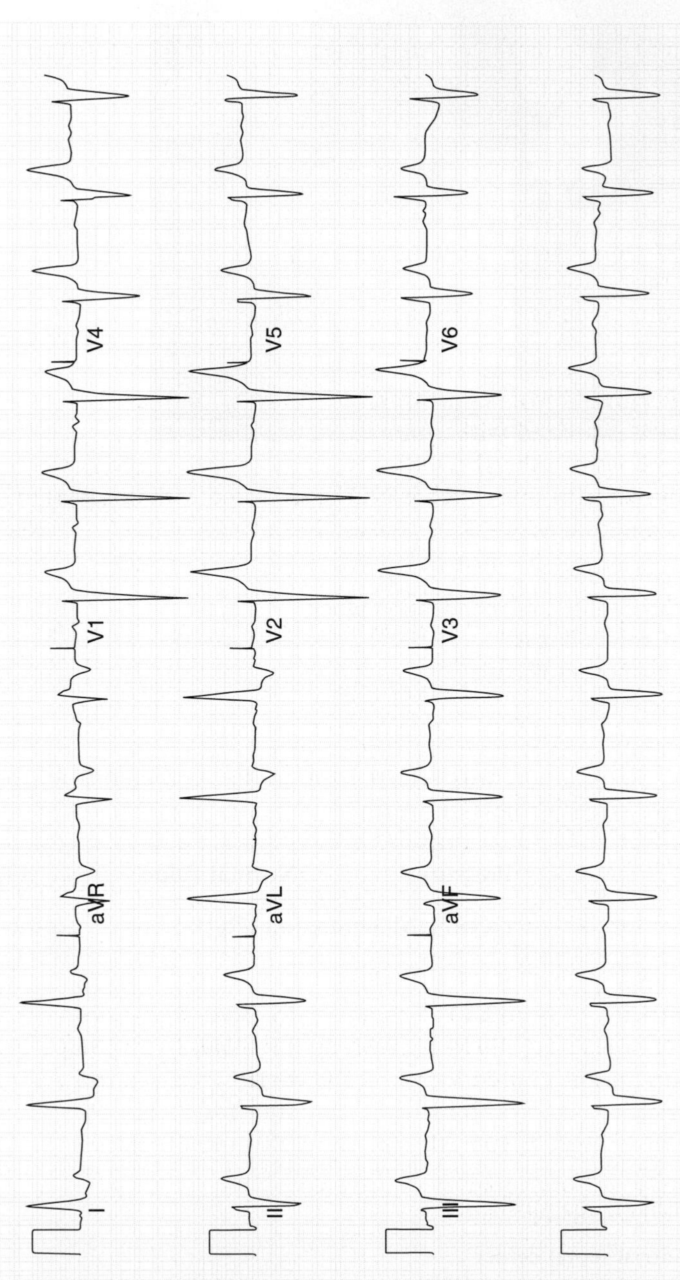
I
aVR
V1
V4
II
aVL
V2
V5
III
aVF
V3
V6

2.20 A 71-year-old woman was found collapsed at home. She could not remember what had happened and complained of some discomfort in her chest and arms.

Her pulse was 60 regular and blood pressure 100/62. Chest and abdominal examinations were normal. ECGs were performed (A) before and (B) a few hours after she was given treatment.

The treatment likely to have changed the ECG appearances is:

A calcium gluconate
B intravenous amiodarone
C intravenous potassium supplements
D rewarming
E thrombolysis with tissue plasminogen activator

2.21 A 39-year-old woman known to suffer from depression and schizophrenia was admitted with vomiting, urinary and faecal incontinence and blurred vision. She also had a headache and felt light headed. Her husband thought she had taken an overdose but did not know of what.

On examination she was alert but uncooperative. Her temperature was 36.9°C, pulse 80 regular and blood pressure 100/69. Her JVP was not elevated and heart sounds were normal. Her chest was clear but she had vague abdominal tenderness. She had a tremor at rest and jerky movements of her upper and lower limbs. Her reflexes were brisk and plantar responses were equivocal.

The most likely overdose this patient has taken is:

A amitriptylline
B haloperidol
C lithium
D lorazepam
E propanolol

2.22 A 46-year-old woman with alcoholic liver cirrhosis was referred because of a non-pruritic, blistering rash on her hands, which left scarring. She also complained of increased facial hair growth. (Figure 2.22, page 377.)

The most likely diagnosis is:

A bullous pemphigoid
B epidermolysis bullosa
C pemphigus vulgaris
D porphyria cutanea tarda
E scleroderma

2.23 A 55-year-old woman was admitted with central crushing chest pain lasting 2 h. Her ECG showed atrial fibrillation and T wave inversion in leads II, III and aVF. She was not given thrombolysis. Her pain responded to diamorphine and glyceryl trinitrate.

On examination she was pale but apyrexial. Her pulse was 60 irregular and blood pressure 130/60. Her chest was clear and heart sounds were normal.

Bloods				
	Hb	12.5	WCC	9.6
	Platelets	270	MCV	86.8
	Na	140	K	3.9
	Urea	4.7	Creatinine	90
	TSH	0.4	Free T_4	6

The most likely explanation for these results is:

A primary hyperthyroidism
B primary hypothyroidism
C secondary hypothyroidism
D sick euthyroid syndrome
E surreptitious treatment with thyroxine

2.24 A case control study was performed to see if there was an association between overhead power cables and development of leukaemia. One hundred and sixty subjects were included, of whom 50 had leukaemia and 110 control patients who did not. Ten leukaemia patients had lived near power cables, as had 30 control patients.

The odds ratio (OR) is:

A (10 x 30)/(40 x 80)
B (10 x 40)/(30 x 80)
C (10 x 50)/(30 x 110)
D (10 x 80)/(30 x 40)
E (10 x 110)/(30 x 50)

2.25 A 60-year-old homeless man presented to Accident & Emergency with confusion. He smelt of alcohol, was verbally abusive but could answer questions.

On examination his GCS was 14/15. He was apyrexial and not jaundiced. His speech was slurred and he was disorientated in time and place but there was no tremor or flap. His pulse was 70 regular and blood pressure 150/100. Chest examination was normal. His abdomen was soft, not tender and mildly distended with shifting dullness. Bowel sounds were present and rectal examination revealed some stool but no melaena.

Bloods	Hb	12.4	WCC	11.3
	Platelets	100	INR	1.4
	Na	135	K	3.9
	Urea	4.5	Creatinine	56
	Protein	60	Albumin	30
	Bilirubin	20	ALT	55
	ALP	230		
Chest X-ray	No abnormality detected			
Urinalysis	Normal			

The next **THREE** steps in his immediate management would be:

A diagnostic ascitic tap
B fresh frozen plasma
C intravenous ranitidine
D intravenous terlipressin
E intravenous thiamine
F intravenous vitamin K
G oral antibiotics
H oral diazepam
I oral neomycin
J oral prednisolone
K oral propanolol
L rectal phosphate enema
M therapeutic paracentesis with albumin cover
N upper gastrointestinal endoscopy

2.26 A 75-year-old man originally presented 10 years ago with sore eyes which were gradually getting worse. Five years ago he started to experience diplopia on upgaze. This had now progressed to blurred vision in his left eye. (Figure 2.26, page 377.)

The **MOST** likely diagnosis is:

A carotico-cavernous fistula
B lacrimal gland neoplasm
C orbital arteriovenous malformation
D orbital cellulitis
E thyroid eye disease

2.27 A 45-year-old woman was referred because of dysphagia and weight loss. There was no haematemesis or melaena. She had no abdominal pain or bowel problems. She had smoked 20 cigarettes a day for over 20 years and drank 4 units of alcohol a night.

On examination she was not jaundiced or pale. Her pulse was 88 regular and blood pressure 120/69. Respiratory and abdominal examinations were normal. An endoscopy was performed and oesophageal biopsies were taken. (Figure 2.27, page 378.)

The most likely diagnosis is:

A Barrett's oesophagus
B normal oesophageal mucosa
C oesophageal candidiasis
D oesophageal adenocarcinoma
E squamous cell carcinoma

2.28 A 19-year-old woman presented with a 5-day history of fever, lethargy and cough. Following this she had some abdominal pain and had noticed frank haematuria. She had returned from Malawi a week ago where she had been on safari. She had no other medical problems and had taken mefloquine malaria prophylaxis. She had one regular sexual partner and did not drink alcohol or smoke.

Her temperature was 38.0°C, pulse 100 regular and blood pressure 130/80. Physical examination was normal except for some cervical lymphadenopathy.

Bloods	Hb	12.7	WCC	10.9
	Neutrophils	8.4	Lymphocytes	1.4
	Eosinophils	1.0	Platelets	210
	Na	130	K	5.0
	Urea	12.1	Creatinine	200
	Protein	70	Albumin	36
	Bilirubin	10	ALT	28
	ALP	120		
Malaria films	Negative			
Urinalysis	Protein 1+, blood 3+			
Chest X-ray	Normal			

The most likely diagnosis is:

A blackwater fever
B brucellosis
C dengue haemorrhagic fever
D schistosomiasis
E typhoid

2.29 A 47-year-old man presented with wasting of the muscles of the hand. This problem had developed gradually over the last 12 months. He also had paraesthesia in his hands and feet. He had no problems with vision or speech.

On examination he looked well. There was wasting of the small muscles of the hand with some clawing and decreased pinprick sensation. There was also wasting of the distal lower limb muscles and pes cavus. Dorsiflexion was weak. Tone was normal but the ankle and plantar reflexes were absent. There was decreased pinprick sensation up to the ankle. His gait showed dragging of both feet.

The most likely diagnosis is:

A Charcot–Marie–Tooth disease (HSMN)
B Friedreich's ataxia
C subacute combined degeneration of the cord
D syringomyelia
E tabes dorsalis

2.30 A 21-year-old woman was admitted with shortness of breath of 1 day's duration.

Arterial blood gases on air	pH	7.51	PCO_2	3.1
	PO_2	14.3	Bicarbonate	25
	Base excess	–0.5		

These blood gases show:

A metabolic alkalosis and respiratory acidosis with no respiratory failure
B metabolic alkalosis with no respiratory failure
C mixed respiratory and metabolic alkalosis with no respiratory failure
D respiratory alkalosis and metabolic acidosis with no respiratory failure
E respiratory alkalosis with no respiratory failure

2.31 A 70-year-old man presented with a 2-month history of worsening oedema and shortness of breath on exertion. His GP had recently started him on furosemide. Rheumatoid arthritis was diagnosed a number of years ago and had resulted in deformity of his hands. He was on hydroxychloroquine but was no longer under hospital follow-up. He did not smoke or drink alcohol.

On examination he had pitting oedema up to the sacrum with some facial puffiness. His pulse was 88 regular and blood pressure 160/90. His JVP was elevated +4 cm and heart sounds were normal. There was decreased air entry at both lung bases. His abdomen was distended with shifting dullness and 4 cm hepatomegaly. Examination of his hands revealed bilateral 'swan neck' deformities of his fingers.

Bloods	Hb	9.9	MCV	88.2
	WCC	4.9	Platelets	248
	Na	138	K	4.7
	Urea	14.5	Creatinine	210
	Protein	53	Albumin	18
	Bilirubin	18	ALT	35
	ALP	80	Calcium	1.98
	Glucose	5.6	ESR	45
	CRP	30		
Urine dipstick	Protein 3+, no blood			
Chest X-ray	Bilateral pleural effusions			

The most likely diagnosis is:

A AA amyloidosis
B analgesic nephropathy
C constrictive pericarditis
D drug-induced glomerulonephritis
E restrictive cardiomyopathy

2.32 A 69-year-old woman was referred because of lethargy.

As part of the examination, the following was the appearance of her mouth.(Figure 2.32, page 378.)

The clinical findings are most consistent with:

A acromegaly
B amyloidosis
C hypothyroidism
D vitamin B12 deficiency
E vitamin C deficiency

2.33 A 57-year-old woman presented with a 6-week history of progressive dysphagia and weight loss.

The most likely diagnosis is:

A achalasia
B benign stricture due to gastro-oesophageal reflux disease
C carcinoma of the oesophagus
D oesophageal candidiasis
E oesophageal varices

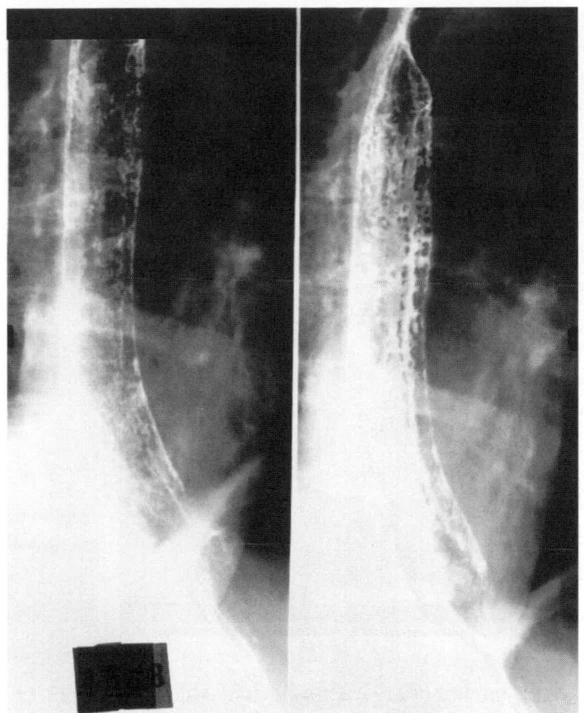

2.34 A 44-year-old woman was referred with a 3-day history of worsening headache, photophobia, nausea and confusion. There was no rash. She had no other medical problems and was not on any medication. She was allergic to penicillin.

On examination she was unwell. Her temperature was 38.1°C, pulse 98 regular and blood pressure 100/60. She was disorientated in time and place but not in person. She had poor short-term memory and her mental test score was 1/10. Kernig's sign was negative. There were no focal neurological signs and plantar responses were flexor. An MRI brain scan was performed.

Bloods	Hb	13.7	WCC	11.0
	Platelets	170	Na	135
	K	4.1	Urea	8.4
	Creatinine	100	Glucose	4.5
	INR	1.2		
CSF	RBC	50	WCC	30
	Neutrophils	14.5%	Lymphocytes	14.5%
	Protein	0.8	Glucose	3.1

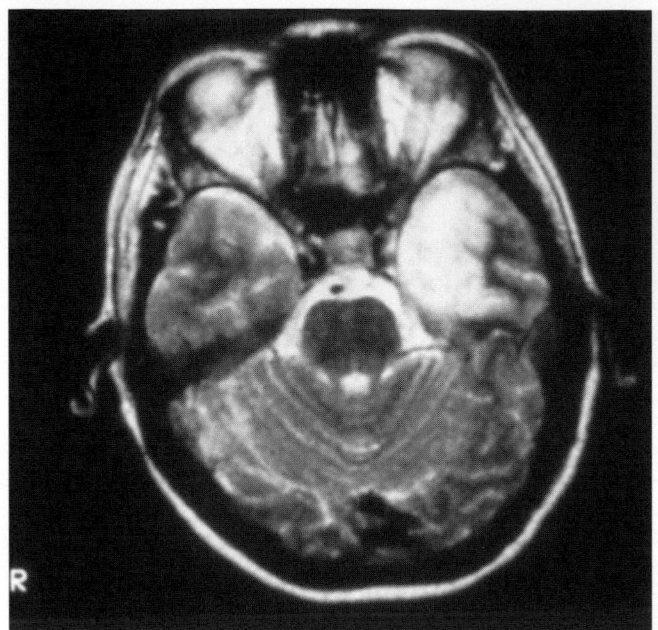

The most appropriate drug treatment for this patient is:

A aciclovir
B cefotaxime
C chloramphenicol
D pyrimethamine and sulphadiazine
E rifampicin, isoniazid and pyrazinamide

2.35 A 59-year-old woman was admitted with pleuritic chest pain and pyrexia. She had no cough, shortness of breath or leg swelling. Four weeks ago she suffered an anterior myocardial infarction, which was treated with thrombolysis, and she had made an uneventful recovery. She had no other previous medical problems. She was taking, since discharge: aspirin, atenolol, simvastatin and isosorbide mononitrate. She did not smoke or drink alcohol.

On examination she was not in pain. Her temperature was 37.6°C, pulse 72 regular and blood pressure 110/70. Her JVP was not elevated. There was an additional heart sound but no murmurs. Her chest was clear. Examination of both lower limbs was normal.

Bloods	Hb	13.0	WCC	11.0
	Platelets	368	INR	1.1
	Na	138	K	4.5
	Urea	4.2	Creatinine	88
	ESR	32	CRP	28
ECG	Q waves in V_{2-6} Minimal ST elevation in V_{2-6} unchanged when compared to previous ECGs			
Arterial blood gases on air	pH	7.43	PCO_2	4.3
	PO_2	11.3	Bicarbonate	25.4
	Base excess	1.1		

The most appropriate treatment for this patient is:

- A amoxicillin
- B diclofenac
- C furosemide
- D nicorandil
- E warfarin

2.36 A 64-year-old man was admitted with palpitations and collapse. He had a previous medical history of hypertension but was not on any medication. He did not drink alcohol or smoke.

His temperature was 37.3°C and blood pressure 110/68.

The ECG shows:

- A atrial fibrillation with aberrant conduction
- B supraventricular tachycardia with aberrant conduction
- C torsades de pointes
- D ventricular fibrillation
- E ventricular tachycardia

2.37 A 42-year-old man was referred with a 3-week history of an ulcerating lesion on his left leg. He was not on any medication.(Figure 2.37, page 378.)

Of the following conditions the THREE **NOT** associated with this skin lesion are:

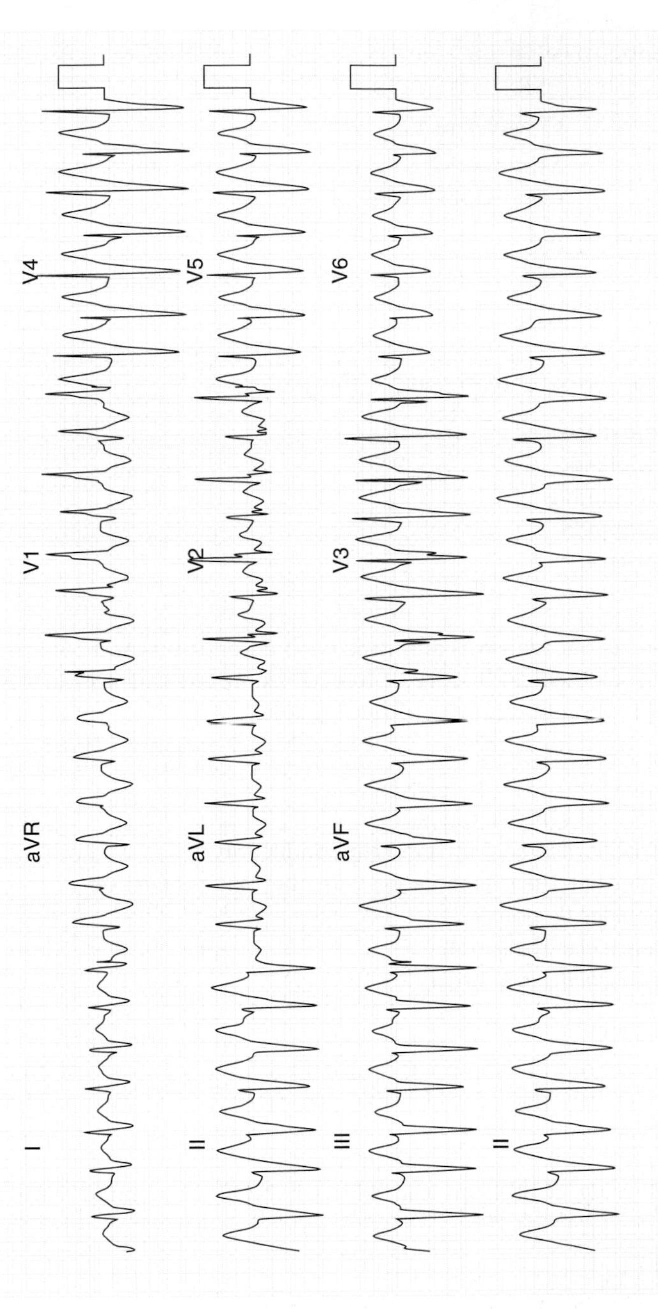
I
aVR
V1
V4
II
aVL
V2
V5
III
aVF
V3
V6
II

A acute myeloid leukaemia
B ankylosing spondylitis
C carcinoid syndrome
D Crohn's disease
E polycythaemia rubra vera
F porphyria cutanea tarda
G rheumatoid arthritis
H sarcoidosis
I tuberculosis
J tuberous sclerosis
K ulcerative colitis
L Wegener's granulomatosis

2.38 An 18-year-old man with learning difficulties presented with numbness and muscle cramps. He had the following blood results:

Bloods	Calcium	1.95	Phosphate	1.6
	Albumin	40	ALP	100
	PTH	7.0	25-Vitamin D_3	75
	1,25-Vitamin D_3	45		

These blood results are most consistent with

A cirrhosis
B hypomagnesaemia
C hypoparathyroidism
D pseudohypoparathyroidism
E pseudopseudohypoparathyroidism

2.39 A 55-year-old female Jehovah's Witness was found to have a carcinoma of the colon at colonoscopy. The colorectal surgeon recommended a total colectomy but informed the patient that this would incur substantial blood loss. The patient was adamant that she did not want a 'blood transfusion' even if she were to exsanguinate on the operating table.

Which one of the following would be acceptable to her and allow the surgeon to perform the operation?

A fresh frozen plasma
B intraoperative autotransfusion of blood collected during operation
C packed red cells
D platelet transfusion
E pre-donation of her own blood with autologous transfusion if necessary

2.40 A 20-year-old woman was referred because of a 6-month history of weight loss and abdominal discomfort. She had an upper gastrointestinal endoscopy with duodenal biopsies suggestive of coeliac disease. She was instructed to follow a gluten-free diet but has concerns about what she can and cannot eat.

Of the following types of food it is safe for her to eat:

A barley
B maize
C oats
D rye
E wheat

2.41 A 29-year-old woman was admitted with palpitations. She had no previous medical history. She did not drink or smoke and was not on any medication.

An ECG was performed.

Of the following drugs the ONE that should be avoided is:

A adenosine
B amiodarone
C flecainide
D sotalol
E verapamil

2.42 A 28-year-old man presented with a 1-week history of progrcssively worse haemoptysis associated with shortness of breath. Subsequently he had passed frank blood in his urine. He had no bowel problems and there was no abdominal pain or haematemesis. He had no joint or skin problems. There was no previous medical history or significant family history. He smoked 20 cigarettes a day and drank 4 units of alcohol at the weekend.

On examination his temperature was 37.3°C, pulse 110 regular and blood pressure 115/80. His JVP was not elevated and heart sounds were normal. There was decreased air entry at his lung bases but no crackles or wheeze. Abdominal examination was normal.

Bloods	Hb	11.5	MCV	80.1
	WCC	9.6	Platelets	245
	Na	135	K	6.3
	Urea	32.4	Creatinine	452
	Protein	70	Albumin	32
	Bilirubin	15	ALT	28
	ALP	65	Calcium	2.24
Urine dipstick	Protein 2+, blood 3+			
Chest X-ray	Bilateral patchy densities			

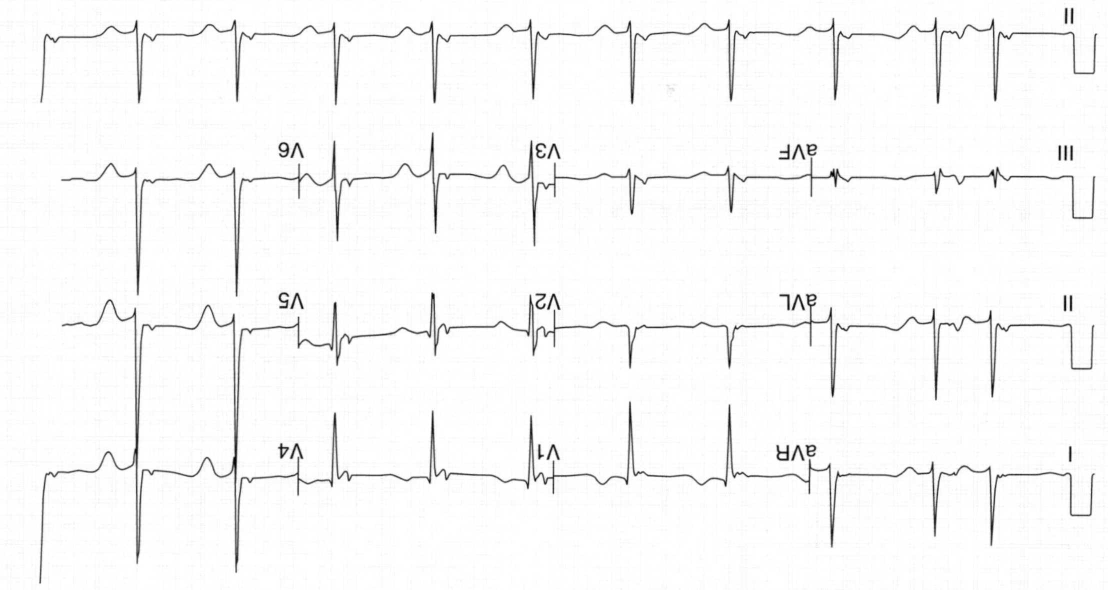
I
aVR
V1
V4
II
aVL
V2
V5
III
aVF
V3
V6
II

The blood test that would be most helpful in establishing the diagnosis is:

A antiglomerular basement membrane antibodies
B antinuclear antibodies (ANA)
C cryoglobulins
D p-ANCA
E rheumatoid factor

2.43 A 47-year-old woman presented with a 1-month history of an ulcer on her left shin that did not appear to be healing. She also complained of decreased sensation in the soles of her feet. For the past 6 months she had been having recurrent attacks of sinusitis and epistaxis. She had now developed a cough associated with blood-tinged sputum. She had a decreased appetite and had lost some weight. She had no previous medical history. She did not smoke or drink alcohol.

On examination her temperature was 37.6°C, pulse 78 and blood pressure 157/79. Her JVP was not elevated and both heart sounds were normal. Her respiratory rate was 20 breaths/min and she had bilateral crackles in her chest. Abdominal examination was normal. There was a 3 cm ulcer on her left shin that appeared 'punched out' with surrounding erythema. She had decreased sensation to light touch and pinprick up to the level of the ankle. There was normal lower limb tone and power but absent ankle and plantar reflexes.

Bloods	Hb	11.9	MCV	92.4
	WCC	7.6	Platelets	459
	Na	138	K	4.8
	Urea	12.4	Creatinine	150
	Protein	74	Albumin	38
	Bilirubin	15	ALT	55
	ALP	100	ESR	65
	CRP	58	C_3	100
	C_4	35		
Rheumatoid factor	Negative			
Antinuclear antibody	Negative			
Hepatitis A, B, C serology	Negative			
Urine dipstick	Blood 2+, protein 3+, red cell casts +			
Chest X-ray	Bilateral infiltrates			
	No consolidation, no pulmonary oedema			

The most likely diagnosis is:

- A Goodpasture's syndrome
- B mixed cryoglobulinaemia
- C polyarteritis nodosa
- D systemic lupus erythematosus
- E Wegener's granulomatosis

2.44 A 72-year-old male smoker complained of headaches. He also had pain in his back and hips.

A skull X-ray was performed.

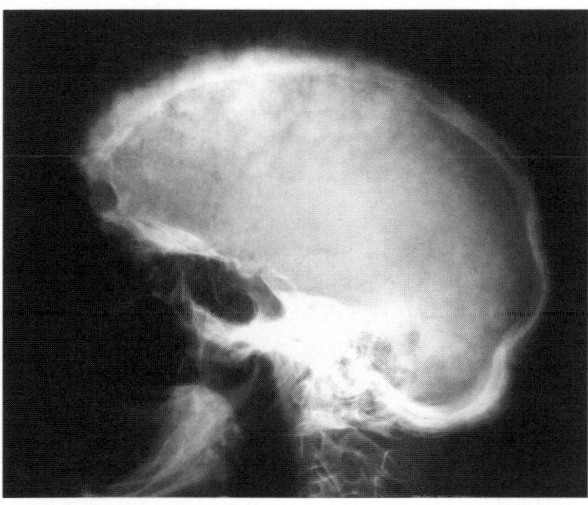

The most likely diagnosis is:

- A acoustic neuroma
- B hypoparathyroidism
- C metastatic lung carcinoma
- D multiple myeloma
- E Paget's disease of bone

2.45 A 58-year-old woman was referred with ulceration of her right index finger. (Figure 2.45, page 379.)

The most likely diagnosis is:

- A dermatomyositis
- B psoriatic arthropathy
- C rheumatoid arthritis
- D systemic lupus erythematosus
- E systemic sclerosis

2.46 A 49-year-old woman presented with weakness affecting all her muscles, including those of her face. This problem had been getting progressively worse over several years. She had also noticed some slurring of her speech. Diabetes mellitus had been diagnosed recently. She had smoked 20 cigarettes a day for 30 years.

On examination she had a left ptosis. There was bilateral wasting of her facial, temporalis, sternocleidomastoid and quadriceps muscles. She had normal tone but reduced power and reflexes. She has difficulty opening her eyes. Sensation and gait were normal. Her cardiovascular and respiratory systems were normal.

The most likely diagnosis is:

A diabetic amyotrophy
B dystrophia myotonica
C Eaton-Lambert syndrome
D motor neurone disease
E myasthenia gravis

2.47 A 65-year-old homeless man was brought to Accident & Emergency suffering from self-neglect. He denied any medical problems and was not on any medications.

He was alert and orientated but was cachexic and dehydrated. The rest of the physical examination was normal.

It was decided to give him intravenous dextrose, insert a nasogastric tube and feed him via this route. Three days later, he became acutely short of breath and very oedematous. His temperature was 37.2°C, pulse 110 regular and blood pressure 140/80. His JVP was elevated +6 cm and he had bilateral crackles in his chest.

Bloods				
	Hb	12.5	WCC	6.8
	Platelets	245	Na	132
	K	2.9	Urea	6.4
	Creatinine	58	Albumin	24
	Protein	50	Bilirubin	17
	ALT	24	ALP	90
	Glucose	4.5	Calcium	1.98
	Magnesium	0.65	Phosphate	0.6

The most likely cause for his deterioration is:

A aspiration pneumonia
B fluid overload with intravenous dextrose
C kwashiorkor
D protein-losing enteropathy
E refeeding syndrome

2.48 A 65-year-old man was referred because of worsening tremor and poor mobility. The tremor was so bad he could not hold a cup without spilling the contents. His handwriting was getting progressively smaller.

On examination he had no facial abnormalities. There was increased tone in his upper limbs and an obvious resting tremor that became worse when he was asked to lift an object. He had normal power and reflexes but his gait was shuffling.

The drug treatment that is contraindicated in his condition is:

A apomorphine
B baclofen
C bromocriptine
D entacapone
E tetrabenazine

2.49 A 72-year-old woman was discharged from hospital after being admitted with an exacerbation of chronic obstructive pulmonary disease (COPD). She had had COPD for 5 years and it was gradually getting worse: she had been admitted four times over a year with the same problem. She had salbutamol and ipratropium bromide nebulisers at home and oxygen cylinders to be used on an 'as needed' basis. She had stopped smoking last year, but prior to that had smoked 30 cigarettes a day for 50 years.

On examination her pulse was 100 regular and blood pressure 145/98. Her JVP was not elevated and both heart sounds were normal. Her respiratory rate was 18 breaths/min and her chest was clear to auscultation.

Arterial blood gases on air	pH	7.35	PCO_2	5.6
	PO_2	7.1	Bicarbonate	38.5
	Base excess	12.4		

Of the following a determinant in deciding whether this patient did NOT need long-term oxygen therapy would be:

A exercise tolerance <5 m
B $FEV_1 \leq 1.5$ L
C $PO_2 \leq 7.3$ kPa on air
D $PO_2 \leq 8.0$ kPa on air with evidence of pulmonary hypertension
E stopping smoking completely

2.50 A 45-year-old woman with Crohn's disease was referred with pain in her left hip for the past 6 weeks. The pain was localized to the buttock, groin, medial thigh and knee, and made her walk with an antalgic gait. There was no back pain or stiffness or other joint pains. She had a normal appetite and no weight loss. She did not smoke or drink alcohol. Her current medication was mesalazine and prednisolone, and she had had numerous courses of steroids in the past. There was no history of trauma.

On examination she was in pain. Her temperature was 37.0°C, pulse 88 regular and blood pressure 125/88. Respiratory and abdominal examinations were normal. The left hip did not appear obviously inflamed but all movements caused severe pain. There was normal sensation and all peripheral pulses were palpable.

Bloods	Hb	13.4	WCC	5.8
	Platelets	260	Na	138
	K	4.0	Urea	4.9
	Creatinine	88	Protein	70
	Albumin	37	Bilirubin	10
	ALT	25	ALP	75
	Calcium	2.20	Phosphate	0.74
	ESR	12	CRP	26
Rheumatoid factor	Negative			
DEXA scan of total hip	T score −0.8			
	Z score −0.5			

The most likely diagnosis is:

- A fibromyalgia
- B osteoarthritis
- C osteomalacia
- D osteonecrosis
- E osteoporosis

2.51 A 52-year-old woman had an MRI scan because of difficulty walking and lack of coordination. She had a normal appetite and no weight loss. She had no previous medical history and was not on any medication. There was no significant family history.

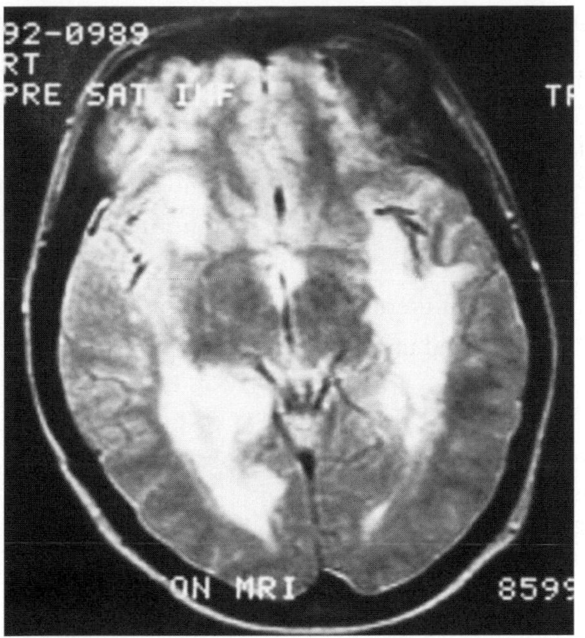

The scan results are most consistent with a diagnosis of:

- A Huntington's chorea
- B metastatic disease
- C multiple sclerosis
- D normal pressure hydrocephalus
- E variant Creutzfeld–Jakob disease

2.52 A 36-year-old woman was referred with a pigmented mole that had increased in size. (Figure 2.52, page 379.)

Of the following features of the pigmented mole the one associated with a **BETTER** prognosis:

- A <1.5cm thick
- B <4 cm in diameter
- C located in the anorectal region
- D located in the buccal mucosa
- E located on upper thigh

2.53 A 16-year-old girl presented with her mother, complaining of primary amenorrhoea. She had been brought up as a girl. She had normal breast development but no axillary or pubic hair. She had no previous medical history and had had a normal development up until now. She was not on any medication.

On examination she was of normal height and weight for her age. Her pulse was 78 and blood pressure 110/70. She had normal breasts. She had normal female external genitalia.

Chromosome analysis	46 XY	
Bloods	17-OH progesterone	7.0 (normal <10 nmol/L)
	FSH	3.5 (normal 1–8 U/L)
	LH	10.4 (normal 1–6 U/L)
Pelvic ultrasound	Absent uterus	
	Bilateral undescended testes	

The most likely diagnosis is:

A 11-β-hydroxylase deficiency
B androgen insensitivity
C gonadal dysgenesis
D Kallman's syndrome
E Klinefelter's syndrome

2.54 A 55-year-old man was found to have a colonic carcinoma on barium enema affecting the caecum. There was no other mass in his large intestine and abdominal ultrasound revealed no liver metastases. He had a right hemicolectomy.

Histology of the mass revealed poorly differentiated adenocarcinoma with invasion through to the muscularis propria and invasion of five regional lymph nodes.

The likely 5-year survival for this patient with treatment would be:

A 20%
B 40%
C 60%
D 75%
E 85%

2.55 A 17-year-old girl was referred with primary amenorrhoea. Since childhood she had had poor growth despite proper care from her parents. Her father was 1.80 m tall and her mother was 1.65 m tall. She had suffered from recurrent urinary tract infections in the past.

On examination she was 1.30 m tall and her weight was 40 kg. There was no breast development and no secondary sexual characteristics. The rest of her appearance was normal.

Bloods	FSH	40 (normal 2.5–10 U/L)
	LH	27 (normal 2.5–10 U/L)
	17-β-oestradiol	45 (normal 70–370 pmol/L)
	17-OH progesterone	7 (normal <14 nmol/L)
	Progesterone	1.5 (normal <5 nmol/L)
	Prolactin	400
Pelvic ultrasound	Small uterus	
	Ovaries not seen very well	
	Duplex kidneys	

Of the following statements concerning her likely diagnosis it is true that:

- A as her progesterone level is normal she only needs cyclical oestrogen therapy
- B growth hormone therapy may improve her stature
- C cardiac abnormalities would be expected in the majority of patients
- D there is an abnormality on chromosome 13
- E this is a form of congenital adrenal hyperplasia

2.56 A 48-year-old man presented with a 1-week history of persistent dull upper abdominal pain and fever. He also complained of pale stools and episodic dark urine. He had decreased appetite, some weight loss and looked yellow. Eighteen months earlier he had undergone laparoscopic cholecystectomy for gallstones and ERCP 4 months ago to remove sludge from the common bile duct. He drank 10 units of alcohol per week and smoked 15 cigarettes a day. He was not on any medication.

On examination he was jaundiced, had a temperature of 39.1°C, pulse 120 regular and blood pressure 120/60. There was right upper quadrant abdominal tenderness but no hepatosplenomegaly and no ascites. Rectal examination was normal. He was not encephalopathic.

Bloods	Hb	12.5	WCC	15.6
	Platelets	345	INR	1.5
	Na	136	K	4.5
	Urea	5.9	Creatinine	120
	Bilirubin	62	Albumin	30
	Protein	60	AST	60
	ALP	360	GGT	140
Chest X-ray	Normal			
Urinalysis	Bilirubin 1+, no protein, no white cells			

The most likely diagnosis is:

A ascending cholangitis
B cholangiocarcinoma
C primary biliary cirrhosis
D primary sclerosing cholangitis
E secondary biliary cirrhosis

2.57 A 57-year-old man was referred with severe abdominal pain, worse after eating but no vomiting. Three months ago a duodenal ulcer had been diagnosed and a proton pump inhibitor started but his symptoms had returned. He had decreased appetite and had lost some weight. He also complained of watery diarrhoea, which woke him from sleep. He was not on any medication.

On examination there were no abnormal findings apart from epigastric tenderness. He was admitted for investigation.

Bloods	Hb	10.5	WCC	5.6
	Platelets	450	Na	140
	K	4.3	Urea	5.5
	Creatinine	79	Chloride	100
	Amylase	120	Calcium	2.24
	Albumin	39		
Fasting serum gastrin	250			
Serum gastrin after secretin infusion	340			
Repeat upper GI endoscopy	Two chronic duodenal ulcers			
CT abdomen	Mass arising from pancreas			

The most likely diagnosis is:

A gastrinoma
B glucagonoma
C insulinoma
D somatostatinoma
E VIPoma

2.58 A 55-year-old Bangladeshi woman was being treated for pulmonary tuberculosis. She was started on rifampicin, isoniazid, ethambutol and pyrazinamide. After 2 months of treatment she complained of tingling in her fingers.

On examination she had sensory loss in a glove distribution in both upper limbs up to the level of the metacarpophalangeal joints and in a stocking distribution up to her ankles. She had no loss of power, tone or reflexes. She also had some glossitis.

The vitamin deficiency she is likely to have is:

A vitamin B_1
B vitamin B_2
C vitamin B_6
D vitamin B_{12}
E vitamin C

2.59 A 38-year-old man was referred because of repeated episodes of chest pain and shortness of breath.

On examination his pulse was 80 regular and blood pressure 126/80. His JVP was not elevated and there was a loud systolic murmur. His chest was clear.

Echocardiogram

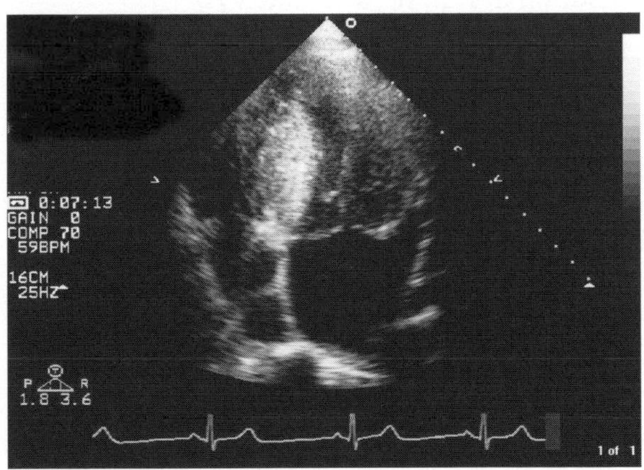

The most likely diagnosis is:

A aortic stenosis
B atrial septal defect
C hypertrophic obstructive cardiomyopathy
D myxoma
E ventricular septal defect

2.60 A 70-year-old woman on the orthopaedic ward developed oliguria 10 days after an emergency operation for a fractured neck of femur. She had a previous medical history of osteoarthritis and was on diclofenac. She had been receiving intravenous fluids and cefuroxime and gentamicin postoperatively.

On examination she had minimal ankle oedema. She was apyrexial, pulse 95 regular and blood pressure 120/80. JVP was elevated +2 cm and she had a soft third heart sound. Breath sounds were decreased in both lung bases. Her abdomen was soft and with no organomegaly. She had passed 100 ml of urine in the preceding 12 h.

Bloods	Hb	12.9	WCC	10.5
	Platelets	360	Na	135
	K	6.5	Urea	50.1
	Creatinine	1100	Protein	66
	Albumin	35	Bilirubin	11
	ALT	23	ALP	110
	Calcium	2.22	Phosphate	2.1
Arterial blood gases on air	pH	7.19	PCO_2	3.7
	PO_2	11.5	Bicarbonate	13
	Base excess –14			
Urinalysis	Red cells 2+			
ECG	ST elevation in I, II, III, aVF and V_{1-6}			
Chest X-ray	No pulmonary oedema			

The most appropriate treatment for this patient is:

A calcium gluconate
B furosemide infusion
C haemodialysis
D pericardiocentesis
E thrombolysis

2.61 A 15-year-old girl with Crohn's disease was seen in the clinic. Her disease affected the proximal small bowel and terminal ileum, confirmed on barium follow through. She did not have colonic involvement on colonoscopy. Her current medication included iron tablets, vitamin B_{12} injections and oral mesalazine. Two months after starting treatment she was still experiencing attacks of abdominal pain, worse after eating. She opened her bowels twice a day with no blood. She was losing weight despite trying to eat and her growth velocity was <5 cm/year. She did not smoke.

On examination she looked thin and pale. She had right iliac fossa tenderness. Rectal examination was normal.

Bloods	ESR	35	CRP	20

The next step in her management would be:

- A 6-mercaptopurine
- B dietary management (elemental/polymeric diet)
- C infliximab
- D oral steroids
- E small bowel resection

2.62 A 56-year-old woman was referred with abdominal pain and deranged liver function tests. She was on analgesic medication for osteoarthritis in her back.

Physical examination was normal with no jaundice or hepatomegaly.

Bloods	Albumin	34	Bilirubin	20
	ALT	88	ALP	132
Liver ultrasound	Normal			
Liver biopsy	(the arrows 1–4 refer to different abnormalities, as described in the answer.) (Figure 2.62, page 380.)			

The most likely diagnosis is:

- A alcoholic hepatitis
- B autoimmune hepatitis
- C drug-induced cholestasis
- D haemochromatosis
- E α_1-antitrypsin deficiency

2.63 A 48-year-old man was admitted with syncope and chest pain radiating to the back. He then developed shortness of breath. He had a previous medical history of hypertension but was not on any medication.

On examination he still had some chest pain. He was apyrexial. Pulse was 98 regular and blood pressure was 150/100 in the right arm and 120/80 in the left arm. The JVP was elevated +6 cm, and there was a third heart sound and soft early diastolic murmur. There were crackles in both lung bases. Abdominal and neurological examination was normal.

CT chest

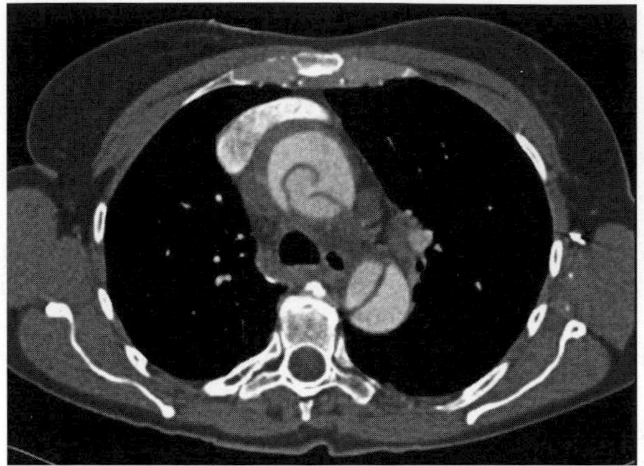

His immediate initial treatment should be with:

A intra-aortic balloon pump
B labetalol
C methyldopa
D nifedipine
E sodium nitroprusside

2.64 A 38-year-old man was admitted to Accident & Emergency with a 3-week history of cough productive of yellow sputum, breathlessness and chest discomfort. He had presented to his GP 2 weeks previously and had been given a course of antibiotics which had not helped his condition. He complained of night sweats but had not travelled abroad and had not knowingly come into contact with anyone who was ill. He had lost his appetite and some weight. He had smoked 20 cigarettes a day for 20 years.

On examination his temperature was 38.9°C, pulse 100 and blood pressure 105/60. He had decreased breath sounds on the right. His respiratory rate was 25 breaths/min and oxygen saturation was 92% on 2 L of oxygen. Cardiovascular and abdominal examination was normal.

Bloods	Hb	13.3	WCC	20.9
	Neutrophils	17.4	Platelets	130
	Protein	55	Albumin	32
	LDH	320	Glucose	6.0
Pleural fluid	pH	7.18	Protein	42
	Glucose	2.2	LDH	1100
	Purulent fluid appearance			
Chest X-ray	Right pleural effusion			
Chest ultrasound	Multi-loculated fluid collection on right			

Of the following statements concerning this patient's management the one that is correct is:

A culturing Gram-positive bacteria from pleural fluid is associated with an increased likelihood of requiring surgical management
B a large bore (24–32 French) intercostal drain should be inserted
C his condition is most likely due to anaerobic bacteria
D if a CT chest were performed and thickened pleura were seen, there would be an increased need for surgical drainage
E intrapleural fibrinolytic therapy should be routinely used to aid drainage

2.65 A 35-year-old Caucasian woman was admitted from Accident & Emergency with a severe headache and collapse. She had a history of headaches but this one was the worst ever. CT head scan showed no evidence of an intracranial lesion. Lumbar puncture the next day showed no evidence of xanthochromia. She was discharged on the following day. A week later she presented again to Accident & Emergency, still with a headache but also feeling very lethargic and dizzy.

On examination she was apyrexial, pulse was 90 regular, blood pressure was 110/70 and GCS was 15/15. The rest of the physical examination was normal and there was no focal neurological deficit.

Bloods	Hb	12.1	WCC	5.5
	Platelets	200	INR	1.0
	Na	118	K	4.5
	Urea	4.3	Creatinine	68
	Glucose	3.0	TSH	<0.1
	Free T_4	7		
	9 am cortisol	80 (Normal 138–690 nmol/L)		
Chest X-ray	Normal			

Of the following statements regarding her diagnosis the one which is correct is:

A a dexamethasone suppression test should be performed
B hyperkalaemia is a recognised complication of the underlying diagnosis
C hyponatraemia is due to hypoaldosteronism
D she may have a high serum prolactin level
E her skin and buccal mucosa will soon become pigmented

2.66 A 55-year-old woman with insulin-dependent diabetes was seen in the clinic. At her last outpatient appointment she had a blood urea of 15.5 and creatinine of 253. Her only medication was insulin and low-dose aspirin. She had pre-proliferative retinopathy but no peripheral neuropathy. She had smoked 15 cigarettes a day for more than 30 years but did not drink alcohol.

On examination her pulse was 92 regular and her blood pressure was 170/100. Apart from mild ankle oedema, the rest of her physical examination was normal.

Bloods	Hb	10.2	WCC	6.4
	Platelets	345	MCV	77.5
	Na	135	K	4.9
	Urea	18.4	Creatinine	280
	Calcium	2.01	Phosphate	1.8
	Albumin	36	Glucose	13.2
Urine	Protein ++, glucose ++			

The most important step in her management is:

A assuming no other cause for her anaemia is found, start on erythropoietin
B consider dialysis once GFR is <5 ml/min
C oral bicarbonate need not be given until the level is <10
D put on a low protein diet <0.5 g/kg/day
E start on an ACE inhibitor

2.67 A 50-year-old woman was referred with pain around her left temple and left eye that was worse with eye movements. It had worsened over the past 10 days. Her vision was previously normal in both eyes but now was blurred in the left eye. She had noticed that colours appeared less vivid in the left eye compared to the other eye. She had no other medical problems but was on hormone replacement therapy. She had smoked 20 cigarettes a day for over 10 years and drank 4 units of alcohol at the weekend. There was no family history of note.

On examination, she was apyrexial and her GCS was 15/15. Cranial nerves were intact apart from a poorly reacting pupil on the left and discomfort on looking laterally, up and down. Fundoscopy was normal. Visual acuity in the left eye was 6/60. Her pulse was 78 regular and blood pressure was 128/88. She had no murmurs or carotid bruits.

The most likely diagnosis is:

A acute angle closure glaucoma
B age-related macular degeneration (wet type)
C anterior ischaemic optic neuropathy
D optic neuritis
E temporal arteritis

2.68 A 35-year-old man presented to Accident & Emergency with severe abdominal pain and vomiting. Earlier in the day he had eaten a beefburger and since then had felt unwell. He had vomited four times and had opened his bowels once with loose motions. The abdominal pain was eased by opening his bowels. He had no other medical problems.

On examination he was apyrexial, his pulse was 98 regular and blood pressure 110/66. Heart sounds and respiratory examination were normal. His abdomen was soft but with generalized tenderness. Rectal examination was normal.

Bloods	Hb	12.4	WCC	11.0
	Platelets	300	Na	133
	K	4.0	Urea	4.6
	Creatinine	70	Amylase	56
	CRP	12		
Chest X-ray	Normal lung fields with no free air under diaphragm			
Abdominal X-ray	No bowel dilatation			

The microorganism most likely to have caused this condition is:

A *Clostridium perfringens*
B enterotoxigenic *Escherichia coli*
C *Listeria monocytogenes*
D Norwalk virus
E *Staphylococcus aureus*

2.69 A 22-year-old man was seen in the genitourinary clinic. He had recently been diagnosed with HIV and was about to start HAART. He was asymptomatic.

His CD_4 count was 120 cells/mm^3. He inquired about vaccinations that may be appropriate for him to receive at this time.

The **TWO** vaccinations that are **CONTRAINDICATED** in this patient are:

A anthrax
B *Haemophilus influenzae* B (Hib)
C hepatitis A
D hepatitis B
E Japanese encephalitis
F meningococcus (MenC)
G poliomyelitis – oral
H rabies
I tetanus–diphtheria
J tuberculosis (BCG)

2.70 A 28-year-old man was referred with swelling and pain in his fingers for the past 2 months. There was associated morning stiffness which could last up to 30 min. For the past 4 years he had suffered with psoriasis, affecting his scalp, elbows, knees and buttocks. His only medication was topical coal tar soap.

On examination there were obvious psoriatic plaques. There was swelling and tenderness of the distal interphalangeal joints of the index, middle and ring fingers of both hands. In the nails there was some pitting and early onycholysis. He was concerned about the prognosis of his arthritis.

The feature associated with a poor prognosis would be:

A development of sacroiliitis
B erosions on hand X-ray
C extensive skin disease
D HLA B22 positive
E low ESR

2.71 A 55-year-old man was referred by his GP with cervical lymphadenopathy and anaemia.

Bloods	Hb	9.3	MCV	98.4
	WCC	6.8	Platelets	85

Blood film

(Figure 2.71, page 380.)

The **MOST** likely diagnosis is:

A acute myeloid leukaemia
B bone marrow infiltration
C chronic lymphocytic leukaemia
D disseminated intravascular coagulopathy
E infectious mononucleosis

2.72 A 56-year-old man with known hepatitis C (HCV) cirrhosis was seen in the hepatology clinic. He complained of anorexia and weight loss of 4 kg. He had not responded to anti-HCV treatment and was no longer on any medication. He reported no haematemesis, abdominal distension or confusion. He did not drink alcohol.

On examination he looked thin. There was no jaundice, pallor, oedema, lymphadenopathy or signs of encephalopathy. Abdominal examination was normal.

Bloods	Protein	65	Albumin	35
	ALT	40	ALP	125
	GGT	35	AFP	580 (Normal 1–7 kU/L)
	INR	1.1		

Ultrasound Small liver with multiple hypoechoic lesions
Normal portal vein flow, no ascites

CT abdomen Four hypervascular lesions (maximum diameter 6 cm) in the right lobe of the liver, which enhance in arterial phase
No extrahepatic lymphadenopathy

The most appropriate management plan for this patient is:

A hepatic resection of the right lobe of the liver
B orthotopic liver transplantation
C percutaneous ethanol injection
D radiofrequency ablation
E transarterial chemoembolization

2.73 A 24-year-old man was admitted to his local hospital with a massive paracetamol overdose. His condition necessitated him being transferred to a liver unit. After 2 days and despite treatment with N acetylcysteine his condition deteriorated and he became very drowsy. He was transferred to the intensive care unit because his GCS was 8/15 and he was intubated and ventilated.

On examination his temperature was 36.4°C. His pulse was 50 regular and blood pressure 160/90. Chest and abdominal examinations were normal. His pupils were dilated. There was general hyperreflexia and he had bilateral ankle clonus. A reverse jugular venous bulb catheter was inserted and revealed a venous O_2 saturation of 85%. The following blood tests were taken on admission to ITU.

Bloods	Hb	10.5	WCC	12.3
	Platelets	75	PT	46
	Na	131	K	3.8
	Urea	15.0	Creatinine	230
	Bilirubin	90	ALT	3500
	ALP	280	Albumin	33

The **MOST** important of the following measures in his management is:

A keep him warm
B treat with hypertonic saline
C nurse him supine
D avoid sedation
E aim to keep PCO_2 >6.0 kPa

2.74 A 43-year-old man presents with chest pain for the past week. Cardiovascular and chest examination were normal. A chest X-ray was performed.

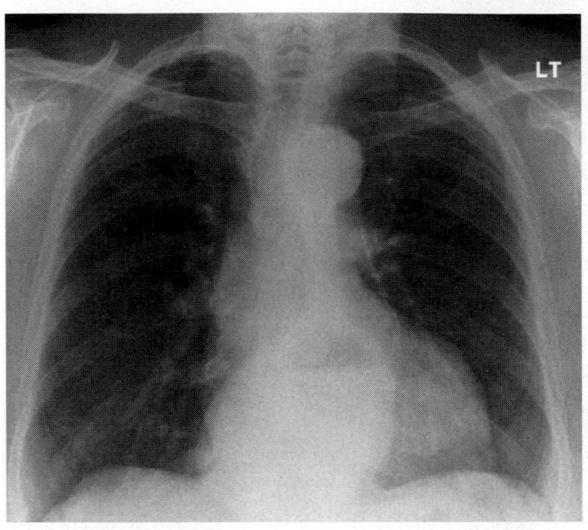

The **MOST** likely diagnosis is:

A hiatus hernia
B left ventricular aneurysm
C lung carcinoma
D pneumonic consolidation
E thoracic aortic dissection

2.75 A 51-year-old man was referred with low back pain. An MRI spine was performed.

The **MOST** likely diagnosis is:

A ankylosing spondylitis
B carcinomatous bony metatases
C multiple myeloma
D paraspinal abscess
E spondylolisthesis

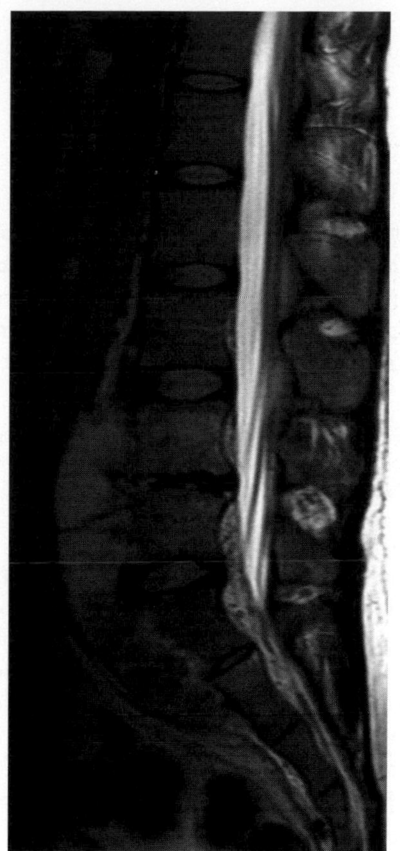

Paper 2

Answers

2.1 **C***** A Type 2 diabetes patient suffers an anterior MI and now has to be put back onto diabetic medication. According to the DIGAMI study, diabetics who suffer an MI have a higher mortality. Patients given intensive intravenous insulin in the acute phase and then put onto 3 months of subcutaneous insulin had an absolute reduction in mortality of 11% at 3.5 years compared to patients left on oral hypoglycaemics.

Malmberg K (1997) Prospective randomised study of intensive insulin treatment on long term survival after acute myocardial infarction in patients with diabetes mellitus. DIGAMI (Diabetes Mellitus, Insulin Glucose Infusion in Acute Myocardial Infarction) Study Group. *BMJ* **314**: 1512–15

2.2 **B***** The ECG trace shows ventricular fibrillation and this patient is in cardiac arrest. If a cardiac monitor or defibrillator were not immediately available (i.e. the patient is outside of the hospital setting), then starting cardiopulmonary resuscitation with a ratio of chest compressions to ventilation of 30:2 would be the next step until the diagnosis of VT/VF is confirmed. In this case, the diagnosis has been confirmed and the most important step in his management is to defibrillate as soon as possible. He should be given 360 J of monophasic shock or 150–200 J of biphasic shock, depending on the type of defibrillator.

2.3 **A***** She has most likely taken a tricyclic antidepressant overdose, as the signs are those of anticholinergic effects, including: sinus tachycardia, pyrexia, dry mouth and tongue, dilated pupils and urinary retention. In severe cases, there may be increased tone and hyperreflexia with extensor plantars.

2.4 **A**** This patient has cutaneous larva migrans, caused by migration of nematode larva through intact skin epidermis. The larvae, which originate from dog faeces, live in damp earth or beaches. The migration shows a characteristic zigzag line. *Borrelia burgdorferi* causes Lyme disease. *Trichophyton mentagrophytes* causes ringworm. *Treponema pertenue* causes yaws, a non-venereal infectious condition similar to syphilis. *Ascaris lumbricoides* causes urticaria, eosinophilia, diarrhoea and transient eosinophilic infiltrates (Löffler's syndrome).

2.5 **E***** An elderly woman presents in a drowsy condition with possible urinary tract infection complicated by high glucose, high sodium and minimal acidosis and ketosis. The clinical presentation may mimic diabetic ketoacidosis (DKA) except that there are few or no ketones in the urine unless the patient has been starving or vomiting. The plasma glucose is very high; it is rare for insulin dependent diabetics (the type who develop DKA) to present with such a high plasma glucose. The plasma osmolality can be calculated from the following formula:

Serum osmolality = 2 x ([Na] + [K]) + [Urea] + [Glucose]

In the present case this would be 373 mosmol/kg. Diabetes insipidus is associated with high serum sodium and high serum osmolality but also a low urinary osmolality, which is not the case here. Cushing's syndrome can present with hyperglycaemia and weakness but there are none of the classical features to suggest this as a viable diagnosis.

2.6 **D**** A cross-sectional study would involve surveying all patients with hepatic encephalopathy at a particular point in time to see if they had raised ammonia, and so generate a possible association between the two. This type of study can be used to assess the prevalence of a disease.

2.7 **C**** The most likely diagnosis in this patient is an acute exacerbation of chronic pancreatitis. Pain is typically epigastric or central, radiating to the back, worse after eating, and can be associated with severe weight loss. Complications with endocrine function lead to diabetes and with exocrine function lead to a failure of the digestion of complex foods and the absorption of digestive products. Fat malabsorption can lead to steatorrhoea, whilst protein malabsorption is much rarer and does not occur until >90% of exocrine function is lost. Twenty to 40% of patients with chronic pancreatitis can develop pseudocysts which are localized collections of pancreatic fluid surrounded by granulation tissue but not an epithelial lining. These can expand to cause pain; biliary or duodenal obstruction; vascular occlusion to splenic and portal veins; fistulae into adjacent structures like the stomach, pleura, ascites and pericardium; to become spontaneously infected and develop into an abscess; to lead to the formation of a pseudoaneurysm through the release of pancreatic enzymes to digest the walls of an adjacent vessel, which can lead to sudden and catastrophic gastrointestinal haemorrhage. These complications can still occur in chronic pancreatitis even in the absence of pseudocysts. Chronic pancreatitis is an independent risk factor for the development of pancreatic cancer.

2.8 **E**** This patient presents with lethargy, weight loss, loss of vision and splenomegaly. The blood results show macrocytic anaemia, lymphocytosis, very raised ESR and raised IgM. Although there is evidence of immunoparesis, the skeletal survey is normal and IgM myeloma is unusual. More likely would be Waldenström's macroglobulinaemia, which is usually associated with a raised IgM gammopathy. As with myeloma, Waldenström's macroglobulinaemia causes a hyperviscosity syndrome that can result in headaches, cerebrovascular accidents and thromboses; the photograph shows central retinal vein thrombosis.

2.9 **B*** HIV attacks CD_4 cells and causes problems with cell-mediated immunity. As a result such patients are at risk of opportunistic infections by viruses, fungi and *Mycobacterium*. By contrast, *Haemophilus influenzae* is an encapsulated bacterium and poses more of a threat to patients who lack humoral immunity (i.e. splenectomy patients), as they are unable to produce opsonizing antibodies.

2.10 **E*** The histology slide shows large bowel and in the centre of the picture is a granuloma with surrounding inflammation; this is characteristic of tuberculous disease. Crohn's disease would give a similar picture but tuberculosis needs to be excluded first. CMV colitis (see **5.6**) and *Giardia* (see **3.9**) are discussed elsewhere. Kaposi's sarcoma typically affects the upper gastrointestinal tract but is not associated with granulomas.

2.11 **A***** Pyrexia, tender hepatomegaly without jaundice and normal liver function tests are characteristic of an amoebic liver abscess. The most likely organism would be *Entamoeba histolytica*, which is a protozoan with a worldwide distribution. This could be a bacterial pyogenic hepatic abscess but patients tend to be older, much more unwell and more associated with enteric symptoms. Hydatid cysts are associated with a much longer history of abdominal distension in patients who rear sheep or cattle. The normal eosinophil count makes schistosomiasis unlikely and there is no history of haematuria. Hepatitis A would be more associated with deranged liver function tests and jaundice.

2.12 **A**** This patient is most likely to have had a cerebral infarct, given his history of atrial fibrillation. There is evidence that he should be started on aspirin 300 mg as an antiplatelet drug. Intracranial thrombolysis is a possible treatment if given within 3 h of the cerebrovascular accident occurring, in the setting of a neurosurgical centre and when there is exclusion by CT scan of haemorrhage. Warfarin is not indicated in the acute setting.

CAST (Chinese Acute Stroke Trial) Collaborative Group) (1997) Randomised placebo-controlled trial of early aspirin use in 20 000 patients with acute ischaemic stroke. *Lancet* **349**: 1641–9.

2.13 **D*** ** This patient is diabetic and has multiple discrete circumscribed laser scars in the peripheries and just within the arcades, but sparing the macular region. The patient has had panretinal photocoagulation for proliferative diabetic retinopathy.

2.14 **E**** This patient has respiratory acidosis, as shown by a low pH and raised PCO_2. The bicarbonate is appropriately raised, suggesting chronic renal adaptation. The PO_2 is low and shows the patient to have type II respiratory failure. For an explanation of arterial blood gas interpretation, see **1.30**.

2.15 **B**** Fibromyalgia is a non-inflammatory diffuse pain syndrome of unknown aetiology. Patients may complain of morning stiffness, fatigue, depression, headache, arthralgia and anxiety. Patients may also have other pain syndromes, like irritable bowel syndrome and migraine. On examination there may be certain tender muscle areas, like the occiput, supraspinatus and trapezius. Blood results are normal. With polymyalgia rheumatica an elevated ESR would be expected.

2.16 **A*** Only Behçet's syndrome is not associated with blue sclera. The other four conditions are heritable disorders of type I collagen, which is necessary for the strength of bone, ligaments, tendons and skin.

2.17 **C**** There is 'eggshell' calcification of the hilar lymph glands and the most likely diagnosis is sarcoidosis. Differential diagnoses for this appearance include silicosis and pneumoconiosis. Hodgkin's lymphoma can produce bi-hilar lymphadenopathy but not calcification.

2.18 **E**** This bariom enema reveals fusion of the vertebral bodies and calcification of the longitudinal ligaments and intervertebral discs consistent with ankylosing spondylitis. Ankylosing spondylitis is associated with iritis, not scleritis.

2.19 **D**** With cardiac catheterisation the oxygen saturation on the right side of the heart should be 65–75%, whereas the saturation on the left side of the heart should be 96–98%. All the oxygen saturations on the right side should be the same: superior vena cava, inferior vena cava, right atrium, right ventricle and pulmonary artery; the oxygen saturations on the left should be the same, only more oxygenated. The first chamber to show a deviation of >5% in the oxygen saturation is the one where the shunt is. In this case there is an increase in the oxygen saturation from the right ventricle to the pulmonary artery consistent with a patent ductus arteriosus. The elevated pulmonary artery pressure suggests that the patient has developed pulmonary hypertension.

2.20 A** On the pre-treatment ECG (A), there are peaked T waves in V_{1-6}, a broad QRS complex and prolonged PR interval, which would be consistent with hyperkalaemia. The treatment of choice would be 10 ml 10% calcium gluconate to protect the myocardium, followed by insulin–dextrose infusion to reduce the hyperkalaemia. The post-treatment ECG (B) shows the reduction in size of the T waves post treatment.

2.21 C** This patient presents with the characteristic features of lithium toxicity: vomiting, incontinence, tremor, myoclonic jerks and restlessness. Other features include hypernatraemia, convulsions, arrhythmias, cerebellar signs and renal failure. There is no specific antidote for lithium overdose but if there are neurological sequelae then haemodialysis should be considered.

2.22 D** Porphyria cutanea tarda (PCT) is a disorder of porphyrin biosynthesis where there is a deficiency of uroporphyrinogen III decarboxylase in the liver; as a result there is increased production of urinary uroporphyrin. In PCT there are no neurological sequelae but it is associated with chronic liver damage. Patients develop characteristic skin lesions: photosensitive skin blisters that heal with scarring, increased skin fragility, hypertrichosis and alopecia, and rarely a 'pseudoscleroderma' where there is extensive sclerosis and thickening of the skin. Epidermolysis bullosa involves blistering of the skin in parts of the body exposed to trauma or friction, like hands and soles of feet.

2.23 D** This patient has suffered a myocardial infarction. Her thyroid function tests show a slightly low TSH and a slightly low free T_4. Given the fact that she has undergone a major physical stress, it is very difficult to interpret her true thyroid status. The thyroid function tests should return back to normal after she recovers.

2.24 D* Odds ratio (OR) is a measure of risk by comparing the odds or probability an event will occur in an experimental group compared to a control group. The closer the value is to 1, the smaller the difference in effect between the two groups' exposure to the risk factor. When an event is rare, OR is equivalent to the relative risk.

	Leukaemia +	**Leukaemia –**	
Exposure to power cables	10 (a)	30 (b)	40
Non-exposure to power cables	40 (c)	80 (d)	120
	50	110	160

Odds for developing leukaemia = number exposed to risk factor/number not exposed = 10/40 = a/c

Odds for controls = number exposed to risk factor/number not exposed = 30/80 = b/d

OR = (a/c)/(b/d) = (ad)/(bc) = (10 x 80)/(30 x 40) = 0.67

2.25 A, E, L** A patient with decompensated liver disease, presumably due to alcoholic liver disease, presents with mild ascites, jaundice and early encephalopathy. He is homeless and so is likely to have poor nutrition, and hence thiamine deficiency is a distinct possibility. Intravenous thiamine (Pabrinex) is a very effective method of correcting any deficiency and certainly this should be started before giving dextrose, as dextrose may precipitate encephalopathy. Rectal phosphate enema and oral lactulose will treat constipation and so reduce the bowel flora, and thus should be given to any patient with decompensated liver disease to prevent encephalopathy. Spontaneous bacterial peritonitis (SBP) must be excluded in any patient with ascites and fluid should be sent for culture and white cell count; a value of 250 cells/cm^3 is diagnostic of SBP and antibiotics should then be started.

2.26 E** The typical features of endstage thyroid eye disease are seen here: scleral show, lid retraction, exophthalmos and ophthalmoplegia. The blurred vision is due to optic nerve compression and requires urgent treatment, initially with high dose steroids. A caroticocavernous fistula classically causes pulsatile proptosis with rapid onset and engorged conjunctival veins; it does not cause lid signs, and the fundal changes include dilated veins, disc oedema, retinal haemorrhages and venous stasis retinopathy. Orbital cellulitis is usually unilateral and painful and it is characterised by proptosis, a reduction in eye movements and optic nerve dysfunction, in addition to periorbital cellulitic features. An orbital arteriovenous malformation can also cause proptosis, but is usually slow growing and unilateral; again, there are no associated lid signs such as lid lag or any diplopia initially. A lacrimal gland neoplasm would cause non-axial proptosis, which would force the eye medially and downwards in the orbit.

2.27 A* The slide shows surface villi with goblet cells, which stain light blue with mucin. As this shows intestinal metaplasia of the normal squamous epithelium, this is Barrett's oesophagus (see **5.15**). Carcinoma would show invasion. Candida is not seen in glandular epithelium; it would be found with squamous epithelial cells showing the hyphae.

2.28 D** A patient with fever, haematuria, dry cough and eosinophilia should suggest a worm infestation. None of the other options is associated with eosinophilia (>0.4). The most likely organism is *Schistosoma haematobium* contracted while swimming. Patients may also complain of pruritus, urticaria and diarrhoea and have patchy pneumonia on chest X-ray. Diagnosis involves microscopy of terminal urine and treatment is with mebendazole.

2.29 A** He has a motor and sensory neuropathy with wasting of the small muscles of the hand, pes cavus and absent ankle and plantar reflexes. The gait is due to bilateral foot drop and so patients appear to drag their feet. This is Charcot–Marie–Tooth disease or hereditary motor and sensory neuropathy, and it is a form of peripheral neuropathy. Classically, patients are said to have 'inverted champagne bottles' to describe the pattern of muscle wasting in the legs and thickened lateral popliteal and great auricular nerves. There may be a family history.

2.30 E*** This patient has respiratory alkalosis, as shown by a raised pH and low PCO_2. Her bicarbonate and base excess are normal so there is no evidence of metabolic alkalosis. The PO_2 is normal, so there is no respiratory failure. These results would be consistent with hyperventilation. For an explanation of arterial blood gas interpretation, see **1.30**.

2.31 A*** Amyloidosis is a protein misfolding disorder in which soluble proteins aggregate and become insoluble amyloid fibrils which are deposited in the extracellular tissue of organs leading to structural and functional damage. Any organ can be involved but the heart, kidneys and peripheral nerves are mainly affected. It can be acquired or inherited, and can have localized or systemic effects. There are four main types: AL, AA, dialysis related/β_2 microglobulin and hereditary amyloidosis. AA amyloidosis occurs as a rare complication of persistent inflammation in patients with chronic rheumatic diseases, long-lasting infections, hereditary periodic fevers, i.e. familial Mediterranean fever, and neoplasms. This patient still has active rheumatoid arthritis (increased ESR and CRP despite treatment) and has now developed nephrotic syndrome, ascites secondary to hypoalbuminaemia, hepatomegaly and bilateral pleural effusions. Neither restrictive cardiomyopathy nor constrictive pericarditis can explain the renal impairment. Hydroxychloroquine does not cause a drug-induced glomerulonephritis.

2.32 A* The photograph shows large separation between the individual teeth characteristic of acromegaly. Amyloidosis, vitamin B_{12} deficiency and hypothyroidism affect the tongue. Vitamin C deficiency causes bleeding and ulcerated gums.

2.33 D** This patient is most likely to complain of odynophagia (pain on swallowing), as her predominant symptom. There are multiple small filling defects in long columns. (see also **5.32**).

2.34 A* This patient has a history and blood results suggestive of encephalitis. Encephalitis may follow a viral prodrome but can present acutely as well. The MRI shows involvement of the left temporal lobe, accounting for her memory problems. The treatment is high dose aciclovir.

2.35 B** This patient presents with low grade fever and pleuritic chest discomfort and has an extra heart sound, which could be a pericardial rub. The diagnosis is Dressler's syndrome, which is an acute pericarditis of unknown aetiology that may complicate myocardial infarction. It tends to present 10 days to 2 months post infarct. Patients may also present with pleural and pericardial effusions and arthralgia. The most effective treatment is anti-inflammatory drugs.

2.36 B** The ECG shows a regular broad complex tachycardia with right bundle branch block. He has no history of ischaemic heart disease and is haemodynamically stable. There are no features of ventricular tachycardia (see **3.35**).

2.37 F, I, J* This patient has pyoderma gangrenosum, which is a chronic ulcer with a necrotic ulcer base and dark red or violaceous border. It is associated with all the conditions mentioned, including other malignancies, endocrinopathies like diabetes mellitus and hypothyroidism, and liver diseases like primary biliary cirrhosis.

2.38 D* This patient with hypocalcaemia has pseudohypoparathyroidism. In this condition patients have raised parathyroid hormone (PTH) because it is ineffective at the target organ. Vitamin D_3 is converted to 25-vitamin D_3 in the liver and then to 1,25-vitamin D_3 in the kidney. In cirrhosis there are decreased levels of 25-vitamin D_3 and also albumin, which is produced by the liver. Patients with pseudohypoparathyroidism have a short stature, short fourth and fifth metacarpals and mental retardation. Pseudopseudo hypoparathyroidism has the clinical features of pseudohypoparathyroidism but serum calcium and other biochemical values are normal.

2.39 **B*** Jehovah's Witnesses are forbidden from having certain transfusions and these include red cells, white cells, platelets and plasma. They cannot receive their own blood even if they donated it prior to an operation. However, they can receive their own blood if it is transfused back into them during an operation, provided that the blood has been through a salvage machine or cell saver whereby the red cells have been separated and 'washed out'. Other blood products that are acceptable include albumin, clotting factors like factors VIII and IX, erythropoetin and immunoglobulins.

2.40 **B***** Coeliac disease is a malabsorption syndrome associated with sensitivity to gluten. Patients should try to cut out foods containing wheat, oats, rye and barley. Those with untreated disease may also have a lactase deficiency secondary to the surface epithelial cell damage already present; before starting a gluten-free diet, patients should avoid milk and milk products. All beers, lagers and ales should be avoided as they are made from barley. Rice, corn, maize, buckwheat, potato, soybean and tapioca are safe in coeliac patients.

2.41 **E**** This patient has Wolff–Parkinson–White (WPW) syndrome, which is a form of atrioventricular (AV) re-entry tachycardia. WPW is caused by an accessory AV pathway (bundle of Kent), which connects atrial and ventricular myocardium and bypasses the AV node and bundle of His. Patients with WPW may develop paroxysmal tachycardias and atrial fibrillation. Drugs like verapamil and digoxin block the AV node and can increase the frequency of conduction in the accessory pathway, so leading to faster ventricular rate. The other drugs slow conduction in the accessory pathway.

2.42 **A**** The likely diagnosis is Goodpasture's syndrome. This is a type II hypersensitivity condition characterized by circulating anti-glomerular basement membrane (GBM) antibodies and linear deposition of immunoglobulin and complement in the GBM, resulting in pulmonary haemorrhage and renal failure. Additional aetiological factors are that he is a young male smoker presenting with severe acute renal failure. A less likely diagnosis is Wegener's granulomatosis but this is characterised by positive c-ANCA.

2.43 **E**** This patient presents with chronic sinusitis, lower respiratory tract inflammation, renal impairment, sensory neuropathy, vasculitic skin lesion and characteristic chest X-ray signs. The serum ANCA is not given but the most likely diagnosis is Wegener's granulomatosis. SLE is unlikely as she is ANA negative and has normal serum complement, also making a diagnosis of mixed cryoglobulinaemia unlikely. Goodpasture's syndrome is characterised by pulmonary haemorrhage and glomerulonephritis but cannot explain the other findings.

2.44 E*** In Paget's disease there is uncontrolled bone metabolism. There is bone resorption due to osteoclast activity and in the skull this can produce a honeycomb appearance, 'osteoporosis circumscripta'. There is bone demineralisation resulting in a sharp contrast being seen between normal and abnormal bone. There is also increased osteoblastic activity which can give a 'cotton wool' appearance. Other deformities that may occur include basilar invagination and platybasia. Myeloma and metastases would show a skull with punched-out lesions, not bone sclerosis (except with some prostate cancers).

2.45 E*** This patient has soft tissue loss of the terminal phalanges of the right index and middle fingers. This type of destruction is characteristic of systemic sclerosis.

2.46 B** This patient has a myopathy with wasting of facial, shoulder and girdle muscles. The reflexes are absent because of muscle atrophy. The ptosis and slurred speech are all consistent with dystrophia myotonia. Other features include percussion dystonia, inability to relax a clenched fist and frontal baldness. Associated clinical features include endocrinopathies; diabetes due to end-organ unresponsiveness to insulin; testicular atrophy and infertility; cardiomyopathy and conduction defects; oesophageal dysmotility; and cognitive impairment. Compare this with myasthenia gravis (see **4.11**).

2.47 E* A severely malnourished person is suddenly given large amounts of kilocalories in the form of intravenous dextrose and nasogastric feed. This has caused salt and volume overload, resulting in low levels of potassium, phosphorus and magnesium. The way to avoid this is to give less than his calculated nutritional requirements and slowly to build up his energy intake. Simple fluid overload is unlikely to cause electrolyte imbalances. Kwashiorkor is a form of protein–calorie malnutrition characterised by fatigue, irritability, decreased immunity, loss of muscle bulk and generalized oedema.

2.48 E* This patient has Parkinson's syndrome. The treatment that should not be given to this patient would be a dopamine depleter like tetrabenazine or reserpine. Baclofen can be used to treat dystonia, especially that caused by levodopa. Entacapone is a catechol-o-methyl transferase inhibitor, which prevents the degradation of dopamine. Apomorphine and bromocriptine are dopamine agonists.

2.49 **A**** Long-term oxygen therapy (LTOT) has been shown to improve mortality in patients with COPD if they have continuous delivery of oxygen via nasal prongs or mask for at least 15 h/day. The oxygen concentration given via a FiO_2 28% mask is 1–3 L/min. However, the benefits have only been shown in patients who have an FEV_1 ≤1.5 L and who have a PO_2 ≤7.3 kPa (or 8.0 kPa if there is evidence of pulmonary hypertension). The oxygen status needs to be assessed at least 30 days after recovery from an acute exacerbation of COPD and must be done on room air. Patients must not smoke in case they ignite themselves but exercise tolerance does not determine whether or not patients should receive LTOT.

Medical Research Council Working Party (1981) Long-term domicillary oxygen therapy in chronic hypoxic cor pulmonale complicating chronic bronchitis and emphysema. *Lancet* **1**: 681–6.

2.50 **D*** The most likely diagnosis is steroid-induced osteonecrosis or avascular necrosis of the femoral head. Her DEXA scan is normal (for DEXA scan interpretation, see **1.7**), and she has no biochemical evidence of osteomalacia. It would be unusual to have osteoarthritis affecting only one hip without a history of trauma. Collapse of the articular surface is characteristic of osteonecrosis.

2.51 **C**** There are multiple foci with increased signal in the periventricular white matter. This would be consistent with multiple sclerosis. A differential diagnosis would be multiple cerebral infarcts. The ventricles are not increased in size. A definitive diagnosis of multiple sclerosis would require looking for oligoclonal bands in the CSF.

2.52 **E**** This patient has a black-pigmented nodule that has an irregular margin, which looks like a malignant melanoma. Poor prognostic features include: lesion diameter ≥2.0 cm; Breslow lesion thickness ≥ 0.75 cm; lesions involving mucosae, anorectal and vulval regions because such areas are not routinely checked and so lesions have become deeply penetrated at time of diagnosis; amelanotic malignant melanomas are more difficult to diagnose and are also more aggressive tumours. Males tend to present with tumours on their face and back rather than females who tend to develop them on the sun-exposed parts of their legs.

2.53 **B*** This girl presents with primary amenorrhoea. She has normal breast development and normal female external genitalia but male internal genitalia. She is genotypically a male but phenotypically a female. This is complete androgen insensitivity. Breasts develop normally because excess testosterone secretion is converted to oestrogen. Development of male external genitalia depends on normal testosterone synthesis, conversion to dihydrotestosterone and normal androgen receptors. Because of her karyotype the patient produces Müllerian inhibitory factor, so there is no uterus, cervix or ovaries. With gonadal dysgenesis there is maldevelopment of the testes. As there is the risk of malignancy with intra-abdominal or maldeveloped testes, orchidopexy should be performed. Klinefelter's syndrome patients would usually have a karyotype of 47,XXY. She does not have the phenotypic features of Kallman's syndrome (see also **1.55**). The normal 17-OH progesterone excludes 11-β-hydroxylase deficiency.

2.54 **B**** This patient has Dukes' C_2 carcinoma of the colon. For a description of the grading system, see **1.14**. The five-year survival rate with treatment depends on the Dukes' grading of the tumour: A is 95–100%, B_1 is 85%, B_2 is 75%, C_1 is 65%, C_2 is 40%, and D is 5–10%.

2.55 **B*** This patient has Turner's syndrome, which is associated with karyotype 45,XO, but many patients have a mosaic form such as 46,XX/45,XO especially if they do not display many of the distinctive features such as cubitus valgus (wide carrying angle), epicanthic folds, low set ears, neck webbing and shield-like chest with widely spaced nipples. Only 20% of patients have cardiac abnormalities like coarctation of the aorta; over 60% have renal anomalies. Patients will require oestrogen sex hormone replacement but unopposed this can lead to endometrial hyperplasia and possibly carcinoma; progesterone will also have to be prescribed with cyclical oestrogen to ensure a withdrawal bleed. Growth hormone may improve longitudinal growth and final height.

2.56 **A***** This patient has all the hallmarks of ascending cholangitis (see also **4.7**). Even though the gallbladder has been removed there is still the possibility that gallstones may occur in the common bile duct.

2.57 **A***** This patient has a gastrinoma. The watery diarrhoea along with the excessive gastrin production is associated with the Zollinger–Ellison syndrome. Normally secretin infusion should cause a decrease in gastrin secretion but with gastrinomas, there is a paradoxical increase. Verner–Morrison syndrome is due to a tumour secreting vasoactive intestinal peptide (VIP) and is associated with watery diarrhoea, hypokalaemia and achlorhydria (WDHA syndrome). All of these tumours can arise from the pancreas.

2.58 **C***** This patient has developed pyridoxine (vitamin B_6) deficiency due to her isoniazid treatment. It might possibly have been avoided if she had been co-prescribed this at the start of her antituberculosis treatment.

2.59 **C**** The echocardiogram shows a thick interventricular septum and dilated left ventricle consistent with hypertrophic obstructive cardiomyopathy.

2.60 C** An elderly woman develops acute renal failure in the postoperative period after being treated with NSAIDs and antibiotics. She has clinical evidence of pericarditis, as shown by ECG changes and extra heart sounds. She has a number of indications for haemodialysis: raised potassium, metabolic acidosis and uraemic pericarditis. Other indications for haemodialysis include resistant fluid overload, multiorgan failure, hypercalcaemia, hypercatabolic states and drug toxicities. An echocardiogram would need to be done to exclude a pericardial effusion but unless the patient clinically had tamponade, pericardiocentesis should not be attempted.

2.61 B** Twenty to 25% of all new cases of Crohn's disease are diagnosed in patients aged younger than 18 years. It can present with abdominal pain, weight loss, failure to thrive, anaemia and diarrhoea. Long-term management of the disease is usually with 5-aminosalicylates, but this patient's disease is clearly not under control. Steroids are excellent drugs to induce remission but the disadvantage is that they could impair her growth even further. Another approach would be to stop her normal diet and institute an elemental, semi-elemental or even polymeric (whole protein) diet. This may be unpalatable and she may not be able to cope with the volume required, in which case it should be administered via nasogastric tube. The other options of azathioprine, 6-mercaptopurine and infliximab could all be used, but not as first line treatment. Surgery should be considered early, especially in children to prevent long-term growth retardation.

2.62 A* The biopsy shows the characteristic features of alcoholic hepatitis: steatosis (1), parenchymal inflammation composed of neutrophils (2), ballooning of hepatocytes (3), and Mallory bodies (4). These features may also be seen in non-alcoholic steatohepatitis.

2.63 E** This patient has a dissecting thoracic aortic aneurysm on the CT chest. A distinct dissection flap can be seen in the ascending and descending aorta, making this a Stanford type A dissection. The priority is to control the blood pressure as this will reduce the shear forces on the arterial wall. The aim is to reduce the systolic blood pressure to 100–120 mmHg. A vasodilator such as nitroprusside, which can be given as a controlled infusion, would be the optimum treatment. Labetalol can also be used but β-blockers would be contraindicated in this patient who is showing signs of pulmonary oedema. The intra-aortic balloon pump requires a competent aortic valve for it to work and is contraindicated in patients with aortic regurgitation.

2.64 D*** The pleural fluid results suggest this patient has an empyema: pH ≤7.20, low glucose, high protein and LDH. This is most likely secondary to a parapneumonic effusion. Sixty per cent of community-acquired empyemas are due to aerobic bacteria. A chest drain needs to be inserted but this can be done using small bore catheters (8–14 French), provided they are flushed with saline every 6 h. Routine use of fibrinolytics has not been shown to improve the drainage of infected material. Patients whose effusions do not resolve with drainage can be treated with streptokinase or urokinase but they require referral to a cardiothoracic centre for video-assisted thoracoscopic surgery (VATS). If the empyema is particularly organised on CT, then this is an indication to refer to cardiothoracic surgeons for decortication and drainage. Gram-negative organisms and pleural thickening increase the proportion of patients requiring thoracotomy and surgical decortication of their empyema.

Davies CWH, Gleeson FV, Davies RJO (2003). BTS guidelines for the management of pleural infection. *Thorax* 2003; **58** (Suppl II): ii18–ii28.

2.65 D** The cause of this patient's initial severe headache and collapse may well have been pituitary apoplexy. This could have been due to haemorrhage into a pre-existing macroadenoma that may have been too small to be seen on a CT head. MRI specifically looking at the pituitary probably would have detected it. The hyponatraemia, low cortisol and low TSH/T_4 are all consistent with hypopituitarism. Usually the functions of the posterior pituitary are spared and there are decreased levels of ACTH, TSH, LH and FSH. (The hypothalamus negatively inhibits the secretion of prolactin and with apoplexy there may be loss of this inhibition on the pituitary, resulting in increased prolactin levels.) Hyponatraemia is most likely due to glucocorticoid and thyroid hormone deficiency; secretion of aldosterone is primarily regulated by the renin–angiotensin axis and this is not affected by secondary adrenal failure. For this reason patients do not develop hyperkalaemia. Hyperpigmentation with Addison's disease (primary adrenal failure) is due to increased ACTH production, which stimulates production of melanin. The synacthen test and not the dexamethasone suppression test could be considered here.

2.66 E*** This patient with diabetes is developing endstage renal failure. She has untreated hypertension, which can exacerbate proteinuria and the progression of her renal failure. Patients undergoing haemodialysis have an increased risk of developing cardiovascular disease and anaemia will contribute to left ventricular hypertrophy. For these reasons, the best drug for the patient to be started on would be ACE inhibitor. Aggressive management of blood pressure has been shown to be more effective than a low protein diet. The aim would be to keep protein intake to about 0.75 g/kg/day and improve caloric intake as malnutrition is an indication to start dialysis. Although the PTH is not mentioned, she probably has secondary hyperparathyroidism, which would be consistent with the low calcium and raised phosphate. She should be treated with a calcium-based phosphate binder like calcichew and a low phosphate diet to keep the phosphate below 1.9. 1α-Calcidol will raise phosphate and contribute to vascular calcification, which will already be an issue in a diabetic with renal failure. Oral bicarbonate is given to keep this in the normal range. Dialysis should be a planned decision and should be considered when the GFR is approximately 14 ml/min. Erythropoietin is used to treat the anaemia of chronic renal failure but this does not need to be started yet; anaemia first should be treated with oral or intravenous iron (Venofer).

2.67 D* Optic neuritis can present in a patient as pain around the eye and with eye movements, decreased visual acuity and altered colour perception. There is decreased pupil reaction to light and a relative afferent pupillary defect. A pale optic disc seen on fundoscopy is a sign of previous optic neuritis; an acute optic neuritis presents as a unilateral swollen disc, or if retrobulbar, fundoscopy is normal. Optic neuritis is more prevalent in younger patients and is associated with demyelination diseases, like multiple sclerosis. Temporal arteritis is associated with jaw claudication, scalp tenderness and temporal artery tenderness, thickening and loss of pulsation. It can cause sudden visual loss in one eye and then the other eye within a short space of time (due to anterior ischaemic optic neuropathy). It is associated with an elevated ESR and CRP. Ischaemic optic neuropathy can also be associated with hypertension. Acute glaucoma often presents with a red painful eye with a fixed, mid-dilated pupil and blurred vision. Age-related macular degeneration can be subdivided into two types: dry/non-exudative type, which is more insidious in onset and painless, with drusen often seen on fundoscopy; and wet/exudative type, which is due to leakage of blood and fluid into the subretinal space leading to sudden, central visual loss.

2.68 E** The main presenting feature of this patient's gastroenteritis is vomiting rather than diarrhoea after a short incubation period. This would be consistent with *Staphylococcus aureus*, *Bacillus cereus* and Norwalk virus, which produce toxins even before the food is consumed. Norwalk virus usually has a longer incubation period and is more associated with raw seafood. *Clostridium perfringens* and enterotoxigenic *Escherichia coli* produce toxins after food ingestion but have a longer incubation time and are more associated with watery diarrhoea. *Listeria monocytogenes* can cause inflammatory watery diarrhoea along with fever as the predominant symptoms and has an incubation period of about 24 h.

2.69 G, J* Traditionally, all live vaccines were contraindicated in patients with HIV. However, the introduction of HAART causing immune reconstitution has shifted the risk–benefit ratio in favour of vaccination. All live vaccines are now only contraindicated in patients with symptomatic HIV infection or CD_4 counts <200 cells/mm^3. The live vaccines that are contraindicated are poliomyelitis – oral; cholera; influenza – intranasal; typhoid – Ty21a; tuberculosis; smallpox (vaccinia); measles, mumps and rubella (MMR); varicella; and yellow fever. The inactivated vaccines are safe in all HIV patients: anthrax, cholera, hepatitis A and B, *Haemophilus influenzae* B, influenza – parenteral, Japanese encephalitis, meningococcus, pneumococcus, rabies, tetanus–diphtheria, tick-borne encephalitis and typhoid.

2.70 B*** A patient with psoriasis and arthropathy affecting the distal interphalangeal (DIP) joints with nail changes is most likely to have psoriatic arthritis. In about 15–20% of cases the arthritis precedes the skin disease. The extent and the severity of the skin disease have no bearing on the course and prognosis of the joint disease. There are five main clinical patterns of arthritis: (1) distal arthritis usually affecting the DIP; (2) asymmetric oligoarthritis affecting fewer than five joints; (3) symmetric polyarthritis, which is associated with a worse prognosis; (4) spondyloarthropathy associated with sacroiliitis and spondylitis; and (5) arthritis mutilans, which is characterised by deformity and destruction of the joints. X-rays showing erosions and destruction of the joints are associated with a worse prognosis. HLA B27, B39 and DQw3 are associated with progressive disease, while DR7 and B22 are seen as protective. A low ESR has a better prognosis.

2.71 B* The blood film shows anaemia and thrombocytopaenia along with a nucleated red cell and a myelocyte. These are consistent with a leuco-erythroblastic reaction seen with extramedullary haemopoiesis and bone marrow infiltration. Bone marrow infiltration can be due to invasion by carcinoma, fibrosis or infections like tuberculosis.

2.72 E** This patient most likely has primary hepatocellular carcinoma (HCC). Confirmatory histological evidence is not necessary to diagnose HCC if there is an elevated AFP (>400) and at least two imaging modalities showing focal lesions >2 cm and arterial hypervascularisation. Although this patient has cirrhosis, he does not have decompensated liver disease. The tumours are too multifocal and too large to be considered for orthotopic liver transplantation (OLT), let alone hepatic resection. To be considered for OLT there must be no more than three lesions and these must have diameters <3 cm, or a single lesion with a diameter of 5 cm. Percutaneous ethanol injection (PEI) involves injection of absolute alcohol under CT/US guidance directly into the tumour. Radiofrequency ablation (RFA) passes alternating current to heat the tumour via a needle introduced into the tumour under guidance. Both RFA and PEI would be useful in patients with smaller tumours who had other systemic disease, or as a bridge in patients awaiting transplantation. Transarterial chemoembolization relies on the fact that HCCs derive their blood supply from the hepatic artery, whereas the surrounding liver receives both portal and arterial blood. A catheter is inserted into the hepatic artery and chemotherapeutic agents are injected directly into the artery, which increases he contact time between drugs and tumour cells. Oral chemotherapy has not been shown to be effective in HCC.

Bruix J, Sherman M, Llovet J (2001) Clinical management of hepatocellular carcinoma. Conclusions of the Barcelona-2000 EASL Conference. *J Hepatol* **35**: 421–430.

2.73 **B*** This patient has developed cerebral oedema as a complication of his worsening hepatic encephalopathy secondary to acute liver failure. This is characterised by the signs of raised intracranial pressure (ICP): bradycardia, hypertension, irregular respirations (not all mentioned here but collectively described as the Cushing's triad), pupillary disturbances, hyperreflexia and clonus. Normal jugular venous O_2 saturation would be <70%; the high value in this case paradoxically suggests that oxygen is not being taken up by the brain. Patients should typically be nursed at 20–45° to facilitate venous drainage and to reduce cerebral blood volume. Sedation can decrease ICP by reducing metabolic demand and the sympathetic responses of hypertension and tachycardia. Hyperventilation and keeping PCO_2 to <5 help by reducing CO_2-induced cerebral vasodilation. Relative hypernatraemia maintains the osmotic gradient across the blood–brain barrier and reduces the risk of cerebral oedema. This should be treated with mannitol but can be supplemented with boluses of hypertonic (30%) saline. Fever results in increased metabolic demand and increased cerebral blood flow; this can be reversed by inducing hypothermia (<35°C).

2.74 **A***** The most obvious abnormality is the presence of a fluid level just behind the heart, which is characteristic of hiatus hernia. There is no mediastinal widening, although the film is slightly rotated.

2.75 **D***** The MRI shows soft tissue lesion with involvement of the disc between L4 and L5. Infection can result in abscess formation and vertebral osteomyelitis by haematogenous spread from a distant site, from direct spread at the site of trauma or surgery, or from an area of surrounding soft tissue infection or cellulitis. The same organisms that cause this can also cause discitis (see **1.75**).

Paper 3

Questions

3.1 A 63-year-old woman was admitted with central chest pain lasting 40 min. Two years ago she had been fitted with a permanent pacemaker and on this admission, this was found to be working well. Her ECG showed a paced rhythm with left bundle branch block.

Pulse was 80 paced rhythm and blood pressure 145/68. JVP was not elevated but there was an early diastolic murmur heard best with the patient leaning forward. Troponin T was normal 12 h after onset of pain.

The next day she was pain free and it was decided that she should have an exercise stress test.

Exercise testing would be contraindicated if this patient:

- A developed a febrile illness
- B had a permanent pacemaker
- C had aortic regurgitation
- D had left bundle branch block on a resting ECG
- E was on β -blockers

3.2 A 74-year-old woman collapsed at home and was brought to the Accident & Emergency department.

Her ECG shows:

- A first-degree AV block
- B complete heart block
- C Mobitz type I second-degree AV block
- D Mobitz type II second-degree AV block
- E sinus bradycardia

3.3 A 52-year-old farmer was admitted to Accident & Emergency with an overdose of an insecticide taken 18 h ago. He complained of lethargy, dizziness, headache, vomiting and abdominal pain, followed by shortness of breath and non-productive cough. Now he could not speak in full sentences.

On examination he was alert but breathless. His temperature was 36.9°C, pulse 55 regular and blood pressure 110/65. His JVP was not elevated and heart sounds were normal. His respiratory rate was 26 breaths/min and there was bilateral wheeze. He had generalized abdominal tenderness.

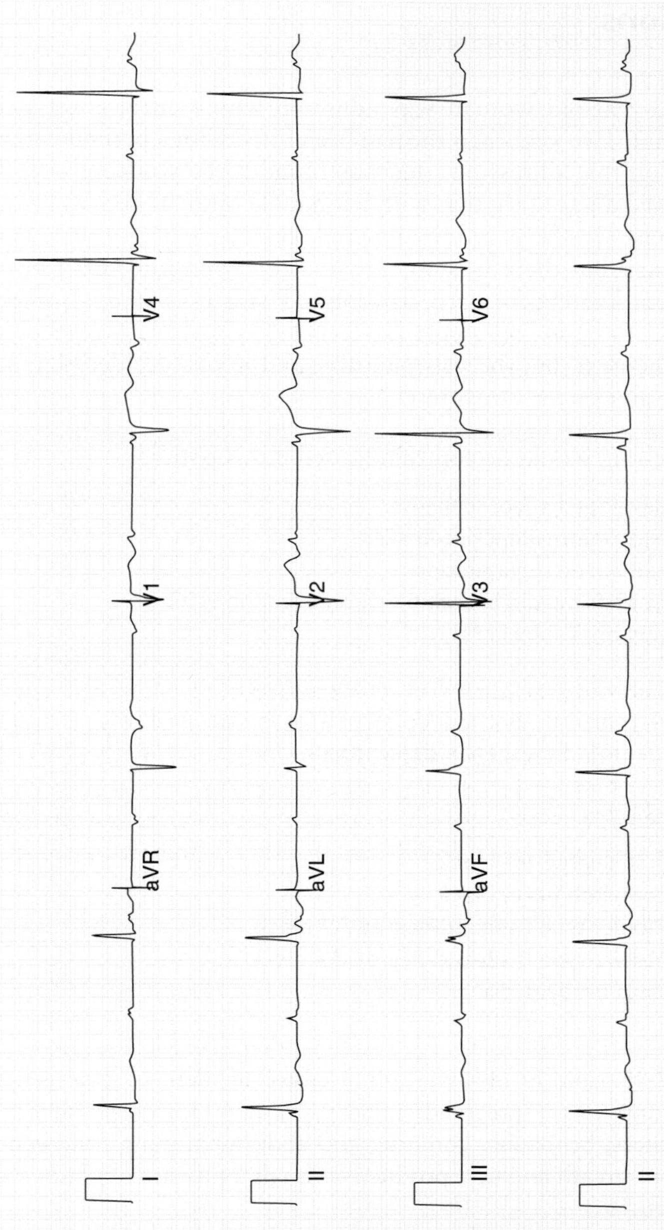
I
II
III
II
aVR
aVL
aVF
V1
V2
V3
V4
V5
V6

Arterial blood gases on air	pH	7.45	PCO_2	3.4
	PO_2	9.9	Bicarbonate	20.9
	Base excess	–3.1		

The correct antidote for this patient is:

A atropine
B bicarbonate
C dimercaprol
D glucagon
E procyclidine

3.4 A 35-year-old farmer presented with a tender itchy lesion on his right index finger that had developed 5 days ago after feeding lambs. He had no other symptoms. (Figure 3.4, page 380.)

The most likely diagnosis is:

A anthrax
B herpetic whitlow
C *Molluscum contagiosum*
D orf
E *Tinea manuum*

3.5 A 65-year-old man presented with headaches and worsening lower limb pain, making walking difficult. He felt that his problems had been worse over the last several months. He had smoked 20 cigarettes a day for nearly 50 years. His appetite was normal but he had lost some weight.

On examination he was apyrexial. Cardiovascular and respiratory examination was normal. There was no focal neurological deficit.

Bloods	Hb	14.2	WCC	8.5
	Platelets	246	Na	142
	K	3.9	Urea	7.8
	Creatinine	80	Calcium	2.30
	Phosphate	1.0	Albumin	39
	ALP	130	Protein	68

Pelvic X-ray

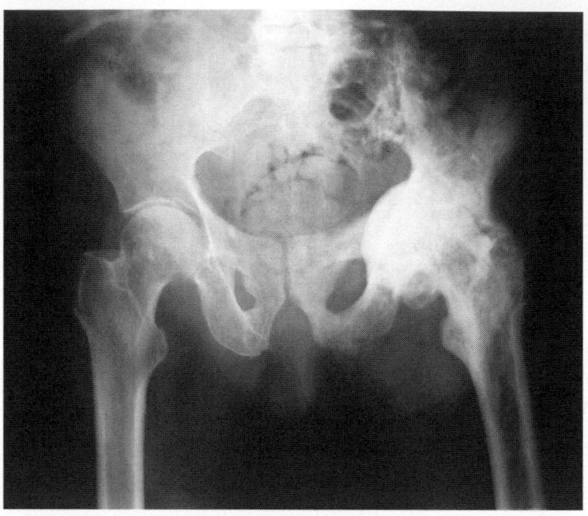

The most likely diagnosis is:

- A multiple myeloma
- B osteomalacia
- C Paget's disease
- D primary hyperparathyroidism
- E secondary metastases from lung carcinoma

3.6 It has been reported that living close to mobile phone masts is associated with an increased risk of developing brain tumours. You have been asked to design a study to investigate this possibility.

The most appropriate study design would be:

- A case control study
- B case reports
- C cohort study
- D cross-sectional study
- E randomised controlled trial

3.7 A 22-year-old woman presented with pain on eye movements and a progressive reduction in vision in the right eye over the last 10 days.

Fundoscopic examination of the right eye was performed. (Figure 3.7, page 381.)

The fundoscopic appearance is of:

A anterior ischaemic optic neuropathy
B central retinal vein occlusion
C myelinated nerve fibres
D optic disc drusen
E optic neuritis

3.8 A 13-year-old boy was referred with recurrent attacks of abdominal pain and jaundice. This was the fourth time it had happened but previously these attacks had resolved spontaneously. Three days ago he had developed a sore throat, myalgia and headache. He had no previous medical history and was not on any medication.

On examination he was mildly jaundiced. His temperature was 37.3°C, pulse 98 regular and blood pressure 100/65. Cardiovascular and respiratory examinations were normal. On palpation of his abdomen he had 4 cm splenomegaly.

Bloods	Hb	11.5	MCV	100.1
	WCC	3.9	Platelets	150
	Protein	70	Albumin	40
	Bilirubin	43	ALT	25
	ALP	600	GGT	35
Urinalysis	Urobilinogen 2+, no bilirubin			
Direct Coombs' test	Negative			

The most helpful test to determine the definitive diagnosis would be:

A bone marrow aspirate and trephine
B haemoglobin electrophoresis
C Ham's test
D osmotic fragility studies
E Schumm's test

3.9 A 46-year-old man was referred with abdominal pain and chronic diarrhoea. He opened his bowels 3–4 times per day and his stools were loose and occasionally associated with mucus. His symptoms started 5 months ago after he had returned from working in Sri Lanka for the past 3 years. His appetite was decreased and he had lost some weight. He had no other medical problems and was not on any medication. He did not smoke or drink alcohol.

On examination he was apyrexial, pulse 78 regular and blood pressure 134/79. Abdominal examination revealed general tenderness. Rectal examination was normal. A duodenal (D2) biopsy was taken at endoscopy. (Figure 3.9, page 381.)

The most likely diagnosis is:

A coeliac disease
B Crohn's disease
C giardiasis
D tropical sprue
E Whipple's disease

3.10 A 24-year-old man presented with epistaxis, haematemesis and melaena for 1 day. Since arriving back in the UK from Burma 5 days ago he had been having a flu-like illness associated with abdominal pain. He had taken malaria prophylaxis before he went. He had no significant previous medical history and was not on any medication except mefloquine.

On examination he looked unwell and jaundiced. There were non-blanching erythematous bruises on his skin. His temperature was 39°C, pulse 110 regular and blood pressure 96/64. Respiratory examination was normal. He had diffuse abdominal tenderness but no organomegaly or lymphadenopathy. Rectal examination revealed melaena.

Bloods	Hb	11.1	WCC	3.0
	Neutrophils	1.4	Lymphocytes	1.1
	Eosinophils	0.1	Platelets	90
	Na	130	K	5.0
	Urea	12.1	Creatinine	200
	Protein	58	Albumin	28
	Bilirubin	75	ALT	80
	ALP	130		
Malaria films	Negative			
Urinalysis	Protein 3+, blood 3+			
Chest X-ray	Normal			

The most likely diagnosis is:

A blackwater fever
B dengue haemorrhagic fever
C hepatitis A
D typhoid
E yellow fever

3.11 A 50-year-old man presented with progressive weakness. He had difficulty walking and climbing stairs, and more recently combing his hair. Over the last few months he had noticed decreased appetite, some weight loss and some dysphagia for solids. There was no previous medical history. He did not smoke or drink alcohol.

On examination he had bilateral wasting of both shoulders and quadriceps. There were no ocular or facial abnormalities. He had normal tone, power and reflexes. Apart from atrial fibrillation with a rate of 88, no other abnormality was found on examination.

The most likely diagnosis is:

A limb-girdle muscular dystrophy
B myasthenia gravis
C motor neurone disease
D polymyalgia rheumatica
E polymyositis

3.12 A 38-year-old diabetic man was referred to the eye clinic by the optician. Fundoscopy was performed. (Figure 3.12, page 382.)

The fundoscopic appearance is most likely due to:

A choroidal melanoma
B coloboma
C preretinal haemorrhage
D retinal detachment
E toxoplasma scar

3.13 A patient was referred for lung function tests.

	Absolute	Predicted (%)
FEV_1	1.8	51
FVC	2.4	55
TLC	3.0	52
DLCO	12.0	53
KCO	5.0	99

These results are consistent with **TWO** of the following diagnoses:

A asthma
B bronchiectasis
C chronic bronchitis
D emphysema
E fibrosing alveolitis
F lymphangitis carcinomatosa
G patient post-pneumonectomy for lung carcinoma
H primary pulmonary hypertension
I pulmonary haemorrhage
J sarcoidosis

3.14 A 51-year-old woman was referred because of worsening joint pain affecting her hands. The problems started about 4 months ago causing pain in both wrists and now the fingers were involved. She was unable to perform her job as a typist. Simple analgesics had not helped her symptoms. She had no previous medical history and was only on codeine phosphate.

On examination she was in pain. She had bilateral swelling and tenderness affecting the wrists, metacarpophalangeal joints and proximal interphalangeal joints. Sensation was normal. She was unable to oppose her fingers.

Of the following the one which is associated with a **BETTER** prognosis for her condition is:

A acute onset
B early erosions on imaging
C presence of HLA-DR4 genetic marker
D presence of subcutaneous nodules
E rheumatoid factor seropositivity

3.15 A 65-year-old man presented with a long history of progressive weakness. (Figure 3.15, page 382.)

The most likely diagnosis is:

A Becker's muscular dystrophy
B dystrophia myotonica
C hypothyroidism
D myasthenia gravis
E Parkinson's syndrome

3.16 A 64-year-old man was referred because of alternating constipation and diarrhoea over the past 4 weeks.

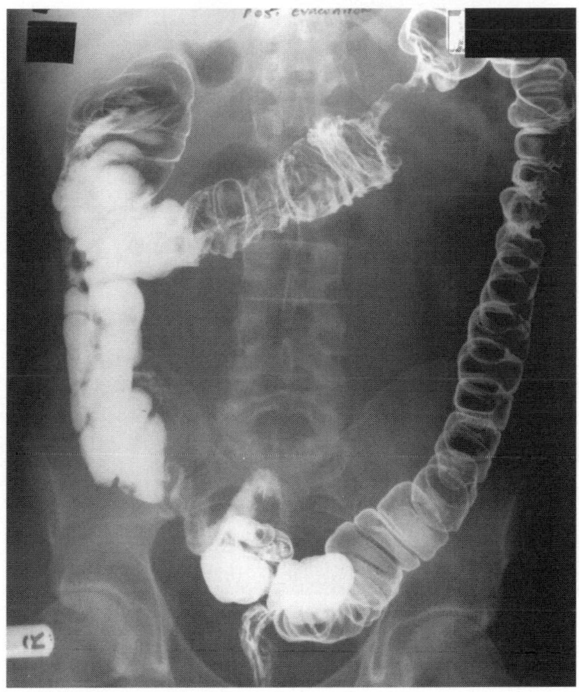

The most significant abnormality on the barium enema is:

A colonic carcinoma
B Crohn's colitis
C diverticular disease
D osteoporosis of the spine
E ulcerative colitis

3.17 A 59-year-old man was referred because of progressive jaundice and weight loss.
An ERCP was performed. (See overleaf)

The most likely diagnosis is:

A carcinoma of the head of the pancreas
B gallstones obstructing the common bile duct
C normal ERCP
D primary biliary cirrhosis
E primary sclerosing cholangitis

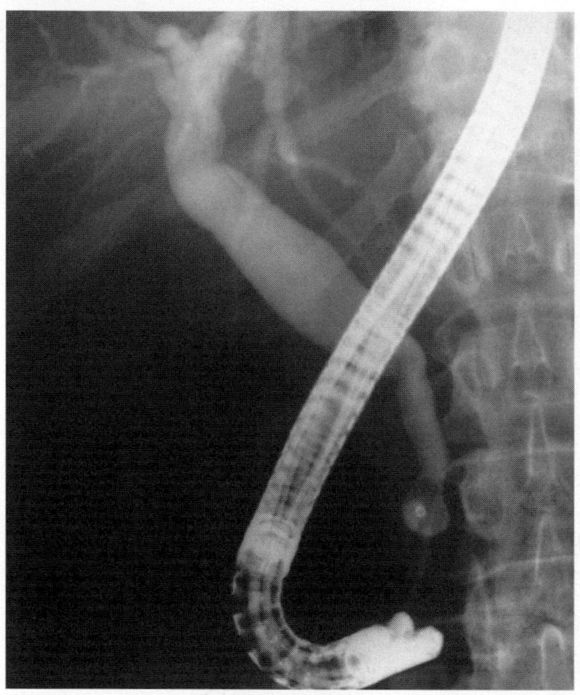

3.18 A 12-year-old boy was referred for cardiac catheterisation because of progressive shortness of breath.

	Pressure (systolic/diastolic [mmHg])	Normal value	O_2 saturation (%)
Right atrium	8	0–8	75
Right ventricle	35/11	15–30/0–8	84
Pulmonary artery	45/15	15–30/0–8	85
Left atrium (mean)	12	1–10	96
Left ventricle	132/12	100–140/3–12	97
Aorta	135/70	100–140/60–90	97

The most likely diagnosis is:

- A atrial septal defect
- B coarctation of the aorta
- C Fallot's tetralogy
- D patent ductus arteriosus
- E ventricular septal defect

3.19 A 56-year-old man was admitted with an inferior MI for which he was treated with thrombolysis. Three hours later he became cold, clammy and short of breath. He continued to have a pulse.

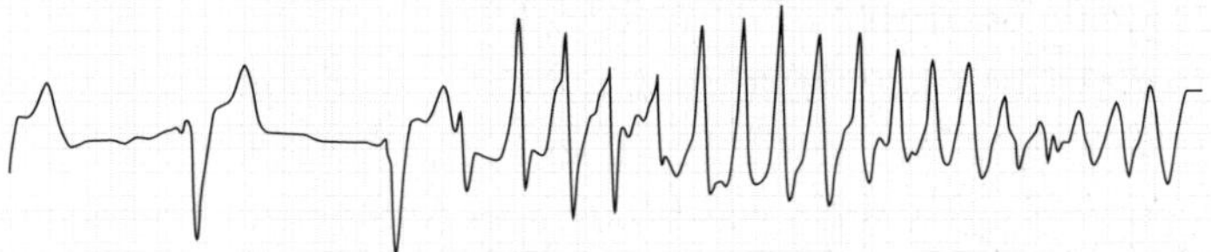

The ECG shows:

A supraventricular tachycardia with aberrant conduction
B atrial fibrillation with aberrant conduction
C torsades de pointes
D ventricular fibrillation
E ventricular standstill

3.20 A 59-year-old vagrant was admitted with abdominal pain, vomiting, dizziness and blurred vision. He was a chronic alcoholic and confirmed he had drunk methylated spirits about 5 h ago. He had no other medical problems and was on no medication.

On examination his GCS was 14/15. His temperature was 37.2°C, pulse 86 regular and blood pressure 138/90. His respiratory rate was 26 breaths/min and his chest was clear. There was diffuse abdominal tenderness. He was uncooperative with the neurological examination but appeared to have decreased visual acuity.

Arterial blood gases on air	pH	7.18	PCO_2	3.4
	PO_2	10.1	Bicarbonate	12.4
	Base excess	−13.5		

Of the following statements concerning this patient's management the one which is **FALSE** is:

A activated charcoal should be given
B haemodialysis is indicated if mental or visual features are present
C intravenous bicarbonate should be given
D ipecacuanha is contraindicated
E oral ethanol should be given

3.21 A 25-year-old man was admitted with community-acquired pneumonia. Two days later he developed a non-pruritic skin rash on both legs, both arms and in his mouth. (Figure 3.21, page 383.)

The skin lesion is most likely to be:

A drug reaction
B erythema multiforme
C erythema nodosum
D guttate psoriasis
E pyoderma gangrenosum

3.22 A 70-year-old woman was brought to Accident & Emergency in a confused state. She was found collapsed at home and was unable to provide a reliable history. Her old notes documented a history of ischaemic heart disease and treatment with radioiodine. She denied any chest pain but did complain of a non-productive cough. She was taking low dose aspirin and a glyceryl trinitrate spray.

On examination she was pale and had a temperature of 33.4°C. Her pulse was 55 regular and blood pressure 95/40. She had bilateral crackles in both bases of her chest. Abdominal examination revealed some generalised tenderness.

Of the following statements concerning the diagnosis and management of this patient it is true that:

A antibiotics are not indicated in the acute situation
B increased TSH and normal free T_4 excludes hypothyroidism
C intravenous hydrocortisone should be given
D she should be actively re-warmed using peritoneal lavage
E Lugol's iodine solution should be given

3.23 Four hundred patients who had suffered myocardial infarction (MI) were followed up to see if continued smoking post-MI was associated with increased risk of dying at the end of 5 years; 100 patients continued to smoke and of these 10 had died compared to 20 deaths in patients who had stopped smoking.

The relative risk (RR) is:

A (10 x 30)/(90 x 370)
B (10 x 100)/(20 x 300)
C (10 x 280)/(20 x 90)
D (10 x 300)/(20 x 100)
E (10 x 370)/(30 x 90)

3.24 A 46-year-old woman was referred with progressive abdominal swelling for the past 2 weeks and increasing lethargy. Following this it was noticed that she looked yellow. She had no other medical problems. She did not smoke, drink alcohol or take any other medication. She had no relevant family history.

On examination she was jaundiced and had scratch marks on her forearms and abdomen. She was apyrexial, pulse 68 regular and blood pressure 110/55. She had 2 cm hepatomegaly and moderate ascites.

Bloods	Hb	13.4	WCC	4.5
	Platelets	110	MCV	85.4
	Na	132	K	4.8
	Urea	3.9	Creatinine	80
	Protein	70	Albumin	28
	Bilirubin	80	ALT	85
	ALP	105	GGT	39
	INR	1.4		
Antinuclear antibodies		1 in 80		
Smooth muscle antibodies		1 in 160		
Antimitochondrial antibodies		1 in 16		
Anti-double stranded DNA		Negative		
Hepatitis A, B, C serology		Negative		
Caeruloplasmin		245		
Liver ultrasound	Hepatomegaly but no focal liver lesion Spleen, pancreas, gallbladder and kidneys normal Moderate ascites No common bile duct dilatation			

The most likely diagnosis is:

A autoimmune hepatitis
B primary biliary cirrhosis
C primary sclerosing cholangitis
D systemic lupus erythematosus
E Wilson's disease

3.25 A 58-year-old man complained of chest tightness and shortness of breath. He had just had an emergency operation for an aortic aneurysm repair and had been transfused 4 units of blood. Apart from hypercholesterolaemia, he had no previous medical history and was on no medication, nor was he allergic to any drugs.

On examination he appeared distressed. His temperature was 40.1°C, pulse 110 regular and blood pressure 90/60. His chest was clear with a respiratory rate of 22 breaths/min. His abdomen was generally tender.

ECG Sinus tachycardia
Chest X-ray Normal
Urinalysis Haemoglobin 2+, blood 1+

The most likely complication to have occurred is:

A acute coronary syndrome
B bowel perforation
C fluid overload
D pulmonary embolus
E transfusion reaction

3.26 A 56-year-old man was admitted with worsening abdominal pain associated with vomiting that had been going on for the past 10 days. He had decreased appetite and some weight loss. For the past 4 months he had had a change in his bowel habit with increased frequency, but had not opened his bowels for a week. He had no previous medical history and was on no medication.

On examination he had bilateral ankle oedema. His temperature was 37.4°C, pulse 100 regular and blood pressure 130/80. His abdomen was distended and generally tender with no bowel sounds heard.

Abdominal X-ray Dilated loops of small bowel

A laparotomy was performed and biopsies were taken: (A) high power; (B) low power stained with synactophysin. (Figures 3.26A and B, page 383.)

The most likely diagnosis is:

A adenocarcinoma
B carcinoid tumour
C coeliac disease
D Crohn's disease
E ischaemic bowel

3.27 A 16-year-old boy was admitted with a 2-week history of fever, malaise, headache and night sweats. He had no cough or shortness of breath. He had some abdominal discomfort and back pain but no bowel or urinary symptoms. His appetite was decreased and he had lost some weight. He had no other medical problems and was on no medication. Two months ago he returned from his native Morocco where he had stayed on his uncle's farm.

On examination he had cervical lymphadenopathy. His temperature was 37.8°C, pulse 98 and blood pressure 95/60. Heart sounds and chest were clear. There was hepatosplenomegaly but no ascites. There was no neurological deficit.

Bloods	Hb	11.4	WCC	3.3
	Neutrophils	1.6	Lymphocytes	1.2
	Eosinophils	0.2	Platelets	150
	INR	1.0	Na	140
	K	4.2	Urea	3.5
	Creatinine	65	Protein	65
	Albumin	35	Bilirubin	10
	ALT	40	ALP	110
	ESR	60	CRP	48
Malaria films	Negative			
Chest X-ray	Normal			

The most likely diagnosis is:

A brucellosis
B Hodgkin's lymphoma
C hydatid cyst
D schistosomiasis
E strongyloidiasis

3.28 A 40-year-old woman on the psychiatric ward was referred because of increased thirst, dizziness and polyuria. She was on medication for her depressive illness.

No abnormality was found on examination. A water deprivation test was performed:

Time (h after starting)	**Plasma osmolality (mosmol/kg)**	**Urine osmolality (mosmol/kg)**
0	285	310
2	292	350
4	296	418
6	302	498
DDAVP 2 μg given intramuscularly		
8	305	580
Plasma$_{ADH}$ post-water deprivation test	4 (normal 3–5 pg/ml)	

Paper three questions

The most likely diagnosis in this patient is:

A complete central diabetes insipidus
B complete nephrogenic diabetes insipidus
C partial central diabetes insipidus
D partial nephrogenic diabetes insipidus
E primary polydipsia

3.29 A 34-year-old woman presented with shortness of breath. She was a non-smoker.

Arterial blood gases on air	pH	7.51	PCO_2	3.9
	PO_2	8.5	Bicarbonate	24
	Base excess	−1.2	O_2 saturation	90%

These results would be most consistent with:

A acute exacerbation of chronic obstructive airways disease
B athlete just finishing a half marathon
C insulin dependent diabetic not taking insulin because feeling unwell
D pulmonary embolus
E salicylate overdose 24 h post ingestion

3.30 A 55-year-old woman was referred because of a 1-week history of headache and blurred vision. She had had no fits or photophobia. She had a normal appetite and no weight loss. She had no other medical problems.

On examination she was not in pain. Her pulse was 90 regular and blood pressure 145/88. Her JVP was not elevated and both heart sounds were normal. Respiratory and abdominal examinations were normal. She did have some scalp tenderness but there was no cranial nerve abnormality and fundoscopic examination was normal. The rest of the nervous system examination was unremarkable.

The most useful investigation to establish the diagnosis would be:

A carotid Doppler ultrasound
B CT head
C lumbar puncture and oligoclonal bands
D MRI head
E temporal artery biopsy

3.31 A 32-year-old woman was referred for flexible sigmoidoscopy complaining of alternating constipation, for which she took lactulose and senna, and loose stools. Her problems had been going on for 6 months. Her appetite was normal, weight was stable and there was no rectal bleeding. Abdominal and rectal examinations were normal. (Figure 3.31, page 384.)

The sigmoidoscopy findings are most consistent with:

A Crohn's disease
B familial adenomatous polyposis
C melanosis coli
D pseudomembranous colitis
E ulcerative colitis

3.32 A 76-year-old Vietnamese man presented with recent haemoptysis and weight loss. He had smoked 20 cigarettes a day for over 30 years.

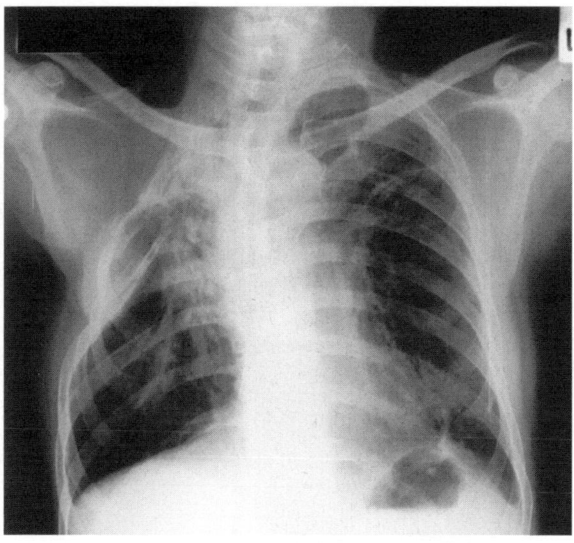

His chest X-ray findings are most likely to be due to:

A aspergilloma
B bronchiectasis
C bronchogenic carcinoma
D mesothelioma
E tuberculosis

3.33 A 53-year-old man presented with shortness of breath and cough. Five days ago he had been to Belgium and returned to the UK yesterday. Since arrival his breathing had got worse. He also had been having abdominal pain, muscle pains and loose stools. He had no previous medical history and he did not smoke or drink alcohol. He had not been started on any medication.

On examination he was in distress and using his accessory muscles of respiration. His temperature was 39.0°C, pulse 100 regular and blood pressure 95/58. His respiratory rate was 32 breaths/min and he had bronchial breathing and coarse crackles in the right upper zone of the chest. His abdomen was generally tender.

Bloods	Hb	11.8	WCC	20.2
	Neutrophils	18.2	Platelets	300
	Na	131	K	3.5
	Urea	15.6	Creatinine	220
	Albumin	29	Protein	56
	Bilirubin	34	ALT	79
	ALP	137	Calcium	2.55
	Phosphate	0.9	CRP	332
Arterial blood gases on 10 L/min O_2	pH	7.19	PCO_2	3.8
	PO_2	6.9	Bicarbonate	8.9
	Base excess	–16		

Chest X-ray

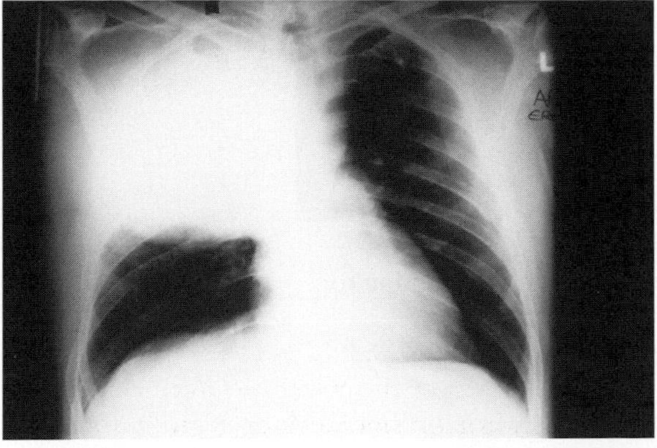

Apart from ventilatory support, the most appropriate medication would be:

A ceftriaxone and clarithromycin
B ciprofloxacin and gentamicin
C clarithromycin and rifampicin
D flucloxacillin and gentamicin
E rifampicin, isoniazid, pyrazinamide and ethambutol

3.34 A 28-year-old woman was admitted with pyrexia and confusion. Two days ago her family had noticed her acting strangely, including an inability to name objects. She did not have a cough or any urinary problems. There was no headache, neck stiffness or photophobia but there was a rash. She had had no obvious contact with illness.

On examination she had a temperature of 39.0°C. Her pulse was 110 regular and blood pressure 134/79. Her JVP was not elevated but she had a loud pansystolic murmur in the apex that radiated to the axilla and carotids. There were some bilateral basal crackles in her chest. Abdominal examination was normal. She had an abbreviated mini-mental test score of 3/10. There was also some expressive dysphasia. Cranial nerve examination was normal and she was moving all four limbs. She had flat, red, non-tender, blanching spots on her hands.

Bloods	Hb	13.1	WCC	17.5
	Platelets	376	INR	1.2
	Na	139	K	4.7
	Urea	3.8	Creatinine	78
	Albumin	32	Protein	65
	Bilirubin	12	ALT	25
	ALP	67	Calcium	2.22
	ESR	76	CRP	234
Chest X-ray	Enlarged heart			
	No pulmonary oedema			
ECG	Voltage criteria for left ventricular hypertrophy			

The most helpful test to establish the diagnosis would be:

A electroencephalogram
B Herpes simplex serology
C lumbar puncture
D transoesophageal echocardiogram
E vaginal swab

3.35 A 68-year-old woman was admitted with palpitations and collapse. She had a previous medical history of hypertension but was not on any medication. She did not drink alcohol or smoke. Her temperature was 37.4°C and blood pressure 115/74.

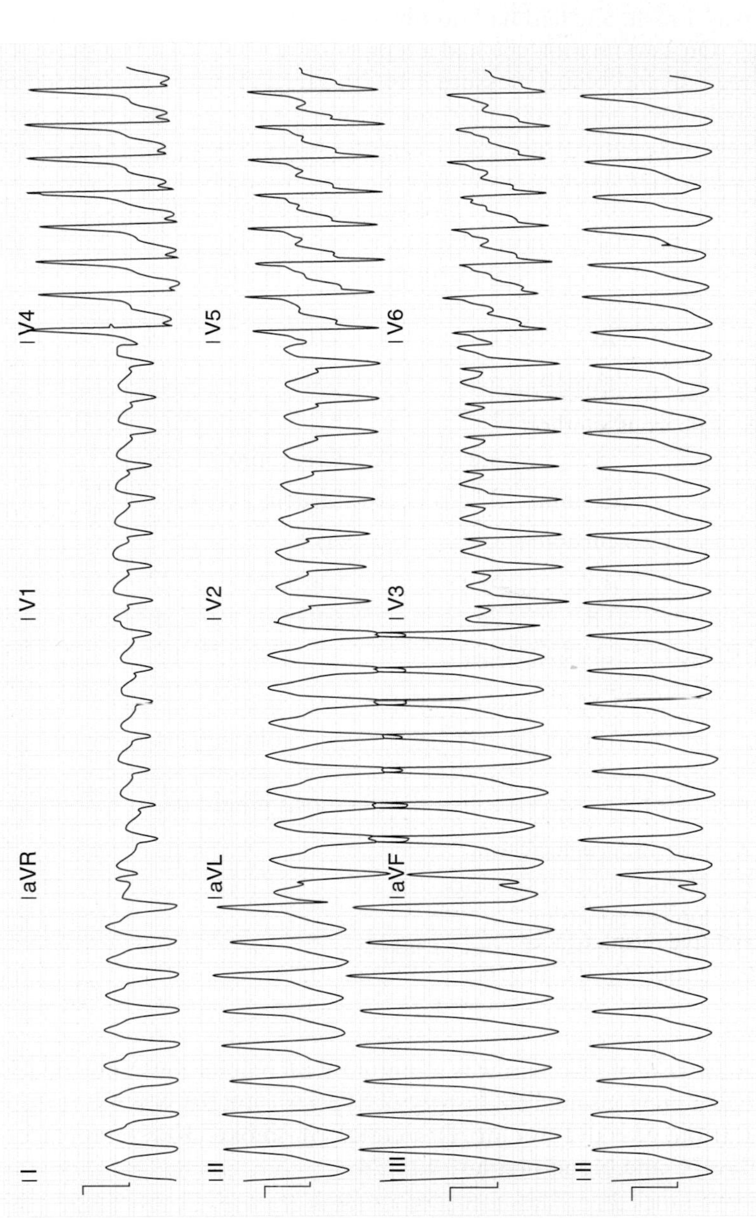

I
aVR
V1
V4
II
aVL
V2
V5
III
aVF
V3
V6
II

The ECG shows:

- A atrial fibrillation with aberrant conduction
- B supraventricular tachycardia with aberrant conduction
- C torsades de pointes
- D ventricular fibrillation
- E ventricular tachycardia

3.36 A 37-year-old woman was referred with a 4-month history of skin changes to both legs. (Figure 3.36, page 384.)

The skin rash is due to:

- A erythema nodosum
- B granuloma annulare
- C lipoatrophy
- D necrobiosis lipoidica
- E tuberous xanthoma

3.37 A 50-year-old man complained of headaches that were getting progressively worse.

MRI head 2 cm mass in sella turcica

Of the following complications the one which is **LEAST** likely to occur is:

- A amaurosis fugax
- B failure to adduct right eye
- C left complete ptosis and dilated pupil
- D loss of sensation of lower face and anterior two-thirds of tongue
- E vertical diplopia on descending stairs

3.38 A 63-year-old man was admitted with a stroke that caused complete expressive dysphasia and right hemiparesis. Initially he was treated with intravenous fluids and then with nasogastric tube feeding. A speech therapist had concluded that 4 weeks after developing the stroke he was still at significant risk of aspiration and that PEG feeding would be advisable. The patient, although aphasic, was able to understand commands and was repeatedly warned that his condition would deteriorate if he did not have feeding. Despite this he kept removing the nasogastric tubes and refused to tolerate further insertions. His family was concerned that the patient appeared to be deteriorating and wanted the PEG tube to be inserted.

The correct management plan for this patient would be:

- A ask psychiatrist to ascertain mental capacity of the patient before deciding
- B insert the PEG tube as requested by the family
- C obtain a court order to insert the PEG tube against the patient's wishes
- D respect the patient's wishes and do not insert PEG tube or nasogastric tubes
- E wait until the patient becomes unresponsive and then insert PEG tube

3.39 A 13-year-old boy was brought in with abdominal pain and jaundice. Over the past 2 days he had had diarrhoea and vomiting. Prior to this he had never been ill.

On examination he was apyrexial. He was jaundiced but there was no lymphadenopathy. His pulse was 98 regular and blood pressure 110/70. Respiratory examination was normal. He had mild abdominal tenderness but no organomegaly.

Bloods	Hb	14.0	WCC	5.2
	Platelets	250	INR	1.0
	Bilirubin	60	Albumin	40
	Protein	70	ALT	20
	ALP	500	GGT	20
	Amylase	24		
Urinalysis	Urobilinogen 2+, no bilirubin			

The most likely diagnosis is:

- A biliary atresia
- B Dubin–Johnson syndrome
- C Gilbert's syndrome
- D hereditary spherocytosis
- E Rotor syndrome

3.40 A 38-year-old woman presented with a 4-day history of severe pain and paraesthesia in her back radiating down her leg. It came on suddenly and she could not walk. Specifically it affected the buttocks, back and lateral aspects of the thigh and leg and dorsum of the foot. The right side was worse than the left.

On examination she had weakness of her hamstrings, peroneus longus and toe extensors. Tone was normal but power was reduced. Knee and ankle reflexes were intact, and plantar responses were flexor. There was decreased sensation to light touch and pinprick over the dorsum of the foot and anterolateral aspect of the leg.

The lesion is most likely to be at the following root level:

A L3
B L4
C L5
D S1
E S2

3.41 A 61-year-old man in the intensive care unit had become acutely dyspnoeic and hypotensive 2 days after an aortic aneurysm repair. Apart from this operation the patient had no previous medical history and did not smoke or drink alcohol. He was still being ventilated.

On examination he appeared distressed with intercostal recession. His skin was cold, cyanosed and clammy. His temperature was 36.5°C, pulse 110 regular and blood pressure 98/64. His respiratory rate was 26 breaths/min and there were bilateral crackles in his chest. Abdominal examination was normal. A Swan–Ganz catheter was inserted and his pulmonary artery wedge pressure was 12 mmHg. His urine output for the last 3 h was 60 ml.

Bloods	Hb	11.5	WCC	16.7
	Neutrophils	12.8	Platelets	279
	Na	132	K	4.0
	Urea	15.7	Creatinine	176
	Protein	56	Albumin	23
	Bilirubin	16	ALT	45
	ALP	110	ESR	29
	CRP	220		
Chest X-ray	Bilateral infiltrates			
	Heart size normal			
ECG	Sinus tachycardia			
	No ischaemic changes			
Arterial blood gases on 60% O_2	pH	7.52	PCO_2	3.6
	PO_2	7.9	Bicarbonate	22.4
	Base excess	–2.2		

The next step in his management should be:

A aerosolized synthetic surfactant
B intravenous furosemide
C intravenous hydrocortisone
D putting patient prone to improve oxygenation
E thrombolysis with tissue plasminogen activator

3.42 A 39-year-old Caucasian man was referred because of recurrent painful ulceration of his scrotum with no associated urinary or bowel problems. He also had ulcers in his mouth. Last month he had a painful red eye that spontaneously resolved. Apart from some pain in his knee, ankle and elbow joints, which was episodic in nature, he was generally healthy. He had no previous medical history or significant family history.

On examination he had several oral and scrotal aphthous ulcers. There was some swelling and tenderness of his left knee.

Bloods				
	Hb	12.0	WCC	5.7
	Platelets	360	INR	1.0
	Na	134	K	4.0
	Urea	5.6	Creatinine	98
	Protein	72	Albumin	38
	Bilirubin	13	ALT	26
	ALP	60	ESR	28
	CRP	35		

Of the following the one which is **NOT** associated with his condition is:

A acneiform skin eruptions
B arterial thrombosis
C erythema multiforme
D HLA B5
E pathergy

3.43 A 26-year-old HIV-positive man was admitted with headache, neck stiffness and photophobia and decreased conscious level. He was not on any medication.

His temperature was 37.6°C, pulse 100 regular and blood pressure 120/88. A lumbar puncture was performed and his CSF revealed the circular opacities shown. (Figure 3.43, page 384.)

The most likely organism to have caused this is:

A *Cryptococcus neoformans*
B *Listeria monocytogenes*
C *Mycobacterium tuberculosis*
D *Neisseria meningitidis*
E *Toxoplasma gondii*

3.44 A 78-year-old woman presented with pain in her back and hips. She also had a decreased appetite and some loss of weight.

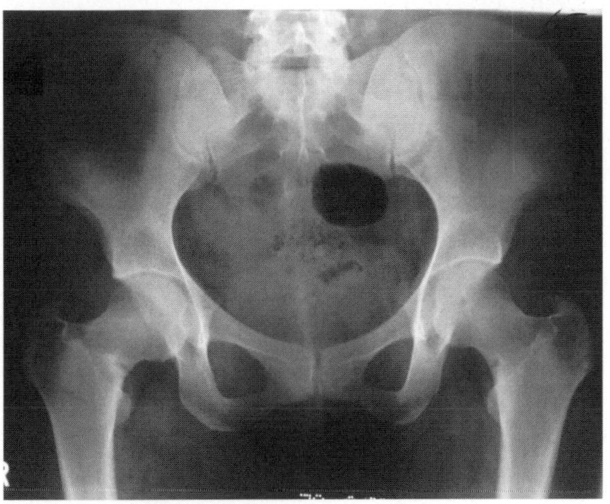

The underlying diagnosis is:

A fibromyalgia
B fractured shaft of femur
C multiple myeloma
D osteomalacia
E Paget's disease of bone

3.45 A 59-year-old woman was admitted with a painful, warm, swollen left leg. (Figure 3.45, page 385.)

The most appropriate treatment for this patient would be:

A dapsone
B flucloxacillin
C furosemide
D indomethacin
E warfarin

3.46 A 55-year-old man was admitted with fits. He had no history of epilepsy or head injury. He had no haemoptysis or shortness of breath but felt very tired and weak. He had smoked 20 cigarettes a day for over 30 years but did not drink any alcohol. He was on no medication.

On examination he looked cachexic but there were no other abnormal findings.

Bloods	Na	115	K	4.0
	Urea	7.0	Creatinine	110
	Glucose	8.0		
Thyroid and adrenal function tests	Normal			
Urine osmolality	420 mosmol/kg			
Urine Na	30 mmol/L			
Chest X-ray	Coin-shaped lesion in left apex			

Which one of the following drugs could be used to treat his condition?

A carbamazepine
B chlorpropamide
C chlorthiazide
D demeclocycline
E vasopressin

3.47 A 60-year-old woman was brought in with acute rectal bleeding. So far today she had passed over 700 ml of fresh red blood. She had mild lower abdominal discomfort but was not vomiting. She had a previous medical history of osteoarthritis but was only taking codeine phosphate. She was not on anticoagulants. She did not drink alcohol or smoke.

On examination she was not in pain. Her temperature was 37.2°C, pulse 110 regular and blood pressure 95/50. Her abdomen was soft, mildly tender but there was no guarding. Bowel sounds were heard. Rectal examination revealed fresh blood but no masses.

Bloods	Hb	8.9	WCC	10.5
	Platelets	550	INR	1.1
	Na	140	K	3.9
	Urea	9.5	Creatinine	90
	Albumin	38	Protein	68
	Bilirubin	15	ALT	25
	ALP	80	Amylase	70
	Glucose	4.5		
Chest X-ray	No free air under diaphragm			
Abdominal X-ray	No obstruction			

Of the following statements concerning this patient's diagnosis and management the one which is true is:

- A an unprepared colonoscopy is the next most appropriate investigation
- B angiodysplasia is the most likely cause of bleeding
- C immediate laparotomy should be considered
- D mesenteric angiography is only useful if she continues to bleed at a rate >2 ml/min
- E the source of bleeding is likely to be proximal to the ligament of Trietz

3.48 A 69-year-old man was referred because of inability to cope at home. He was able to walk with assistance. He lived alone but did not eat much. His carers complained he was persistently drooling and miserable. He had no previous medical history and had had no recent illnesses. He was not on any medication.

On examination he had a resting tremor, worsening when he tried to shake hands. His handwriting was small and illegible. He had increased tone in his upper and lower limbs. There was reduced power but in the lower limbs extensors were stronger than flexors. He had increased reflexes in the lower limbs but plantar responses were flexor. Sensation was normal. His gait was shuffling. Pupil size and fundoscopy were normal but he was unable to look down, although the other ocular movements were normal and there was no nystagmus. The other cranial nerves were normal. He had an abbreviated mental test score of 7/10. He was apyrexial, his pulse was 78 regular and his blood pressure was 120/90 sitting and standing.

The most likely diagnosis is:

- A Huntington's disease
- B multisystem atrophy/Shy-Drager syndrome
- C Parinaud's syndrome
- D Parkinson's disease
- E progressive supranuclear palsy/Steel-Richardson-Olszewski syndrome

3.49 A 60-year-old man was admitted with shortness of breath and chest pain. The symptoms had started 6 days ago but worsened today. Although known to have hypertension, he was not on any medication. He smoked but did not drink alcohol.

On examination he looked unwell and was sweating. His temperature was 36.8°C, pulse 110 regular and blood pressure 95/58 in both arms. His JVP was elevated +4 cm and both heart sounds were normal. He had decreased air entry in both lungs but there was no wheeze or crackles. His respiratory rate was 36 breaths/min. As the patient was becoming increasingly exhausted he was intubated and admitted to intensive care.

Bloods	Hb	12.9	WCC	5.8
	Platelets	256	Na	143
	K	4.2	Urea	6.1
	Creatinine	88	Protein	69
	Albumin	39	Bilirubin	14
	ALT	26	ALP	58
Chest X-ray	No abnormality detected			
ECG	Sinus tachyardia			
Arterial blood on 60% O_2	pH	7.28	PCO_2	6.9
	PO_2	7.6	Bicarbonate	29.1
	Base excess	3.9		
Expired CO_2	1.4			

The most likely diagnosis is:

A dissection of thoracic aortic aneurysm
B inhaled foreign body
C myocardial infarction
D pneumothorax
E pulmonary embolus

3.50 A 23-year-old man with learning difficulties was referred because of severe pain in his back and stiff joints. The joints affected included his hands, knees and spine. As a teenager he had been found to have osteoporosis and last year he suffered a pulmonary embolus and was on warfarin.

On examination he was 200 cm tall. Apart from lens dislocation, his fingers were long and thin, and he had pectus carinatum. His pulse was 88 regular and blood pressure 140/88. His JVP was not elevated and heart sounds were normal with no murmurs. Respiratory and abdominal examinations were normal. There was some spinal tenderness as well as some inflammation of his knees and metacarpophalangeal joints. Neurological examination was normal.

Of the following statements concerning this patient's diagnosis the one which is true is:

A if his urine was left to stand it would turn blue-black
B the condition cannot be diagnosed in the neonatal period
C the condition displays autosomal recessive inheritance
D the major defect is in collagen synthesis
E the most likely diagnosis is Marfan's syndrome

3.51 A 55-year-old woman was referred because of a 3-week history of jaundice and right upper quadrant pain. An ERCP was attempted but was technically difficult so a percutaneous transhepatic cholangiogram (PTC) was performed.

The PTC findings are most consistent with:

- A carcinoma of the head of the pancreas
- B lymphoma at the porta hepatis
- C pancreatic divisum
- D primary sclerosing cholangitis
- E stone in the common bile duct

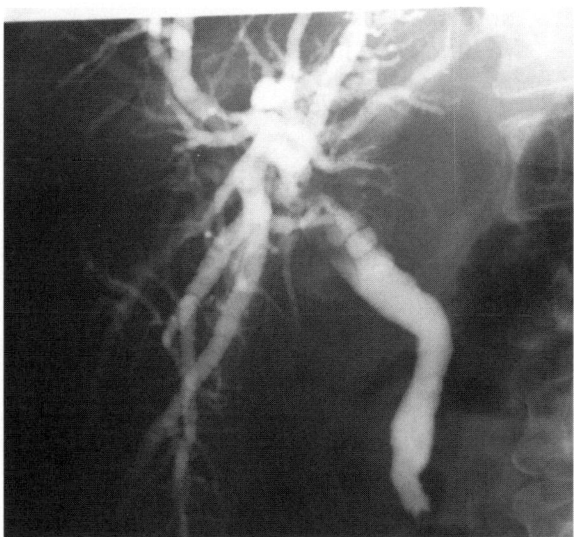

3.52 A 73-year-old man was referred because of a painless lesion on his left lower eyelid that had been getting bigger over the past 9 months. There was no lymphadenopathy. (Figure 3.52, page 385.)

The most likely diagnosis is:

- A Bowen's disease
- B keratoacanthoma
- C nodular malignant melanoma
- D basal cell carcinoma
- E squamous cell carcinoma

3.53 A 17-year-old girl presented with primary amenorrhoea. She performed well at school and was a keen athlete. She had no previous medical history and was not on any medication. She did not smoke or drink alcohol.

On examination she looked well. Her height was on the 30th centile and her weight was on the 20th centile. She had breast buds but no axillary or pubic hair. She had normal female external genitalia.

Chromosome analysis	46,XX		
Bloods	17-OH progesterone	2 (normal <14 nmol/L)	
	FSH	2.0 (normal 2.5–10 U/L)	
	LH	2.0 (normal: 2.5–10 U/L)	
	Testosterone	0.8 (normal 0.5–3.0 mmol/L)	
	TSH	4	Free T_4 20
Pelvic ultrasound	Normal uterus Multicystic changes in the ovaries		

The most likely diagnosis is:

- A 11-β-hydroxylase deficiency
- B 5-α-reductase deficiency
- C constitutional growth delay
- D polycystic ovarian syndrome
- E primary ovarian failure

3.54 A 35-year-old woman presented with tender lesions on both legs. She had no respiratory symptoms and was not on any medication.

On examination she was apyrexial, pulse 90 regular and blood pressure 136/88. Her chest was clear. There were bilateral, erythematous raised lesions on her shins.

Chest X-ray Bi-hilar lymphadenopathy

The most helpful test that would give a definitive diagnosis would be:

- A Kveim test
- B serum angiotensin-converting enzyme
- C serum calcium
- D skin biopsy
- E transbronchial biopsy

3.55 A 48-year-old man presented with sudden onset right loin pain. He had no previous medical history and was not on medication.

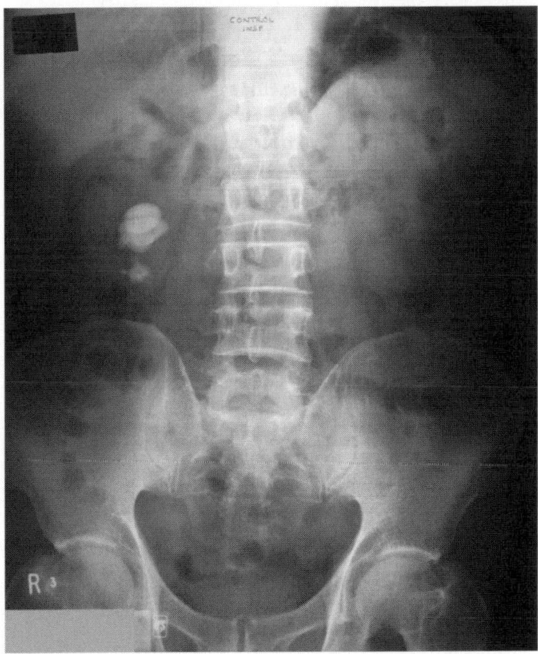

The likely composition of his stone is:

A calcium oxalate
B calcium phosphate
C cholesterol
D cystine
E magnesium ammonium phosphate

3.56 A 55-year-old man presented with a 2-week history of painless, frank haematuria. He reported no abdominal pain or bowel symptoms. He smoked 10 cigarettes a day but did not drink alcohol. He had no recent foreign travel and was not on any medication.

On examination he was apyrexial, pulse 68 regular and blood pressure 120/70. Abdominal examination was normal and rectal examination revealed a smooth prostate.

Bloods	Hb	13.5	WCC	9.5
	Platelets	245	INR	1.1
	Na	140	K	4.2
	Urea	5.6	Creatinine	100
	Protein	68	Albumin	39
	Bilirubin	10	ALT	15
	ALP	118	ESR	15
	CRP	40		
Renal ultrasound	No hydronephrosis			
	Left kidney 11.0 cm, right kidney 10.8 cm			
Chest X-ray	Normal			

The most helpful test to establish the diagnosis is:

A flexible cystoscopy
B intravenous pyelogram
C prostatic specific antigen
D serum ANCA
E transrectal ultrasound

3.57 A 65-year-old man was admitted complaining of severe generalised abdominal pain for the past 2 days, which was worse soon after eating. The pain started off colicky in nature but was now constant. Today he had also passed fresh red blood per rectum. He had a previous medical history of ischaemic heart disease and peripheral vascular disease. He was on aspirin, atenolol and digoxin. He smoked 15 cigarettes a day.

On examination he was in pain with a temperature of 37.0°C, pulse 100 irregular and blood pressure 120/70. Respiratory examination was normal. There was generalised abdominal tenderness but no guarding and no palpable masses were felt. Rectal examination revealed some blood but no masses.

Bloods	Hb	13.5	WCC	12.5
	Platelets	300	Na	140
	K	4.0	Urea	8.5
	Creatinine	100	Albumin	35
	Protein	65	Bilirubin	12
	ALT	35	ALP	100
	GGT	60	Amylase	200
	CRP	140	ESR	35
	Lactate	5		
Arterial blood gases on air	pH	7.31	PCO_2	4.5
	PO_2	10.9	Bicarbonate	18
	Base excess	–7		
Chest X-ray	Normal			
Abdominal X-ray	Normal			

The most likely diagnosis is:

A acute diverticulitis
B acute pancreatitis
C bleeding from aspirin-induced gastric erosion
D mesenteric ischaemia
E ruptured aortic aneurysm

3.58 A 39-year-old woman was referred because of persistent hypokalaemia and hypertension going on for several months. She had no other medical problems and was treated with amlodopine and doxazosin but these had been stopped because they failed to control her hypertension.

On examination her pulse was 90 and blood pressure 190/100. She was admitted overnight for tests.

Bloods	Na	140	K	2.8
	Urea	5.4	Creatinine	80

	Renin	**Aldosterone**
8 a.m. (lying)	0.9	1800
12 p.m. (standing)	1.2	2500

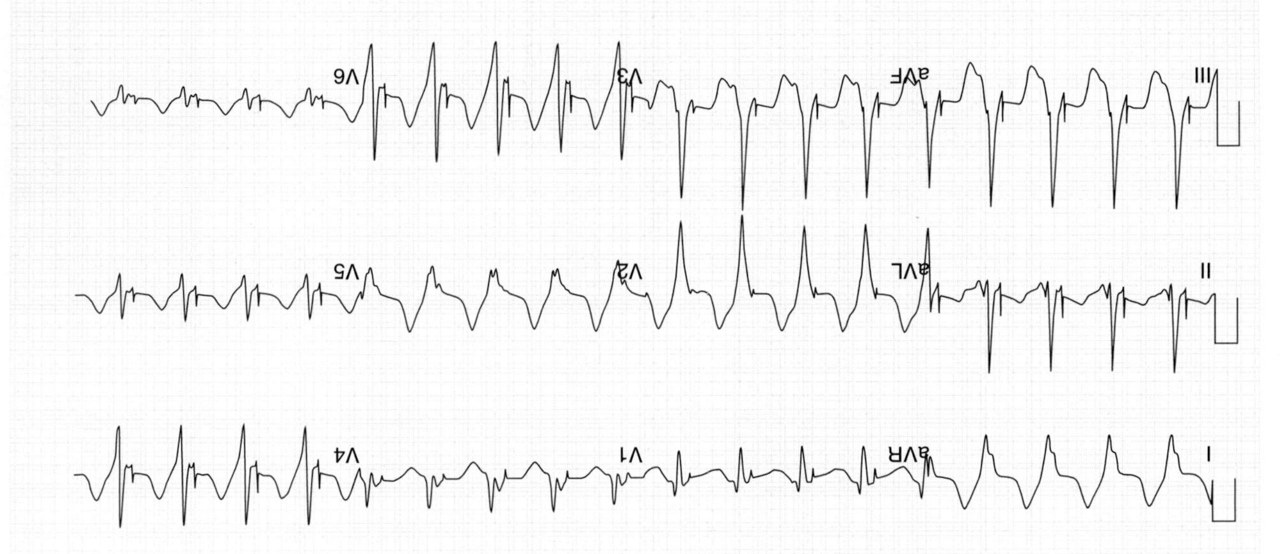
I
aVR
V1
V4
II
aVL
V2
V5
III
aVF
V3
V6

These findings are most consistent with:

A adrenal cortex adenoma
B adrenal medulla adenoma
C bilateral adrenal cortical hyperplasia
D essential hypertension
E renal artery stenosis

3.59 A 30-year-old man was referred with a 3-month history of increasing difficulty swallowing liquids and solids. This was associated with regurgitation of food soon after eating and waking up at night coughing. His appetite was decreased and he had lost weight. He had no previous medical history and was not on any medication.

Physical examination was normal.

The test that is most likely to give the definitive diagnosis is:

A barium swallow
B CT chest
C endoscopic ultrasound
D oesophageal manometry
E upper GI endoscopy

3.60 An 80-year-old man was admitted with collapse. He reported no chest pain or shortness of breath.

On examination his pulse was 38 regular and blood pressure 90/50. His JVP was not elevated and his heart sounds were normal. ECG showed complete heart block and a temporary pacing wire was inserted.

The post-procedure ECG is consistent with the complication of:

A development of acute MI
B electrical break
C electrode displacement
D perforation of the interventricular septum
E too high a threshold

3.61 A 67-year-old homeless man was referred with rectal bleeding and abdominal pain for 3 weeks. Six months ago he was treated for prostate cancer with surgery and radiotherapy.

A flexible sigmoidoscopy was performed which revealed ulceration up to the descending colon.

Colonic biopsy (the arrows 1–3 refer to different abnormalities as described in the answer) (Figure 3.61, 385.)

The most likely diagnosis is:

A cytomegalovirus colitis
B inflammatory bowel disease
C pseudomembranous colitis
D radiation enteritis
E tuberculous colitis

3.62 A 20-year-old man was referred to the clinic because of deranged liver function tests. He had no history of jaundice, haematemesis or pruritis. He had no risk factors for viral hepatitis. For the past 2 years he had suffered with tremor and problems with walking. There was no family history of note and he was an only child. He did not smoke, drink alcohol or take any illicit drugs. He was on no medication.

On examination he had tremor in both hands at rest but no flap and no jaundice. Abdominal examination revealed hepatomegaly. Neurological examination revealed increased tone and rigidity in the upper and lower limbs, flexor plantar response and a clumsy gait. Cranial examination was normal.

Bloods	Albumin	36	Bilirubin	16
	ALT	50	ALP	45
	INR	1.2	Caeruloplasmin	150
	Ferritin	300		
Hepatitis A, B, C serology	Negative			
Liver ultrasound	Hepatomegaly with no focal liver lesion seen			

The **BEST** test to establish the diagnosis is:

A 24-h urinary copper
B gene studies
C hepatic copper concentration
D serum copper
E slit lamp examination

3.63 A 32-year-old woman was referred from the antenatal clinic because of high blood pressure and headache for the past 2 weeks. She was 26 weeks into her first pregnancy. She had no previous medical history and was on no medication. She did not smoke or drink alcohol.

On examination her pulse was 78 regular and her blood pressure was 158/96. Apart from a gravid abdomen there were no other significant findings. There was no protein in her urine.

The treatment of choice for this patient is:

A atenolol
B bed rest
C immediate delivery of fetus
D lisinopril
E methyldopa

3.64 A 48-year-old man was referred by his GP because of poor night-time sleep and excessive daytime somnolence which was affecting his job and had almost caused a road traffic accident. His wife complained that he snored very loudly and that during the night he would periodically stop breathing. He had no other medical problems and was on no medication. He had smoked 20 cigarettes a day for over 30 years and drank 12 units of alcohol a week. He worked in an office and did very little exercise.

On examination he was obese with BMI 36, weight 130 kg and height 1.9 m. His pulse was 94 regular and blood pressure was 155/92. His JVP was not elevated and heart sounds and chest were clear.

This patient is at increased risk of suffering from all the following **EXCEPT**:

A cerebrovascular accident
B hyperlipidaemia
C non-insulin dependent diabetes mellitus
D primary pulmonary hypertension
E ventricular arrhythmias

3.65 A 42-year-old woman with a 20-year history of insulin dependent diabetes was reviewed in the clinic where she complained of frequent hypoglycaemic episodes. She took short-acting insulin with meals and long-acting insulin at bedtime, and had been on the same dose for the past 4 months. She was adamant that she was taking her insulin as prescribed.

Of the following, the **LEAST** likely explanation for her hypoglycaemia is:

A development of Cushing's syndrome
B development of renal failure
C excessive alcohol intake
D increased exercise and weight loss
E persistent injection of insulin into the same site

3.66 A 16-year-old girl presented to Accident & Emergency with a 3-day history of bloody diarrhoea and abdominal pain but no vomiting. She had felt unwell since eating a hamburger almost a week ago. She had not passed any urine today. She had no previous medical history and was not on any medication.

On examination her temperature was 37.4°C, pulse 78 and blood pressure 150/100. Her JVP was not elevated and heart sounds were normal. There was mild abdominal tenderness and rectal examination revealed blood on the glove but no masses. GCS was 15/15 and all cranial nerves were intact with no focal neurological deficit. She was unable to give a urine specimen.

Bloods	Hb	8.0	MCV	96.0
	WCC	14.2	Platelets	75
	Reticulocytes	8%	Haptoglobin	0.05
	LDH	500	INR	1.1
	Na	133	K	5.8
	Urea	20.2	Creatinine	310
	Bilirubin	28	Albumin	30
	ALT	37	ALP	120
Direct Coombs' test	Negative			
Blood film	Schistocytes, thrombocytopaenia, reticulocytes			
Chest X-ray	Normal			
Abdominal X-ray	No large or small bowel dilatation			

The next step in this patient's management would be:

A haemodialysis
B intravenous heparin
C intravenous steroids
D plasma exchange
E platelet transfusion

3.67 A 74-year-old woman was admitted with facial paralysis and an unsteady gait. She was unable to close her right eye or puff out her right cheek. Over the past 5 months her hearing had got worse.

On examination she had drooping of the right side of her mouth and was unable to raise her right eyebrow when looking up. She did have horizontal nystagmus in the right eye and the corneal reflex was absent. There was decreased sensation on the right side of her face from the forehead down to her chin. She had an intention tremor in her right upper limb. In her lower limbs power, tone, reflexes and sensation were intact, but she was unable to run her right heel down her left shin and she had an ataxic gait.

The most likely cause of her condition is:

A cerebellopontine angle lesion
B jugular foramen syndrome
C lateral medullary syndrome
D medial medullary syndrome
E pseudobulbar palsy

3.68 A 57-year-old homeless man was admitted from Accident & Emergency with vomiting, abdominal pain and blurred vision. He also complained of dysphagia but no shortness of breath. He had not opened his bowels today. There was no history of trauma but his symptoms had worsened; he thought they might be related to something he had eaten from a can yesterday. Apart from self neglect he had no previous medical problems.

On examination he was apyrexial and unkempt. His pulse was 98 regular and blood pressure was 126/78. JVP, heart sounds and chest examination were normal. There was generalized abdominal tenderness but bowel sounds were present and rectal examination revealed soft stool. GCS was 15/15. Both pupils were fixed and dilated with bilateral partial ptosis and nystagmus. Examination of the other cranial nerves was not possible due to the patient being uncooperative. There was weakness in the upper limbs with decreased tone but normal reflexes and sensation. Plantar responses were flexor.

Bloods	Hb	12.2	WCC	5.8
	Platelets	200	INR	1.0
	Na	137	K	4.4
	Urea	5.5	Creatinine	69
	Calcium	2.25	Phosphate	1.0
	Glucose	5.8	Albumin	35
	Bilirubin	12	ALT	36
	ALP	120		
Urine	Normal			
CT head	No abnormality detected			
Abdominal X-ray	Some faecal loading			
Spirometry	Normal			

The **NEXT** step in this patient's management would be:

A intravenous gentamicin
B intravenous immunoglobulin
C intravenous penicillin
D intravenous steroids
E sodium phosphate enemas

3.69 A 25-year-old female staff nurse presented to Accident & Emergency having sustained a needlestick injury from a known HIV patient less than 1 h ago. Whilst changing bed sheets she accidentally pricked her thumb with a discarded needle on the patient's bed. She had no previous medical history and was not on any medication.

She was very concerned about contracting HIV and has requested treatment – post exposure prophylaxis (PEP).

Of the following statements concerning this patient the one which is correct is:

- A intravenous immunoglobulin should be given in the first instance
- B PEP treatment should continue for 4 weeks
- C start on zidovudine (AZT) monotherapy
- D the most important initial step is to wash her hands with antiseptic
- E the risk of her contracting HIV from this needlestick injury is 1%

3.70 A 35-year-old woman was referred to the rheumatology clinic with a 3-month history of pain and swelling affecting her knuckles, wrists and elbows. Stiffness in these joints lasted for more than an hour after she woke up in the morning. Her mother had been diagnosed with rheumatoid arthritis aged 50. She had no other medical problems. Currently she only took ibuprofen when the pain was severe. She had recently got married and was planning to start a family soon.

On examination there was swelling and tenderness of the metacarpophalangeal joints, wrists and elbows of both upper limbs. There were no nodules or obvious joint deformities. All other joints were normal.

This patient should be started on:

- A cyclophosphamide
- B infliximab
- C leflunomide
- D methotrexate
- E sulfasalazine

3.71 A 62-year-old man was admitted with a 1-day history of haematemesis. There was no previous medical history of peptic ulcer or liver disease. Over the past 2 months he had also noticed increased lethargy and had lost 3 kg in weight despite a normal appetite. He was not on any medication and did not drink alcohol.

On examination he was not in pain but did look pale. He was apyrexial, pulse was 88 regular and blood pressure was 136/78. Heart sounds and respiratory examination were normal. He had marked hepatosplenomegaly but no signs of chronic liver disease. Neurological examination was normal. An endoscopy revealed two columns of oesophageal varices.

Bloods	Hb	9.9	MCV	96.2
	WCC	5.4	Platelets	88
	Albumin	35	Bilirubin	11
	ALT	38	ALP	120
	Vitamin B_{12}	600	Folate	7.0
	Ferritin	300		
Abdomen ultrasound	Hepatomegaly with no focal liver lesion Splenomegaly with increased flow in portal vein Mild ascites			

Bone marrow (Figure 3.71 page 386.)

The **MOST** likely diagnosis is:

A chronic myeloid leukaemia
B hairy cell leukaemia
C myelodysplastic syndrome
D myelofibrosis
E primary portal hypertension

3.72 A 14-year-old boy was referred to the oncology clinic with Hodgkin's lymphoma. He had disease affecting the mediastinal and para-aortic lymph nodes. Before beginning treatment he and his parents were concerned about long term complications.

Of the following the one which is **NOT** a recognised long-term complication of treatment is:

A hypothyroidism
B impotence
C osteosarcoma
D pneumonitis
E short stature

3.73 A 59-year-old man was admitted to ITU following an accident at home where he suffered significant third-degree burns to his face, neck, chest and upper limbs. He had a previous medical history of ischaemic heart disease. He was intubated and ventilated. He was started on cefotaxime and metronidazole antibiotics.

The next day he became more unwell. His temperature was 37.7°C , with a pulse of 100 regular and a blood pressure of 90/60. His CVP was +4 cmH_2O and heart sounds were normal. Chest and abdominal examinations were normal. An oesophageal Doppler was inserted and the calculated cardiac output was 4 L/min. His mixed venous O_2 saturation was 65%.

The **MOST** likely cause for his deterioration is:

A anaphylactic shock
B cardiogenic shock
C hypovolaemic shock
D neurogenic shock
E septic shock

3.74 A 57-year-old woman was admitted to Accident & Emergency with collapse and unconsciousness. No history was available.

Physical examination revealed a decreased conscious level with GCS of 8/15 and generalised weakness. CT head was performed.

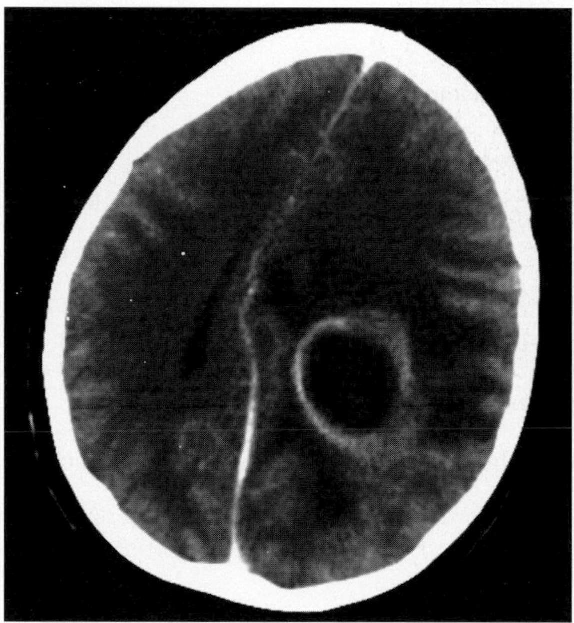

The interpretation of the CT findings is:

A hyperacute haematoma
B cerebral tumour/metastasis
C congenital abnormality
D no significant cerebral oedema
E unilateral hydrocephalus

3.75 A 59-year-old man presented to Accident & Emergency with acute back pain.

An MRI spine was performed.

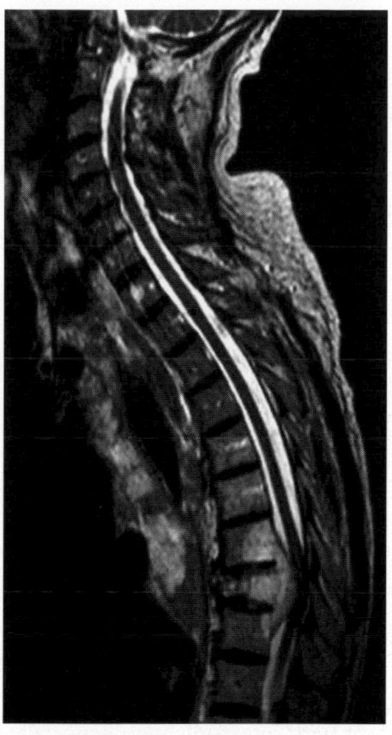

The **MOST** likely diagnosis is:

A discitis
B paraspinal abscess
C spinal cord compression
D spondylolisthesis
E syringomyelia

Paper 3

Answers

3.1 **A**** Contraindications to exercise testing include severe left ventricular outflow tract obstruction, severe aortic stenosis, acute myocarditis or pericarditis, left ventricular failure, unstable angina, ventricular arrhythmias, dissecting aortic aneurysm and febrile illness. Left bundle branch block and a permanent pacemaker may make interpretation more difficult but are not contraindications.

3.2 **B***** The ECG shows regular P waves but occurring independently of the QRS complex characteristic of complete heart block.

3.3 **A*** This patient has taken an overdose of insecticide, of which the commonest is an organophosphate. All these symptoms are characteristic although not specific to organophosphate poisoning. The correct treatment involves oxygen, atropine and, if necessary, pralidoxime to reactivate cholinesterase.

3.4 **D*** Orf or ecthyma contagiosum is a viral infection that begins as an inflamed reddened papule that may enlarge to form a nodule that often resolves spontaneously. It is associated with contact with infected sheep, especially lambs. Anthrax is a bacterial infection that is associated with mild pyrexia, malaise and a malignant pustule.

3.5 **C***** An elderly man presents with headaches and bone pain. The pelvic X-ray shows thickening of the trabeculae due to bone sclerosis. All these findings are in keeping with Paget's disease of bone. Other complications of Paget's disease include progressive deafness due to calcification of the ossicles and compression of cranial nerve VIII in the bony canal, blindness due to optic atrophy, a high output cardiac failure and rarely the development of osteosarcoma. Other bony deformities include bowing of the tibia and enlargement of the skull (see **2.44** and **6.29**). The main differential diagnosis would be secondary metastases. Against this possibility is the thickening of the trabeculae; myeloma and metastases usually cause lytic lesions.

3.6 **A**** The ideal study would be a cohort study, as the subjects could be grouped according to their proximity to the potentially offending source and then followed up at a later date to see if they developed brain tumours. Unfortunately this approach would be ethically unacceptable. Case control studies involve collection of data about patients with the disease and appropriate 'matched' controls without the disease, followed by comparison of the two groups regarding rates of exposure to the possible aetiological factors.

3.7 **E**** Optic neuritis typically affects younger individuals and is associated with pain on eye movements. The picture shows a hyperaemic optic disc with blurred margins but no obvious macular oedema; all these features are consistent with acute optic neuritis. Anterior ischaemic optic neuropathy affects an older age group and causes sudden painless vision loss. The main feature is a pale swollen disc. It can be subdivided into arteritic or non-arteritic forms. Myelinated nerve fibres radiate out from the disc and are not associated with visual symptoms. The clinical features of a central retinal vein occlusion include tortuous engorged veins and haemorrhages in all four quadrants in addition to a swollen disc. Optic disc drusen do not cause progressive visual loss. They give the disc a lumpy appearance, are usually asymptomatic and are an incidental finding in the young.

3.8 **D**** A teenager presents with abdominal pain, jaundice, macrocytic anaemia, and increased urinary urobilinogen, and is Coombs' test/direct antiglobulin test negative. The most likely diagnosis is hereditary spherocytosis. This is a form of hereditary intravascular haemolysis where there is a defect in the red cell membrane spectrin so that all are spherical in shape, as opposed to biconcave discs. The spleen recognises them as abnormal and causes their destruction. Clinical sequelae include anaemia, splenomegaly, leg ulcers and pigment gallstones. Biochemical tests show a raised serum (unconjugated) bilirubin. The Coombs' test is negative and therefore excludes an autoimmune haemolytic anaemia. Osmotic fragility studies will confirm the diagnosis. When red cells are placed in hypotonic solution they swell up and lyse; this is more so with spherocytes. Ham's test is a test for paroxysmal nocturnal haemoglobinuria. Schumm's test is a test for the presence of methaemalbumin.

3.9 **C**** The histology slide shows the *Giardia lamblia* flagellate protozoa between the villi. None of the other options would give such a picture. Although giardiasis is often associated with foreign travel it must always be considered in cases of chronic diarrhoea.

3.10 **B*** Dengue fever begins with symptoms of an upper respiratory tract infection. To diagnose dengue haemorrhagic fever there needs to be fever of recent onset; haemorrhagic manifestations, in this case epistaxis, microscopic haematuria, haematemesis and melaena; low platelet count; and evidence of leaky capillaries, in this case albumin <30. There is no available vaccination and treatment is symptomatic. Yellow fever is another viral haemorrhagic fever and has similar clinical features, but is found only in Africa and South America and a vaccination is available. Hepatitis A is unlikely as the incubation period is normally 2 weeks and would be associated with more deranged transaminases in a patient this unwell. Typhoid and blackwater fever are discussed in **1.11**.

3.11 **E*** The insidious onset symptoms of proximal myopathy with no evidence of nerve involvement are likely to be a form of primary muscle disease. Patients with limb–girdle muscular dystrophy tend to have severe disability much earlier on, i.e. early 20s. Polymyalgia rheumatica does not cause cardiac or swallowing problems although both are associated with elevated ESR and possibly muscle tenderness. Serum creatine kinase levels, electromyography, and muscle biopsy can be used to confirm the diagnosis. The loss of weight, anorexia, dysphagia and atrial fibrillation suggest there may be an underlying oesophageal carcinoma.

3.12 **A**** There is a large, dark, pigmented mass emerging nasal to the optic disc that appears to be invading the optic nerve. This appearance is consistent with a choroidal (below the retina) melanoma. A choroidal melanoma would not cause blurred vision, unless it encroached on the macula, in which case it might cause a field defect.

3.13 **G, I*** From the lung function tests, the patient has a restrictive lung defect as shown by a FEV_1:FVC ratio of 75% and a reduced TLC. The DLCO is the transfer factor and gives an indication of how easy it is for gas to cross the alveolar lining. In restrictive disease this value is decreased. The KCO is very similar to the DLCO but takes into account the effective surface area of the diffusion area. Causes of increased KCO include pulmonary haemorrhage, arteriovenous shunts, asthma and removal of non-functioning lung. The discrepancy between a reduced DLCO and normal KCO would be explained by pulmonary haemorrhage and removal of an effectively dead part of lung.

3.14 **A**** This woman has the signs and symptoms of a bilateral symmetrical arthritis consistent with rheumatoid arthritis. Whilst prognosis is very variable, certain markers are associated with more severe disease: positive rheumatoid factor; presence of extra-articular features, especially nodules and vasculitis; HLA-DR4 genetic marker; female sex; radiographic erosions within 2 years of disease onset; and severe disability at presentation. Insidious onset of the arthritis is also associated with more severe disease as opposed to palindromic rheumatism, which is characterised by episodic attacks followed by complete resolution in between.

3.15 **B***** This patient has frontal balding, wasting of the facial, shoulder and temporalis muscles, and bilateral ptosis. All of these could be explained by dystrophia myotonica (see **2.46**).

3.16 A*** This barium enema shows an 'apple core' lesion in the distal transverse colon. This should be treated as a colonic neoplasm until proven otherwise, even though the stricture is relatively smooth and there is no soft tissue shadow of an obstructing carcinoma. The spine is normal. There are some isolated diverticula but these are not the most salient feature of this X-ray.

3.17 A** This ERCP shows a common bile duct, which is narrow distally and dilated proximally. This would be consistent with compression of the common bile duct by a pancreatic neoplasm. There are no gallstones.

3.18 E*** For explanation of how to interpret cardiac catheterisation values see **2.19**. There is an increase in the oxygen saturation between the right atrium and right ventricle. This suggests that there is a ventricular septal defect as oxygenated blood from the left ventricle is mixing with the deoxygenated blood of the right ventricle. The increased pressures in the right ventricle and pulmonary artery are suggestive of pulmonary hypertension.

3.19 C** After complex 3 on the ECG trace, the R wave of complex 4 coincides with the T wave of complex 3, the so-called 'R-on-T phenomenon'. Following this there is a regular but sinusoidal broad complex tachycardia that is characteristic of torsades de pointes and the patient is still maintaining a pulse.

3.20 A** If patients with methanol poisoning are admitted within 1 h of ingestion then gastric lavage could be attempted. Activated charcoal does not adsorb methanol and ipecacuanha is contraindicated because of the risk of aspiration. The metabolic acidosis is corrected with intravenous sodium bicarbonate to keep the pH >7.20. Indications for haemodialysis or peritoneal dialysis include: presence of mental or visual features; plasma methanol concentration >500 mg/L; and worsening acidosis not responding to intravenous bicarbonate.

3.21 B** This patient has a symmetrical erythematous rash affecting both upper and lower limbs and also the mouth. The diagnosis is erythema multiforme. The rash may be due to penicillin or *Mycoplasma* pneumonia.

3.22 C*** This patient appears to be having a myxoedematous crisis. Increased TSH and normal freeT_4 could still mean that this patient has T_3 hypothyroidism, and so T_3 should be given albeit in small quantities. Such patients may have other endocrine problems such as adrenal failure, and no harm could come from assuming she may be addisonian and treating her with steroids. She needs antibiotics in case there is an underlying infection. Hypothermia can occur with hypothyroidism and it can be dangerous to over correct hypothermia. Passive measures should be started first with removal of wet/damp clothes and use of blankets. This can be followed by giving warmed intravenous fluids but this should be done cautiously in a patient with ischaemic heart disease. Cardiopulmonary bypass and peritoneal or bladder lavage with warmed liquids should be done in comatose patients with severe hypothermia <30°C. Lugol's iodine solution is used to treat thyrotoxicosis.

3.23 D** The relative risk (RR) is the ratio of the incidence of death in the exposed group (i.e. smokers) to the incidence of death in the non-exposed group (non-smokers).

Incidence among smokers = 10/100

Incidence among non-smokers = 20/300

RR = (10/100)/(20/300) = (10 x 300)/(20 x 100) = 1.5

As the RR > 1, this would suggest a positive association between smoking and death.

	Dead	Alive	
Smoker	10	90	100
Non-smoker	20	280	300
	30	370	400

3.24 A** Blood results show elevated autoantibodies and a raised globulin (protein – albumin = 42) consistent with autoimmune hepatitis. There are three main types of autoimmune hepatitis. Type I is associated with elevated antinuclear antibodies and smooth muscle antibodies. To be clinically significant these titres ought to be >1 in 80. Type II is associated with elevated anti-LKM (anti-liver–kidney–muscle antibodies); this form is more associated with other autoimmune conditions such as insulin dependent diabetes, autoimmune thyroiditis and vitiligo. Type III is the least prevalent form and is more associated with antibodies to soluble liver antigen/liver–pancreas (anti-SLA/LP). Liver biopsy typically shows interface hepatitis with disruption of the limiting plate of the portal tract. The antimitochondrial antibody titre is not significant and is not diagnostic of primary biliary cirrhosis. There are no features of systemic lupus erythematosus and anti-double stranded DNA is negative. The normal caeruloplasmin goes against Wilson's disease.

3.25 E** This patient presents with pyrexia, chest tightness, shock and haemoglobinuria, which are consistent with an acute haemolytic transfusion reaction, probably due to ABO incompatibility or bacterial contamination of the blood unit being transfused. Treatment would involve stopping the transfusion, fluid resuscitation and informing the blood bank of the reaction.

3.26 B** All the options could cause small bowel obstruction. The slide shows islands of uniform cells, which are not mitotic and without lots of nuclei that would suggest adenocarcinoma. Synactophysin stains for neuroendocrine tumours and stains the cytoplasm brown. With ischaemic bowel there is normal structure but with a pink, necrotic epithelium; as the ischaemia worsens so does the necrosis as it spreads towards the serosa where it can perforate.

3.27 A** The long history of a flu-like illness, night sweats, pyrexia, cervical lymphadenopathy and hepatosplenomegaly after visiting a Mediterranean country is suggestive of brucellosis. The patient may have handled cattle or ingested unpasteurized dairy products. Hodgkin's lymphoma is a possibility but would be more likely in an older person if there were associated eosinophilia and pruritus. Leishmaniasis is another possible differential diagnosis.

3.28 E* This patient has primary polydipsia. No mention was made of the urine volume produced but it is likely to be >4 L. The urine osmolality is >300 mosmol/kg, thereby suggesting this is not diabetes insipidus. The urine becomes more concentrated as the patient is more water deprived. There is only a modest increase in the urine osmolality with DDAVP (desmopressin) injection. In a normal person the urine osmolality would be expected to be >750 mosmol/kg but due to chronic polydipsia and polyuria there is a reduction in the concentrating power of the nephron due to the washout of solute from the renal interstitium. Partial nephrogenic diabetes insipidus would produce a similar water deprivation test but there would be a higher than normal $\text{plasma}_{\text{ADH}}$ level.

3.29 D** Of all the responses only a pulmonary embolus is likely to cause a respiratory alkalosis in a hypoxic patient. A salicylate overdose may cause respiratory alkalosis compensating for the metabolic acidosis but for that to occur over 24 h post ingestion would be unusual.

3.30 E*** The most likely diagnosis in this patient is temporal or giant cell arteritis. A properly performed biopsy will define the need for therapy in 85% of cases but because the arteritis is patchy, biopsy may miss the area of inflammation. If the clinical condition warranted it, high dose prednisolone should be started before the biopsy is taken to prevent blindness.

3.31 C** The history is of a patient who has a long history of erratic bowel movements. Frequent over-use of laxatives, especially those that are anthracine-derived, can result in generalised pigmentation of the bowel when viewed endoscopically. There is no treatment required.

3.32 **E**** This patient has had a thoracoplasty as collapse therapy for tuberculosis (TB) involving the upper six ribs on the right. The chest wall is deformed because of the surgery performed. There is fibrosis in the right apex and left apical and basal regions; a recrudescence of TB is a possibility that must always be considered, particularly if he was not treated with anti TB drugs.

3.33 **C**** This patient has a history of recent foreign travel, cough, gastrointestinal symptoms, deranged liver function tests and right upper lobe pneumonia. The most likely diagnosis is legionnaire's disease. The most appropriate antibiotics would be an intravenous macrolide and rifampicin. The chest X-ray appearance of legionnaire's disease can vary widely from a ground-glass appearance to a peripheral lobar consolidation.

3.34 **D**** This young woman presents with fever, confusion, Janeway lesions on her hands and a murmur. The murmur could be due to a floppy mitral valve prolapse that had infective vegetations that were embolising to the brain, making infective endocarditis a very real possibility. She does not have any signs or symptoms of meningitis. Encephalitis presents with altered consciousness, personality changes, seizures and paresis and cranial nerve involvement. There is nothing in the history to suggest toxic shock syndrome.

3.35 **E**** The ECG shows broad complex tachycardia, concordance of the chest leads (deep S waves in V_{1-6}), right axis deviation, fusion beat (beat 9) on the rhythm strip and dissociated P waves (see V_5). Fusion beats occur when a supraventricular impulse and an impulse originating from the ventricle depolarise the ventricle simultaneously and resemble a combination of the two beats. Dissociated P waves or independent P wave activity is another characteristic of VT; if they were retrograde P waves, they would look morphologically the same but in this case the P waves appear to be 'buried' within the QRS complex. Other characteristics of VT include: capture beats, QRS complex >140 ms, ventricular rate >160, atypical right bundle branch block and history of ischaemic heart disease.

3.36 **A***** This patient is likely to suffer from a number of conditions like sarcoidosis or secondary to various drugs. The differential diagnosis for this lesion includes pretibial myxoedema, which would be expected to have a raised peau d'orange appearance.

3.37 **D**** This patient has a pituitary tumour. It is possible that it will grow inferiorly to involve the cavernous sinus. Within the cavernous sinus run the internal carotid artery, oculomotor, trochlear, abducens and ophthalmic and maxillary branches of the trigeminal nerve. The mandibular branch of the trigeminal nerve supplies sensation to the lower face and anterior two-thirds of the tongue.

3.38 D** Although this patient was unable to communicate verbally, he understood his condition. The principle of autonomy dictates that he can decide what treatment he wants. Oral feeding and drinking constitute basic care; nasogastric tubes, intravenous fluids, artificial feeding and PEG insertion are considered treatments and so if a patient refuses these, that is his prerogative and he can choose not to have them even though he may die without them.

3.39 C** A young boy presents with abdominal pain and jaundice of short duration. The only abnormal blood result is the raised bilirubin. An ALP <785 in 13-year-old boys is normal and represents adolescent bone growth. Gilbert's syndrome is an asymptomatic congenital hyperbilirubinaemia characterised by a deficiency of bilirubin glucuronidase leading to unconjugated hyperbilirubinaemia. The condition can present itself during times of intercurrent illness, vomiting or fasting. There is no treatment. Diagnosis can be confirmed by finding raised serum levels of unconjugated bilirubin and normal reticulocyte count to distinguish it from haemolysis. With hereditary spherocytosis, the clinical picture may be very similar but often patients have splenomegaly. Dubin–Johnson syndrome is a benign autosomal recessive (AR) condition causing conjugated hyperbilirubinaemia due to defective excretion of bile into the canaliculi. There is no alteration of liver enzymes except raised serum levels of conjugated bilirubin; on liver biopsy the colour is green–black but of normal architecture. Rotor syndrome is another benign AR condition due to defective uptake and storage of organic acids in the liver resulting in conjugated hyperbilirubinaemia; liver biopsy is normal. Biliary atresia is progressive inflammation of the biliary tree leading to a failure to excrete bile which leads to scarring and cirrhosis. Treatment is surgical and the patient may need transplantation.

3.40 C** This could have occurred as result of a prolapsed intervertebral disc. The most common radiculopathies involve roots L4, L5 and S1. L5 lesions involve the toe extensors. Lesions to L3 and L4 would involve the knee jerk. Lesions to S1 would involve the ankle jerk and the plantar flexors. S2 lesions would not result in muscle weakness but may involve the ankle jerk and sensation in the perianal region.

3.41 D* This patient's acute deterioration is most likely to be due to adult respiratory distress syndrome (ARDS), an acute syndrome caused by direct or indirect injury to the lung. The exact pathogenesis is unknown but may be triggered by a number of events, including sepsis, blood transfusions, chest trauma and aspiration of gastric contents. According to the American–European Consensus Conference, to diagnose ARDS three criteria need to be met: (1) new infiltrates on chest X-ray; (2) PAWP ≤ 18 mmHg, i.e. non-cardiogenic pulmonary oedema; and (3) PO_2:FiO_2 (arterial oxygen partial pressure:inhaled oxygen) ratio is >200 mmHg or 40 kPa. In this case the patient is oliguric, has a low PAWP and is hypotensive, so the main principle of treatment is to ensure the patient is well filled; diuresis is likely to cause intravascular depletion and worsen renal failure. Unlike with neonatal respiratory distress syndrome, neither surfactant nor steroids have been shown to improve prognosis of ARDS. There is thought to be an element of right-to-left shunting through atelectatic and consolidated lung units that are not ventilated. Turning patients prone can shift perfusion to previous non-ventilated lung zones.

3.42 C* This patient has Behçet's syndrome, which is a vasculitis that is characterised by recurrent orogenital ulceration, eye lesions, arthritis and skin lesions. The skin lesions include erythema nodosum, thrombophlebitis, acneiform skin eruption and hyperirritability of the skin (pathergy). The condition is more prevalent from the Eastern Mediterranean and Turkey to the Far East and there is an association with HLA-B5 and -B51, but not -B27. Twenty-five per cent of patients may develop arterial or venous thrombosis, which may lead to the formation of aneurysms. Up to a third of these patients have factor V Leiden mutation.

3.43 A** This patient has meningitis secondary to *C. neoformans.* The CSF has been stained with Indian ink and shows the characteristic haloes of *C. neoformans.* The patient should be treated with amphotericin.

3.44 D* This pelvic X-ray shows pseudofractures or 'Looser's zones' in the neck of both femurs. They are characteristic of osteomalacia.

3.45 B** This patient appears to have left lower limb cellulitis. The correct management involves antibiotics against *Staphylococcus aureus*, such as flucloxacillin.

3.46 D** This patient has a serum osmolality of 253 mosmol/kg (serum osmolality = 2 x ([Na] + [K]) + [urea] + [glucose]). He has syndrome of inappropriate ADH secretion (SIADH), as shown by a low serum osmolality, normal concentration of his urine, dilutional hyponatraemia and a probable lung neoplasm. To fully diagnose SIADH, patients have to be euvolaemic, have normal thyroid, renal and adrenal function tests and a urinary Na >20 mmol/L. The normal treatment of SIADH and hyponatraemia is fluid restriction. However, should that fail, then possible treatments include demeclocycline or lithium. Fits in this case should be treated with phenytoin.

3.47 D** A patient presents with large volume fresh red rectal bleeding. The next most appropriate test after resuscitating her would be a prepared colonoscopy. Usually a phosphate enema can be given, otherwise blood and faeces are likely to obstruct the view. Diverticular disease or even neoplasms are more likely than angiodysplasia of the colon. For angiography to detect a lesion there needs to be active bleeding. Bleeding proximal to the ligament of Trietz is likely to present as melaena rather than red blood per rectum.

3.48 E* This patient has Parkinson's syndrome with pyramidal features, thereby making it a Parkinson's plus syndrome. There is no autonomic involvement, which goes against multisystem atrophy. There is a problem with the supranuclear connections of the oculomotor nerve leading to vertical conjugate gaze palsy. Parinaud's syndrome involves damage to the midbrain and superior colliculus, resulting in loss of vertical gaze, nystagmus on attempted convergence, loss of the light reflex, retraction of the eyelids and relative mydriasis.

3.49 E** This patient presents as having had a massive central pulmonary embolism (PE). This is why his arterial PO_2 and PCO_2 are low and consistent with a type I respiratory failure pattern. His expired CO_2 is low because the PE has managed to block the pulmonary artery and therefore very little air with CO_2 is being expired.

3.50 C** Tall stature, downward dislocation of the lens, mental retardation, chest wall deformity, arachnodactyly and evidence of thromboembolism are all features of homocystinuria. This is an autosomal recessive disorder due to deficiency of cystathione β-synthase, leading to increased homocystine in the blood and urine. Newborn homocystine screening is available. Alkaptonuria is associated with urine that turns blue–black on standing. Marfan's syndrome is an autosomal dominant disease of type I collagen and is associated with upward dislocation of the lens and aortic dissection but not thromboembolism or mental retardation.

3.51 E** The scan shows dilated intrahepatic ducts and common bile ducts, suggesting a proximal biliary lesion. There is some beading of the intrahepatic ducts but this is not characteristic of sclerosing cholangitis. There are stones in the distal common bile duct and obstructing the proximal common bile duct.

3.52 D*** There is a crateriform ulcer on the lower lid with a raised, pearly and telangiectatic edge and crusty surface. Basal cell carcinomas hardly ever metastasise but instead cause local infiltration and destruction. Squamous cell carcinomas start off as warty, hyperkeratotic nodules, which can ulcerate and typically have everted edges. They are usually faster growing and can metastasise via the lymph nodes. Keratoacanthomas are benign, rapidly growing tumours that are characterised by having a central horny plug and may resolve spontaneously. Bowen's disease is a form of superficial squamous cell carcinoma in situ that presents as a psoriasis-like or eczema-like lesion.

3.53 C** Primary amenorrhoea is defined as no menses by age 16. Extremely active girls like runners, swimmers, gymnasts and ballet dancers are well known to have delayed puberty and menarche. Her pelvic ultrasound showed normal internal genitalia albeit with multiple cysts on her ovaries, and this is normal for a girl of her age. With polycystic ovarian syndrome she would be expected to be obese and have raised LH and testosterone levels. She has this normal external genitalia thereby excluding 5-α-reductase deficiency and 11-β-hydroxylase deficiency.

3.54 E** Bi-hilar lymphadenopathy and erythema nodosum is highly suggestive of sarcoidosis. Serum ACE would be raised in >70% of patients but would also be seen with TB, lymphoma, asbestosis and silicosis. Serum calcium is raised in >60% but is not specific. Transbronchial biopsy would show infiltration of the alveolar walls and interstitial spaces, with inflammatory cells and granuloma formation in >90%, even in cases where the chest X-ray shows no parenchymal involvement, thereby giving a histological diagnosis. The Kveim test is no longer performed because of the potential risk of transmitting HIV or other prion diseases.

3.55 E** This patient has a 'staghorn' calculus. The most likely composition of these types of stones is 'struvite', which contains magnesium ammonium phosphate and sometimes calcium associated with infection.

3.56 A*** Patients with unexplained painless haematuria need to undergo cystoscopy to exclude a bladder carcinoma.

3.57 D** This patient is an arteriopath, has a history of atrial fibrillation and presents with abdominal pain that is worse after eating, which would be most consistent with mesenteric ischaemia. Patients may often present with vague abdominal symptoms and minimal abdominal findings. The raised lactate is suggestive of ischaemia, which would be unusual in someone with diverticulitis unless perforation had occurred. CT abdomen and/or mesenteric angiogram would be the investigations of choice. Abdominal X-ray may show bowel wall thickening or thumb printing, although this may not present acutely.

3.58 C* This patient has Conn's syndrome, as shown by the low baseline serum renin and elevated serum aldosterone. The patient is admitted for overnight lying and standing renin and aldosterone measurements to differentiate between adrenal cortex adenoma and adrenocortical hyperplasia. When patients with Conn's syndrome are lying down, the serum aldosterone is high and the serum renin is high. When patients stand up and have been ambulating, there is an increase in the serum renin. With patients who have adrenal cortical hyperplasia there is an increase in serum aldosterone after standing because the tissue is still stimulated by renin; patients with adrenal cortex adenomas have a decreased serum aldosterone because the tumour is unresponsive to renin. ACTH stimulates adrenal cortex adenomas; this follows a diurnal variation and is decreased during the day.

3.59 D** A young man with progressive dysphagia, regurgitation and nocturnal cough is most likely to have achalasia. Oesophageal manometry is the 'gold standard' for early diagnosis of the condition and will show failure of the lower oesophageal sphincter to relax, lack of peristalsis and elevated lower oesophageal sphincter pressure. Later upper GI endoscopy may show a large dilated oesophagus. In practice, upper GI endoscopy would be done to exclude >% 'pseudoachalasia' usually due to a tumour below the gastro-oesophageal junction. A barium swallow can be useful in detecting achalasia and does produce a characteristic picture (see **1.18**) but only in a proportion of patients.

3.60 D* The ECG shows a normal electrical capture as each pacing spike is followed by a QRS complex. Normally there should be left bundle branch block following insertion of the pacing wire. In this case there is right bundle branch block suggestive of perforation of the interventricular septum and pacing of the left ventricle.

3.61 B* The biopsy shows the characteristic features of inflammatory bowel disease: (1) chronic active inflammation with lymphocytes and neutrophils; (2) crypt abscesses; and (3) crypt distortion – normally all crypts are regularly arranged and of a similar size but here there is also loss of mucin. This is consistent with ulcerative colitis. Compare this with pseudomembranous colitis (see **1.10**). Radiation colitis can present acutely but strictures and abdominal pain rather than rectal bleeding are characteristic when it presents more chronically; biopsy tends to show more fibrosis in the lamina propria. CMV colitis is more likely in immunosuppressed patients and characteristic inclusion bodies might be seen (see **5.26**). Tuberculous colitis would be associated with granulomas (see **2.10**).

3.62 C* This young man with elevated ALT, decreased caeruloplasmin, hepatomegaly, rigidity, tremor and gait abnormalities almost certainly has

Wilson's disease. Other conditions like nephrotic syndrome, protein-losing enteropathy and chronic liver disease may also be associated with low caeruloplasmin. Slit lamp examination is performed to look for Kayser–Fleischer rings or sunflower cataracts. Total copper stores are increased but total serum copper is usually low as most of it is bound to caeruloplasmin, although this may increase if the unbound fraction rises as in fulminant liver failure. In Wilson's disease there is increased copper in the urine (>5 µmol/24 h) but this may also be seen in other chronic liver diseases. More discriminating is the increase in urinary copper following a penicillamine challenge (>25 µmol/24 h). The 'gold standard' test is liver biopsy (with a copper-free needle) and measurement of the hepatic copper, which would be >250 µg/g dry weight (normal <50 µg/g). Biopsy may reveal similar findings to autoimmune hepatitis and non-alcoholic steatohepatitis. Gene analysis can be performed in families with at least two affected full siblings but would not be useful in this case.

3.63 E*** This patient most likely has gestational hypertension. Her systolic pressure is >140 mmHg and her diastolic pressure is >90 mmHg, both increasing after the first 20 weeks of gestation. If there were evidence of proteinuria, then she would fit criteria for pre-eclampsia. Labetalol and methyldopa are the treatments of choice. Beta-blockers that lack α-blocking activity, like atenolol, have been associated with low placental and birth weight babies at delivery, possibly due to interruptions in placental blood flow. ACE inhibitors and angiotensin II receptor blockers should be avoided in pregnancy because they can cause uterine ischaemia and renal dysfunction in the fetus, but are not teratogenic. There is no evidence that bed rest is beneficial in pre-eclamptic women.

3.64 D*** This patient is most likely to have obstructive sleep apnoea (OSA), as characterised by the snoring, excessive daytime somnolence and apnoeic attacks. The diagnosis could be confirmed by a sleep study showing episodes of respiratory effort ceasing and coinciding with drops in arterial saturation. The development of complications is determined more by neck size and BMI rather than weight per se. OSA is an independent risk factor for stroke. Cardiovascular complications include secondary pulmonary hypertension, right heart failure and cor pulmonale, and arrhythmias: tachycardias, bradycardias and sudden death. By definition, primary pulmonary hypertension cannot be diagnosed until OSA, amongst other causes, has been excluded. There is an association with Type 2 diabetes and the degree of OSA has an inverse relationship with serum HDL.

3.65 A** Hypoglycaemia is a common complication in patients with type I diabetes. Patients who have tight control of their diabetes are more prone to getting hypoglycaemic attacks. Common causes of hypoglycaemia include alcohol, missed meals, excessive exercise and weight loss. Repeated insulin injections into the same site may cause lipohypertrophy leading to unpredictable absorption of insulin into the bloodstream, causing hypoglycaemia. In Cushing's syndrome, where there is relative steroid excess, the insulin requirements usually increase and therefore there is less likelihood of hypoglycaemic attacks. In Addison's disease there is a relative lack of steroids and hence sensitivity to insulin increases with a greater likelihood of developing hypoglycaemia.

3.66 **A*** This patient has haemolytic uraemic syndrome (HUS) which consists of a triad of non-autoimmune microangiopathic haemolytic anaemia, thrombocytopaenia and renal failure. HUS is typically a disease of childhood following a diarrhoeal illness where the child is infected by the *Escherichia coli* 0157:H7 serotype toxin. It can also follow an upper respiratory tract infection, can be caused by other microorganisms like *Shigella*, *Salmonella*, *Yersinia* and *Campylobacter*, and can be made worse by taking antidiarrhoeal agents. Other causes include HIV infection, chemotherapy or bone marrow transplantation. The disease can also develop in pregnancy and early post partum. Patients are subdivided into D^+ and D^- (atypical) depending on whether or not diarrhoea is present. In adults it can also occur as part of the spectrum between thrombotic thrombocytopaenic purpura (TTP) and HUS. The distinction between HUS and TTP is not very clear, but TTP is more common in adults, is associated with fever and neurological sequelae and has a worse prognosis. The process is thought to start with endothelial injury leading to the development of platelet thrombi, which can lead to occlusion of arterioles and capillaries in various organs, including the skin, gastrointestinal tract, spleen, brain and kidneys. The main treatment for HUS is supportive, especially in D^+ disease, and often with haemodialysis. TTP is treated by plasma exchange with fresh frozen plasma to reverse the platelet consumption. Platelet transfusions can make the thrombosis worse. Heparin can induce bleeding, especially as the thrombi are due to platelets rather than fibrin. Steroids and other immunosuppressive agents, such as rituximab, ciclosporin and cyclophosphamide 3 can be considered if plasma exchange fails.

3.67 **A**** This patient has a lower motor neurone V and VII nerve palsy and cerebellar symptoms most likely due to a neoplastic lesion arising in the space between the pons and cerebellum. Meningiomas are the most common cause of this syndrome and can affect cranial nerves VI and VIII as well. Acoustic neuromas tend to present with unilateral deafness and tinnitus; the tumour would have to be quite massive and extend beyond the internal auditory meatus to cause pressure effects on the other cranial nerves and cerebellum. The other options in this question are discussed in **5.39**.

3.68 **E*** *Clostridium botulinum* releases toxins which irreversibly block the presynaptic release of acetylcholine at the neuromuscular junction of peripheral cholinergic nerves. These toxins are absorbed from the stomach and small intestine and are not denatured by stomach acid. Botulism can also occur in infants and in wounds infected with *C. botulinum* spores. The toxins cause hypotonia, flaccid motor paralysis, cranial nerve palsies and smooth muscle paralysis, leading to urinary retention and constipation. Transfer to ITU should be made early because disease progression can lead to diaphragmatic paralysis that may require intubation and mechanical ventilation. Diagnosis is made clinically but can be confirmed by serum analysis for toxin in a mouse bioassay. There is an antitoxin that has been shown to decrease mortality even if given after 24 h, but botulinum immunoglobulin is only given to infants. If there is no evidence of paralytic ileus then enemas are given to remove unabsorbed toxin from the intestine. Magnesium can worsen the effects of toxin-induced neuromuscular blockade. Antibiotics should be avoided in food-borne botulism (as opposed to wound botulism) as this can cause increased lysis of intraluminal *C. botulinum* toxin; aminoglycosides can also induce neuromuscular blockade.

3.69 B** Immediately following any exposure, whether or not from an HIV contact, the site of exposure should be washed thoroughly with copious amounts of soap and water and the wound should be encouraged to bleed. There is no evidence that antiseptics or skin washes are of any benefit and may actually cause more skin irritation and damage to local defences. Similarly, scrubbing is not encouraged as this may cause increased trauma to the exposure site. Ideally PEP should be started within 1 h but there is evidence of it being effective up to 2 weeks post exposure. The risk of transmission is 3 per 1000 where there is percutaneous exposure. The risk is higher where there is deep injury, visible blood on device that caused the injury, exposure of broken skin and exposure of mucous membranes like the eye. Transmission of saliva, urine, vomit and faeces, unless heavily bloodstained, carries a very low risk. Monotherapy with any antiretroviral drug is suboptimal because there is a high rate of resistance and mutation. The current UK guidelines for PEP are treatment for 4 weeks with zidovudine 300 mg b.d., lamivudine 150 mg b.d. and nelfinavir 1250 mg b.d. Following a needle stick injury it is important to check for other blood-borne infections such as hepatitis B and C. There is no role for the use of immunoglobulin in HIV postexposure prophylaxis.

3.70 E*** This patient clinically appears to have rheumatoid arthritis given that she has a symmetrical arthropathy affecting at least three joints and associated with morning stiffness. X-rays may show erosions but even if they did not, she should be started on treatment with disease-modifying drugs. The usual first-line agent is methotrexate but not in this case as she is planning to start a family. The same reason rules out leflunomide and infliximab, although the latter would not be first-line treatment. Cyclophosphamide is also contraindicated in pregnancy but is used more often in the treatment of vasculitis rather than rheumatoid arthritis.

3.71 D** Myelofibrosis is a chronic myeloproliferative disorder characterised by the neoplastic transformation of early haemopoietic cells. It is characterised by anaemia, hepatosplenomegaly, extramedullary haematopoiesis and bone marrow fibrosis. The peripheral blood film may reveal a leucoerythroblastic reaction with megakaryoctyes and tear drop poikilocytes. As in polycythaemia rubra vera, essential thrombocytosis and CML transformation into acute myeloid leukaemia can ultimately occur. Bone marrow examination is important to establish the diagnosis: aspiration may result in a dry tap but trephine will reveal fibrosis, which can be further visualised with reticulin staining. In this case the patient has developed the relatively rare complication of portal hypertension: varices, ascites and thrombocytopaenia due to increased splenic and portal blood flow. Other complications that may occur as a result of extramedullary haematopoiesis are cord compression, seizures, pleural and pericardial effusions and bone pain due to osteosclerosis. CML can present with weight loss and splenomegaly but the bone marrow and peripheral blood film are very different and show increased production of immature and mature granulocytic cells. Unlike myelofibrosis, CML would be positive for Philadelphia chromosome but have a low leucocyte ALP score. With hairy cell leukaemia the bone marrow would show lymphocytes that have a cytoplasm surrounded by fine strands.

3.72 B** There are a number of long-term sequelae associated with the treatment of Hodgkin's disease, and these vary with the treatment given. Chemotherapeutic complications include sterility, pneumonitis (bleomycin), cardiac toxicity (doxorubicin), secondary infections and peripheral neuropathy (vincristine). Radiotherapy can cause hypothyroidism, sterility (not impotence), pneumonitis, cardiac toxicity, and bone and chest wall deformities. There is also an increased risk of secondary tumours such as leukaemia, osteosarcomas, and lung and breast cancer. Growth failure can be due to a number of causes, including radiation to growth centres and spine, inadequate weight gain, hormone deficiency and hypothalamic–pituitary disorders secondary to the treatment and depression.

3.73 C*** Shock is a physiological condition where the circulation is unable to perfuse tissue adequately, resulting in cellular hypoxia. The two major determinants of tissue perfusion are cardiac output (CO) and systemic vascular resistance (SVR). CO depends on heart rate and stroke volume, which in turn depends on myocardial contractility, preload and afterload. SVR depends on blood viscosity, blood vessel length and the diameter of the blood vessel. There are three broad categories of shock and these can be distinguished by their effects on CO and SVR. *Hypovolaemic shock* is due to haemorrhage or fluid loss. There is decreased preload as characterised by decreased pulmonary capillary wedge pressure and CVP, decreased pump function as characterised by cardiac output, increased SVR and decreased mixed venous O_2 saturation. *Cardiogenic shock* results from pump failure and is characterised by decreased CO and increased SVR and preload. *Vasodilatory or distributive shock* often results from decreased SVR and preload with an increased CO. Examples include sepsis, neurogenic shock, anaphylaxis and Addisonian crisis. This patient requires intravenous fluid resuscitation.

3.74 **B***** The CT shows a contrast-enhancing, ring-shaped lesion in the left parietal lobe with surrounding oedema and midline shift – this could not be a congenital abnormality. There is no hydrocephalus. If there was hyperacute haematoma then blood would appear white on CT. The differential diagnosis of this scan is primary or secondary brain neoplasms, toxoplasmosis, lymphoma and cerebral abscess.

3.75 **C*** The MRI shows a high signal mass centred on T8, compressing the cord and extending to the vertebral level above and below. Spondylolisthesis refers to forward slippage of one vertebra on another.

Paper 4

Questions

4.1 A 55-year-old man was noted by his GP to have atrial fibrillation. He had no other medical problems and was not on any medication. He drank alcohol occasionally.

His pulse was 80 irregular and blood pressure 130/78. His JVP was not elevated and his heart sounds and chest were normal.

Bloods				
	Hb	13.8	WCC	6.6
	Platelets	230	Na	140
	K	4.5	Urea	4.2
	Creatinine	89	Magnesium	0.80
	Calcium	2.30	Glucose	4.3
	TSH	2.2	Free T_4	14.6

This patient should be treated with:

A amiodarone
B aspirin
C digoxin
D sotalol
E warfarin

4.2 A 69-year-old man was admitted with dizziness.

His ECG shows:

A first-degree AV block
B complete heart block
C Mobitz type I second-degree AV block
D Mobitz type II second-degree AV block
E sinus bradycardia

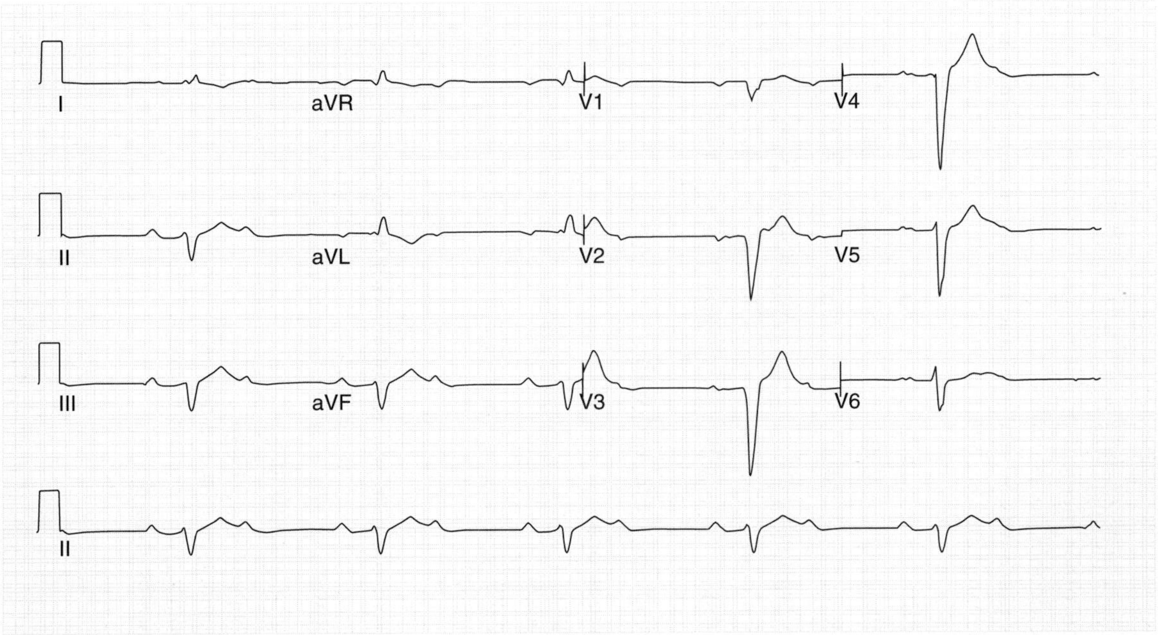
I
aVR
V1
V4
II
aVL
V2
V5
III
aVF
V3
V6
II

4.3 A 16-year-old girl was found collapsed in the toilet of the ward. She was admitted 3 days ago with a paracetamol overdose from which she was making a good recovery. The nursing staff suspected that she had taken another overdose of another drug. The patient complained of dizziness.

On examination she was alert. Her temperature was 37.0°C, pulse 40 regular and blood pressure 78/40. JVP was not elevated and both heart sounds were present. Her respiratory rate was 26 breaths/min and chest was clear. Abdominal examination was normal. Both pupils were dilated.

Bloods	Hb	13.2	WCC	9.9
	Platelets	340	INR	1.0
	Na	135	K	4.0
	Urea	3.8	Creatinine	88
	Protein	70	Albumin	39
	Bilirubin	15	ALT	50
	ALP	100	Calcium	2.22
	Magnesium	0.72		
ECG	First-degree AV block, heart rate 40/min			

The most likely overdose this patient has taken is:

A amitriptylline
B atenolol
C codeine phosphate
D diazepam
E digoxin

4.4 This 16-year-old girl developed a mild fever and a lesion around her mouth 4 days ago. She was not on any medication. (Figure 4.4, page 386.)

The most likely diagnosis is:

A impetigo contagiosa
B gingivostomatitis
C tinea capitis
D seborrheic dermatitis
E rosacea

4.5 A 16-year-old boy presented with a 1-week history of cough, abdominal pain and weight loss. He had recently returned from visiting his family abroad.

On examination he was apyrexial and not jaundiced. Pulse was 90 regular and BP 100/60. His chest was clear but he had some mild, generalised abdominal tenderness.

Bloods	Hb	13.4	WCC	9.8
	Platelets	269	Na	127
	K	6.1	Urea	8.5
	Creatinine	90	Glucose	3.0
	Calcium	2.88	Phosphate	1.1
	Amylase	80		
Blood gases on air	pH	7.31	PCO_2	3.7
	PO_2	10.6	Bicarbonate	18
Urine osmolality	320 mosmol/kg			

The most likely diagnosis is:

- A Addison's disease
- B Cushing's syndrome
- C diabetes insipidus
- D Nelson's disease
- E syndrome of inappropriate antidiuretic hormone secretion (SIADH)

4.6 The research and development committee at the university has to consider applications for research. A number of proposals, all claiming to be randomised controlled trials (RCTs) have been submitted. You have been asked to determine which of the proposals' study designs is most appropriate for an RCT.

Of the following studies the one which would be the most appropriate for an RCT is:

- A whether atenolol can prevent recurrence of stroke
- B whether glucosuria can predict diabetes mellitus
- C whether hypertension is associated with chronic renal failure
- D whether hypertriglyceridaemia is associated with acute pancreatitis
- E whether smoking during pregnancy increases fetal loss

4.7 A 49-year-old man presented with a 1-week history of persistent dull upper abdominal pain and fever. He also complained of pale stools and episodic dark urine. He had decreased appetite, some weight loss and looked yellow. Eighteen months earlier he had undergone laparoscopic cholecystectomy for gallstones and ERCP four months ago to remove sludge from the common bile duct. He drank 10 units of alcohol per week and smoked 15 cigarettes a day. He was not on any medication.

On examination he was jaundiced, had a temperature of 39.1°C, pulse 120 regular and blood pressure 120/60. There was right upper quadrant abdominal tenderness but no hepatosplenomegaly and no ascites. Rectal examination was normal. He was not encephalopathic.

Bloods	Hb	12.5	WCC	15.6
	Platelets	345	INR	1.5
	Na	136	K	4.5
	Urea	5.9	Creatinine	120
	Bilirubin	62	Albumin	30
	Protein	60	AST	60
	ALP	360	GGT	140
Chest X-ray	Normal			
Urinalysis	Bilirubin 1+, no urobilinogen, no protein, no white cells			

The test that would ascertain the diagnosis would be:

A alpha-fetoprotein
B blood culture
C CT abdomen
D ERCP
E liver biopsy

4.8 A 60-year-old man was referred because of pruritus, headache and hypertension. He had no previous medical history and was not on any medication.

On examination he had a plethoric face. His temperature was 37.0°C, pulse 88 regular and blood pressure 165/90. His JVP was elevated to +4 cm and both heart sounds were normal. His chest was clear. Abdominal examination was normal except for a palpable spleen.

Bloods	Hb	18.5	MCV	99.2
	WCC	13.0	Platelets	600
	Haematocrit	56%	Red cell mass	36 ml/kg
	Neutrophils	7.2	Lymphocytes	3.1
	Monocytes	0.3	Na	135
	K	4.0	Urea	5.3
	Creatinine	88		

Of the following features the one which would be **MOST** consistent with a diagnosis of polycythaemia rubra vera is:

A enlarged kidneys on ultrasound
B low neutrophil alkaline phosphatase score
C low serum erythropoetin
D O_2 saturation on air <92%
E packed cell volume <0.40

4.9 A 58-year-old Pakistani man was admitted with shortness of breath associated with a dry cough. His appetite was decreased and he had lost weight. He had smoked 20 cigarettes a day for the last 35 years. He had a previous medical history of pulmonary TB, which had affected the right apical region, and he had completed a course of anti-TB medication. He was not on any medication.

On examination he was cachexic. His temperature was 37.0°C, pulse 88 regular, blood pressure 140/88 and respiratory rate 20 breaths/min. He had decreased air entry and breath sounds in the right lung.

Chest X-ray

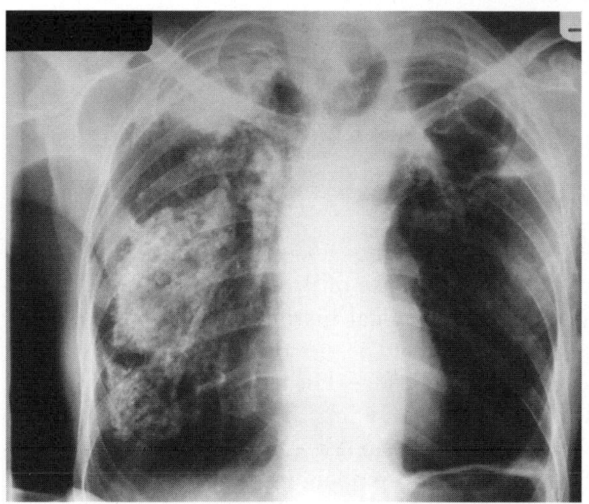

Biopsy of right lung lesion (Figure 4.9B, page 386.)

The most likely diagnosis is:

- A *Aspergillus* sp
- B carcinoma of the lung
- C *Pneumocystis juroveci* (formerly *carinii*) pneumonia
- D pulmonary TB
- E sarcoidosis

4.10 A 35-year-old man with hepatitis C was referred for treatment. Although he still continued to inject heroin, he had cut down and wanted to be treated. He was hepatitis B and HIV negative. He had no other medical or psychiatric problems. He smoked 15 cigarettes a day but did not drink alcohol.

Bloods	Hb	14.5	WCC	5.5
	Platelets	100	INR	1.0
	Protein	72	Albumin	35
	Bilirubin	15	ALT	70
	ALP	100	GGT	95
	AFP	5		
HCV PCR RNA	Positive			
HCV genotype	3a			
Liver ultrasound	Liver normal sized with no focal lesion. Normal blood flow, intrahepatic ducts and common bile duct			
Liver biopsy	Moderate active hepatitis			

Of the following statements concerning treatment of this patient it is true that:

A he should be treated with pegylated interferon and lamivudine
B his chances of a cure are 50–60%
C this level of thrombocytopaenia is a contraindication to starting treatment
D treatment for genotype 3a patients is for 6 months
E treatment should be deferred until he has stopped injecting drugs

4.11 A 35-year-old woman presented with progressive fatigue and weakness. She had had to give up work as a secretary because her hands became uncomfortable after a short period of typing. However, there were no paraesthesia and her symptoms improved with rest. She also complained of some double vision, dysphagia and shortness of breath on exertion. Three years ago she was diagnosed with hypothyroidism and type 1 diabetes but she had good control and regular follow-up at the diabetic clinic. She had had no recent illnesses. She had smoked 20 cigarettes a day for over 15 years.

On examination she had bilateral ptosis and strabismus. The rest of her cranial nerve examination was normal. Her pulse was 72 regular and blood pressure 120/80. Respiratory examination was normal. There was no limb muscle wasting or weakness. Tone, power, reflexes and sensation were normal, as was neck examination.

The most likely diagnosis is:

A dystrophia myotonica
B Eaton–Lambert syndrome
C mononeuritis multiplex
D motor neurone disease
E myasthenia gravis

4.12 A 42-year-old woman was referred with headaches.

As part of the examination, fundoscopy was performed. (Figure 4.12, page 387.)

The fundoscopic appearance is most likely due to:

A coloboma
B myelinated fibres
C neovascularisation
D optic atrophy
E swollen optic disc

4.13 A previously well 25-year-old woman presented with a 2-day history of cough productive of green purulent sputum. She had no allergies and did not keep any pets. She had not been abroad and had not come into contact with anyone else who had an illness. She had a normal appetite and no weight loss.

On examination she had a temperature of 37.4°C. Her pulse was 90 regular, blood pressure 120/75 and respiratory rate was 20 breaths/min. There were crackles and bronchial breathing in the right mid-zone.

Bloods	Hb	14.5	WCC	14.5
	Neutrophils	11.3	Platelets	270
	Na	139	K	4.5
	Urea	4.5	Creatinine	86
	Protein	70	Albumin	38
	Bilirubin	10	ALT	20
	ALP	69	CRP	45
Chest X-ray	Consolidation in the right midzone			

The best antibiotic treatment for this patient is:

A amoxycillin and clarithromycin
B ciprofloxacin and gentamicin
C clarithromycin and metronidazole
D rifampicin and clarithromycin
E rifampicin, isoniazid and pyrazinamide

4.14 A 26-year-old woman was referred with pain and tenderness in both hands for the past few months. In that time she had developed a rash on her face and scalp which had improved but had left her with scarring and alopecia. She was on no medication.

On examination she had bilateral swelling, tenderness and inflammation of the metacarpophalangeal joints and wrists. There was a faint, scarred rash over her nose, forehead and scalp.

The **THREE** blood tests likely to be positive or increased in the majority of such patients would be:

- A anti-La antibody
- B anti-mitochondrial antibody
- C antinuclear antibody (ANA)
- D anti-RNP
- E anti-Ro antibody
- F anti-Sm antibody
- G anti-smooth muscle antibody
- H c-ANCA
- I creatinine kinase
- J CRP
- K ESR
- L HLA B27
- M p-ANCA
- N rheumatoid factor

4.15 A 56-year-old woman was referred complaining of lethargy. (Figure 4.15, page 387.)

The most likely diagnosis is:

- A acromegaly
- B Cushing's syndrome
- C hypopituitarism
- D hypothyroidism
- E Paget's disease

4.16 A 79-year-old woman known to suffer from hypertension and on warfarin for atrial fibrillation was admitted with right hemiparesis and aphasia. There was no history of trauma.

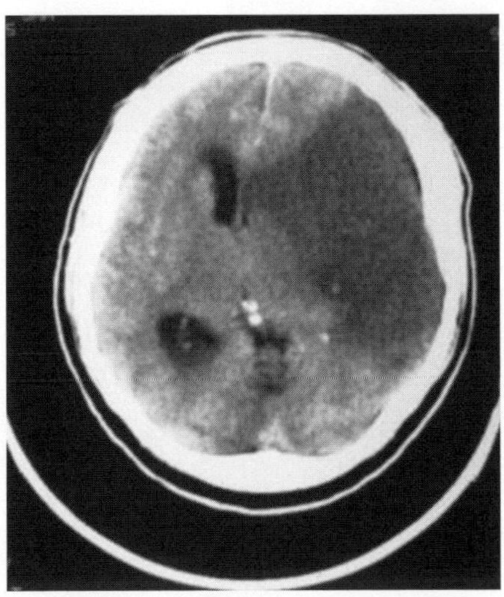

The CT scan shows:

A cerebral infarct
B extradural haematoma
C intracerebral haemorrhage
D subdural haematoma
E subarachnoid haemorrhage

4.17 A 61-year-old woman was referred with a 5-week history of progressive dysphagia and weight loss.

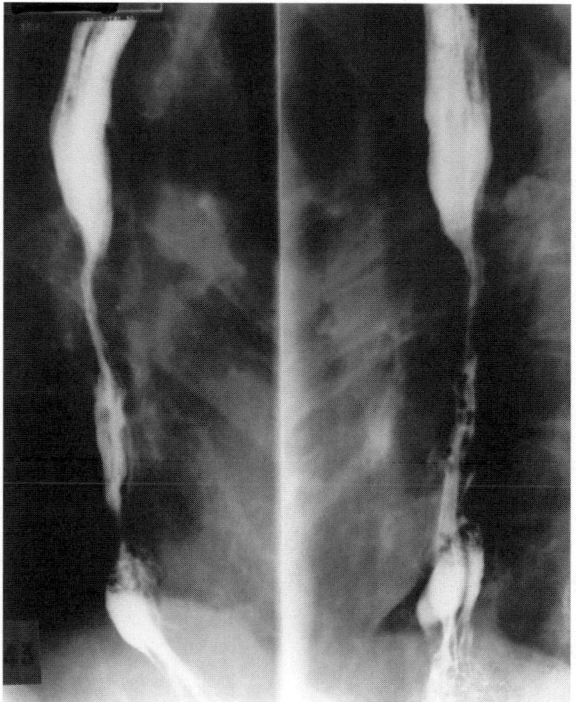

The most likely diagnosis is:

A achalasia
B benign stricture
C carcinoma of the oesophagus
D oesophageal candidiasis
E oesophageal varices

4.18 A 60-year-old man was referred for cardiac catheterisation because of progressive shortness of breath and the presence of a murmur.

	Pressure (systolic/diastolic [mmHg])	Normal value (systolic/diastolic [mmHg])	O_2 saturation (%)
Right atrium	8	0–8	73
Right ventricle	28/8	15–30/0–8	75
Pulmonary artery	30/15	15–30/0–8	75
Left atrium (mean)	12	1–10	96
Left ventricle	165/12	100–140/3–12	97
Aorta	107/88	100–140/60–90	97

The most likely diagnosis is:

A aortic regurgitation
B aortic stenosis
C mitral regurgitation
D mitral stenosis
E ventricular septal defect

4.19 A 35-year-old woman was referred with an 8-month history of recurrent attacks of palpitations. There was no previous medical history and she did not drink or smoke.

On examination she was pain free. Her temperature was 36.9°C, pulse 66 regular and blood pressure 120/84. JVP was not elevated and heart sounds were normal. Chest, abdominal and neck examinations were normal. She had normal blood tests.

Her condition should be managed in the long-term by:

A DC cardioversion
B digoxin
C implantable defibrillator
D permanent pacemaker
E radiofrequency ablation

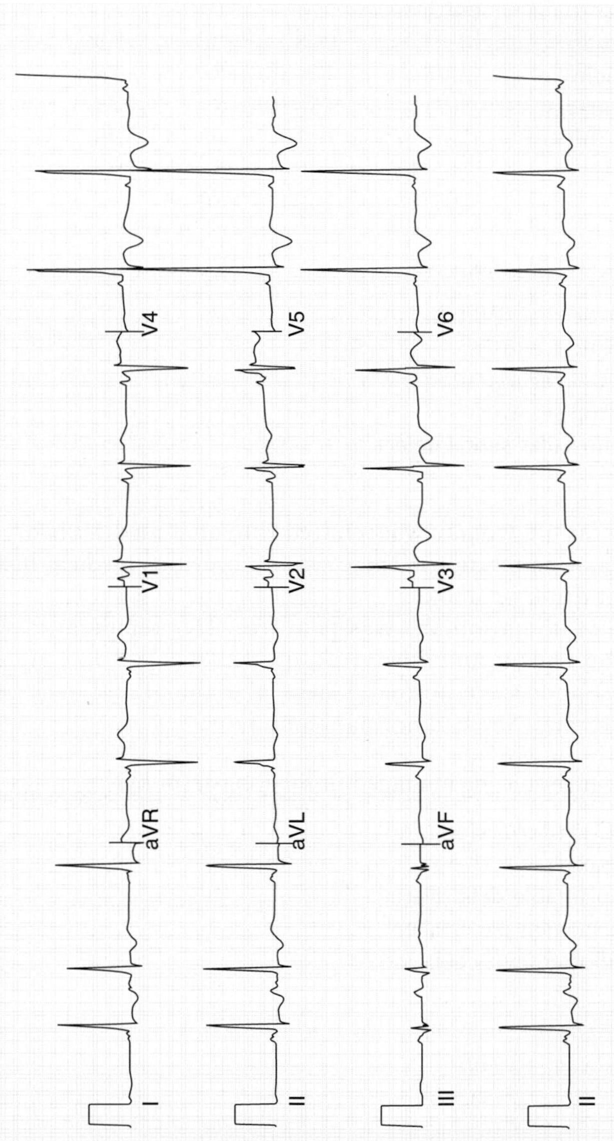
I
aVR
V1
V4
II
aVL
V2
V5
III
aVF
V3
V6
II

4.20 A 21-year-old woman was admitted following a paracetamol overdose. She had been treated with N-acetylcysteine but after 3 days had failed to improve. She had become more confused and disorientated.

She was jaundiced, had a hepatic flap and GCS of 14/15. Her temperature was 37.3°C, pulse 92 regular and blood pressure 105/68. JVP was elevated +2 cm, and heart sounds and chest were clear. Her abdomen was soft and there was no ascites. Her urine output was 25 mL/h.

Bloods	Hb	12.6	WCC	6.5
	Platelets	90	PT	50
	N	134	K	4.0
	Urea	13.8	Creatinine	280
	Protein	64	Albumin	34
	Bilirubin	80	ALT	12 500
	ALP	340		
Arterial blood gases on air	pH	7.30	PCO_2	3.0
	PO_2	10.8	Bicarbonate	15.5
	Base excess	–6.5		

Referral to a liver transplantation unit should be based on her:

A ALT
B bicarbonate
C bilirubin
D creatinine
E platelets

4.21 A 22-year-old woman was referred with a non-pruritic, disfiguring rash on both forearms. She had no previous medical history and was not on any medication. (Figure 4.21, page 388.)

The treatment of choice for this patient is:

A coal tar soap
B hydrocortisone ointment
C observation and follow-up
D oral prednisolone
E topical clotrimazole

4.22 A 55-year-old man was referred with a 4-week history of weight loss, jaundice, dark urine and pale stools, but no abdominal pain. He had no previous medical history. He drank 2 units of alcohol a week and was a non-smoker. He was not on any medication and had not had any blood transfusions in the past. His last trip abroad was over 20 years ago.

On examination he was markedly jaundiced and looked thin. He was apyrexial, pulse 78 regular and blood pressure 120/70. His abdomen was soft and non-tender with 3 cm hepatomegaly below the costal margin.

Bloods	Hb	13.5	WCC	11.3
	Platelets	450	INR	1.1
	Na	135	K	4.2
	Urea	4.5	Creatinine	90
	Glucose	4.6	Bilirubin	96
	Albumin	30	Protein	60
	AST	60	ALP	300
	GGT	30		
Hepatitis A, B, C serology	Negative			
Abdominal ultrasound	Mild hepatomegaly – normal echo texture			
	Normal common bile duct			
	Gallbladder empty with no stones seen			
	Dilated intrahepatic ducts			

The most likely diagnosis is:

A autoimmune hepatitis
B carcinoma of head of pancreas
C lymphoma at porta hepatis
D primary biliary cirrhosis
E sclerosing cholangitis

4.23 It had been proposed that faecal occult blood (FOB) could be used to screen for colorectal carcinoma. A trial using 1000 patients was carried out and 95 cases of carcinoma developed. The FOB detected 80 cases and 65 false-positives.

The sensitivity of FOB as a screening test is:

A 80/145
B 80/95
C 840/855
D 840/905
E 920/1000

4.24 A 50-year-old man in the intensive care unit had a 2-day history of jaundice. He was admitted there following an emergency abdominal aortic aneurysm repair 2 weeks previously and had been slow to wean off ventilation. Five days ago he had developed cellulitis around the insertion of the CVP line in the right groin and for which he had been started on intravenous antibiotics. He used to drink 2 units of alcohol most nights for 10 years. He had a previous medical history of hypercholesterolaemia but was not on any regular medication.

On examination he was alert and not being sedated. He had a tracheostomy and received mechanical ventilation. His temperature was 36.5°C, pulse 78 regular and blood pressure 145/92. His abdomen was soft and there was no organomegaly or distension. Rectal examination was normal. The abdominal wound site looked clean.

Bloods	Hb	12.5	MCV	84.6
	WCC	12.4	Platelets	180
	Albumin	28	Protein	54
	Bilirubin	135	ALT	50
	ALP	250	GGT	150
	INR	1.1		
Urinalysis	Bilirubin 2+, no urobilinogen			

The most likely cause of his deranged liver function is:

A ascending cholangitis
B autoimmune hepatitis
C decompensated liver disease secondary to alcoholic liver disease
D drug-induced cholestasis
E portal vein thrombosis

4.25 A 42-year-old man was referred with hepatomegaly and deranged liver function tests. He drank 2 units of alcohol a day and was a heavy smoker. He had no risk factors for hepatitis. He had a normal appetite and stable weight.

On examination he was not jaundiced or pale. His pulse was 79 regular and blood pressure 140/89. His respiratory rate was 18 breaths/min and his chest was clear. He had 6 cm hepatomegaly but no other signs of chronic liver disease.

Bloods	Hb	13.4	WCC	4.5
	Platelets	110	INR	1.4
	Na	132	K	4.8
	Urea	3.9	Creatinine	80
	Albumin	33	Protein	70
	Bilirubin	30	ALT	85
	ALP	105	GGT	39
	Glucose	5.4		
Hepatitis A, B, C serology	Negative			

Liver biopsy stained with PAS-D (Figure 4.25, page 388.)

The most likely diagnosis is:

A α_1-antitrypsin deficiency
B amyloidosis
C haemochromatosis
D hepatocellular carcinoma
E Wilson's disease

4.26 A 61-year-old man presented with difficulty in walking and weakness in his arms of recent onset. He had no visual or speech problems. His bladder and bowels were normal.

On examination there was generalised weakness and wasting of the muscles of the hands, arms shoulders, with fasciculation. There was reduced tone and upper limb reflexes were decreased. In the lower limbs there was weakness of the muscles with increased tone and reflexes. Plantar responses were extensor. Pinprick, light touch, vibration sense and proprioception were normal throughout. His gait was 'scissors-like'.

The most likely diagnosis is:

A cervical myelopathy
B Charcot–Marie–Tooth disease (HSMN)
C motor neurone disease
D poliomyelitis
E syringomyelia

4.27 A 55-year-old man was admitted with shortness of breath and abdominal pain. He had suffered from osteoarthritis and took diclofenac. He was a heavy smoker but did not drink alcohol.

Arterial blood gases on air	pH	7.11	PCO_2	6.5
	PO_2	10.2	Bicarbonate	12
	Base excess	–14		

These blood gases show:

- A metabolic acidosis and respiratory alkalosis with no respiratory failure
- B mixed metabolic and respiratory acidosis with no respiratory failure
- C mixed metabolic and respiratory acidosis with respiratory failure
- D respiratory acidosis and metabolic alkalosis with no respiratory failure
- E respiratory acidosis with no respiratory failure

4.28 A 30-year-old woman was referred with a 2-month history of fever, arthralgia affecting shoulders and neck, and some weight loss. She also complained of dizziness and some leg and chest pain that occurred with exercise. She had no previous medical history and was not on any medication. She did not smoke or drink alcohol.

On examination she looked well. Her temperature was 37.4°C, her radial pulses were difficult to feel but at the apex her heart rate was 88 regular, and blood pressure 148/90. Her JVP was not elevated and both heart sounds were normal. She had bilateral carotid bruits. Respiratory and abdominal examinations were normal. Her legs looked normal but she experienced pain on elevating them >35°. There was no focal neurological deficit.

Bloods	Hb	12.3	WCC	4.8
	Platelets	259	Na	140
	K	4.1	Urea	5.8
	Creatinine	89	Protein	68
	Albumin	39	Bilirubin	0
	ALT	25	ALP	73
	ESR	58	CRP	38
	PT	12	APTT	25
Rheumatoid factor	Negative			
Antinuclear antibody	Negative			
Chest X-ray	Normal			
ECG	No ischaemic changes			

The most likely diagnosis is:

- A antiphospholipid syndrome
- B Kawasaki's disease
- C polyarteritis nodosa
- D Takayasu's arteritis
- E type A dissection of ascending aorta

4.29 A 55-year-old man was admitted with recent abdominal pain, weight loss, jaundice and ascites. He did not drink alcohol.

On examination he was cachectic and mildly jaundiced. Abdomen was tender with gross ascites. An ascitic tap was performed with the fluid aspirated shown below. (Figure 4.29, page 389.)

The most likely diagnosis is:

A acute pancreatitis
B Budd–Chiari syndrome
C constrictive pericarditis
D lymphoma
E nephrotic syndrome

4.30 A 43-year-old woman had pain in both hands. She was undergoing renal dialysis.

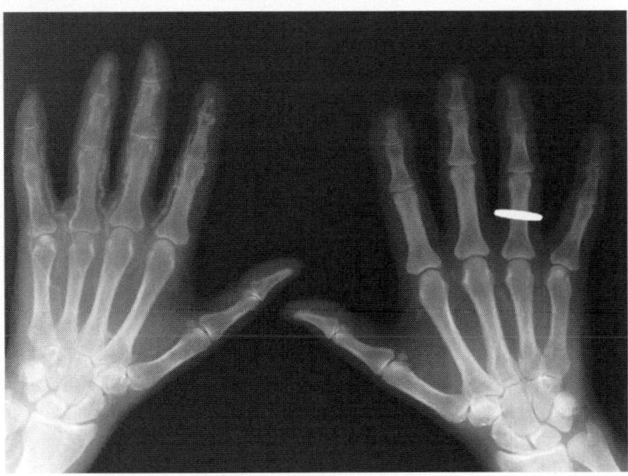

The most likely cause for the pain is:

A gout
B hyperparathyroidism
C Paget's disease
D rheumatoid arthritis
E sarcoidosis

4.31 A 48-year-old Armenian refugee was admitted with shortness of breath and haemoptysis. No previous history was available.

On examination he was unwell and breathless. His temperature was 38.0°C, pulse 90 regular and blood pressure 120/60. His respiratory rate was 30 breaths/min and there were bilateral crackles on auscultation.

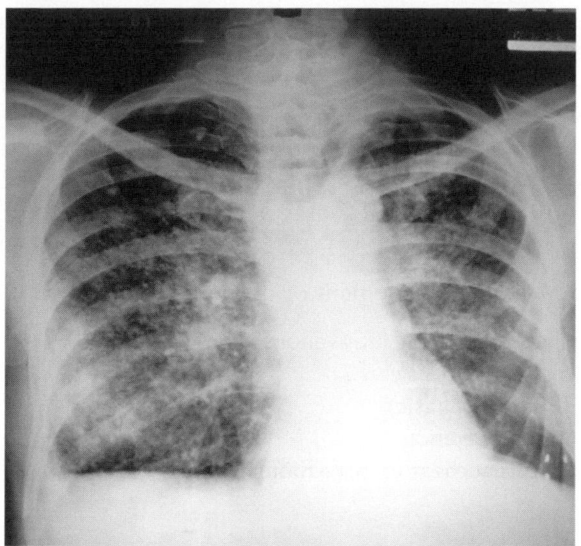

Apart from oxygen, the most appropriate treatment for this patient is:

A aciclovir
B cefuroxime and clarithromycin
C furosemide
D hydrocortisone
E rifampicin, isoniazid, pyrazinamide and ethambutol

4.32 A 61-year-old man was referred with worsening shortness of breath on exertion over the past 5 months with associated attacks of central chest pain that also occurred at rest. He could walk about 200 m before being stopped by dyspnoea. He slept with three pillows but sometimes had breathlessness at night. He did not smoke. He had had rheumatic fever as a child.

On examination he was breathless at rest. His pulse was 74 regular and blood pressure 120/90. His JVP was not elevated and his carotid pulse was difficult to palpate. There was a loud ejection systolic murmur that radiated to both carotids. There were bilateral crackles at both bases.

Of the following statements concerning management of his condition the one which is correct is:

A an ACE inhibitor is the best treatment option
B balloon valvuloplasty is the treatment of choice
C a bioprosthetic rather than mechanical valve replacement would give longer life-expectancy
D the louder the murmur the more severe the condition
E valve replacement should be performed if the surface area of the valve is <0.8 cm^2

4.33 A 73-year-old man was visiting his wife in hospital when he collapsed. A cardiac monitor showed the following trace. There was no palpable pulse.

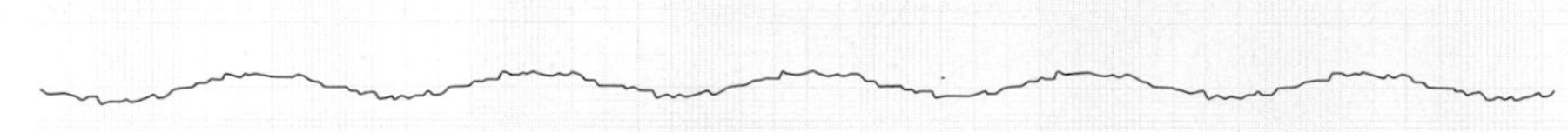

The next step in the immediate management of this patient would be:

- A adrenaline (epinephrine) 1 mg intravenously
- B atropine 300 mg intravenously
- C defibrillate 360 J (monophasic)
- D lignocaine 100 mg intravenously
- E start cardiopulmonary chest compressions 30:2

4.34 A 19-year-old student complained of a painless rash on his penis and some dysuria. (Figure 4.34, page 389.)

The rash shows:

- A chancroid
- B circinate balanitis
- C condyloma accuminata
- D herpes genitalis
- E primary chancre

4.35 A 35-year-old woman was referred with a 10-week history of galactorrhoea and loss of menstrual periods. She also complained of loss of libido and headaches. She was not on any medication.

On examination there was no focal neurological defect. Breast examination was normal.

Bloods	Na	140	K	4.1
	Urea	5.2	Creatinine	78
	TSH	4	Free T_4	20
	Prolactin	1450		
Urine β-HCG	Negative			
MRI pituitary	Microadenoma			

The most appropriate treatment for this patient is:

A amitriptyline
B bromocriptine
C cimetidine
D metoclopramide
E oestrogen

4.36 A 15-year-old girl was admitted with abdominal pain and bloody diarrhoea. She opened her bowels up to 10 times a day, passing blood and mucus. A provisional diagnosis of inflammatory bowel disease was made and the consultant in charge of her care suggested a colonoscopy would help with the diagnosis. The benefits and risks with colonoscopy were explained to the patient who appeared to understand what the procedure involved. She agreed to have the procedure. Unfortunately, her mother objected to the test being performed and refused to allow it.

The correct management plan for this patient would be to:

A explore other options of investigating this patient's bowel condition
B obtain a court order to perform the procedure
C postpone the procedure until the mother changes her mind
D proceed with the colonoscopy as the patient has given informed consent
E proceed with the colonoscopy as the consultant in charge of the patient's care can take full responsibility for inpatient care because she is aged under 16

4.37 A 35-year-old woman was admitted with abdominal pain and increased abdominal distension going on for the past 3 weeks. She had no relevant previous medical history. She did not drink or smoke. She was not pregnant and was on the oral contraceptive pill. She was not on any other medication.

On examination she looked ill but was alert and orientated. She was apyrexial and mildly icteric. Her pulse was 100 regular and blood pressure 95/60. Cardiovascular and respiratory examination was normal. She had gross ascites and generalised abdominal tenderness. Rectal examination was normal.

Bloods	Hb	12.5	WCC	10.5
	Platelets	85	INR	1.5
	Na	135	K	4.5
	Urea	8.5	Creatinine	200
	Albumin	24	Protein	56
	Bilirubin	40	ALT	1200
	ALP	140	GGT	100
	Amylase	58		
Hepatitis A, B and C serology	Negative			
Paracetamol	Not detected			
Salicylate	Not detected			
Chest X-ray	Normal			
Abdominal X-ray	No evidence of obstruction			
Ultrasound abdomen	Gross ascites			
	Hepatomegaly with an enlarged caudate lobe			
	Splenomegaly			
	Portal vein and inferior vena cava patent			

The most likely diagnosis is:

A autoimmune hepatitis
B Budd–Chiari syndrome
C ecstasy overdose
D metastatic disease
E portal vein thrombosis

4.38 A 42-year-old man presented with a 5-week history of severe pain and paraesthesia in his back radiating down his leg. It came on gradually and he found walking difficult. The right side was worse than the left. There were no symptoms in his arms or face. He had no bowel or bladder problems. He had a previous medical history of diabetes mellitus for which he was on insulin. He has no eye or renal complications.

On examination he had weakness of his plantar flexors, peroneus longus, extensor digitorum brevis and hamstrings. Tone was normal but power was reduced. Knee jerk was intact but ankle reflex was absent; plantar responses were flexor. There was decreased sensation to light touch and pinprick over the lateral border of the foot.

His neurological abnormalities are due to:

A myelopathy
B myopathy
C peripheral neuropathy
D radiculopathy
E subcortical lesion

4.39 A 47-year-old smoker was referred with haemoptysis.

Chest X-ray revealed a left hilar lesion. At bronchoscopy an endobronchial tumour was found, which histology confirmed as squamous cell carcinoma. Liver ultrasound showed no evidence of metastases.

Surgical resection of the tumour might still be possible in the presence of:

A dysphagia
B elevated left hemidiaphragm on chest X-ray
C hypercalcaemia
D hoarse voice
E predicted postoperative FEV_1 of 0.7 L

4.40 A 28-year-old male was referred with pain and stiffness in his right knee for about 1 week. Since then that pain had resolved, but now his hands and wrists were painful. He had a rash on his penis and complained of dysuria and a creamy discharge. He was heterosexual but had multiple sexual partners.

On examination his temperature was 37.5°C, pulse 88 regular and blood pressure 130/74. Respiratory and abdominal systems were normal. The right knee joint looked normal. Both wrists and metacarpophalangeal joints were mildly inflamed with some inflammation and tenderness of the tendon sheaths. There was a small, painless ulcer on his penis and small, tender vesicles on the back of the hands and wrists.

Bloods	Hb	12.0	WCC	11.8
	Platelets	480	Neutrophils	7.5
	Na	137	K	4.2
	Urea	5.7	Creatinine	89
	Protein	70	Albumin	40
	Bilirubin	10	ALT	25
	ALP	70	ESR	34
	CRP	40		
Synovial fluid	Slightly turbid appearance			
	WCC	40 000		
	Neutrophils	60%		
	No growth			
	Protein	35		
Urine culture	No growth			
Blood cultures	Awaited			

The most likely diagnosis is:

A ankylosing spondylitis
B Behçet's syndrome
C gonococcal arthritis
D primary syphilis
E Reiter's syndrome

4.41 A 16-year-old girl presented with sudden onset cough and shortness of breath. She suffered from asthma that was well controlled. She had no calf swelling. There was no significant family history and she had not been abroad recently.

On examination she was in some distress using her accessory muscles of respiration. Temperature was 36.5°C, pulse 110 regular and blood pressure 100/60. Her respiratory rate was 30 breaths/min but no wheeze was heard.

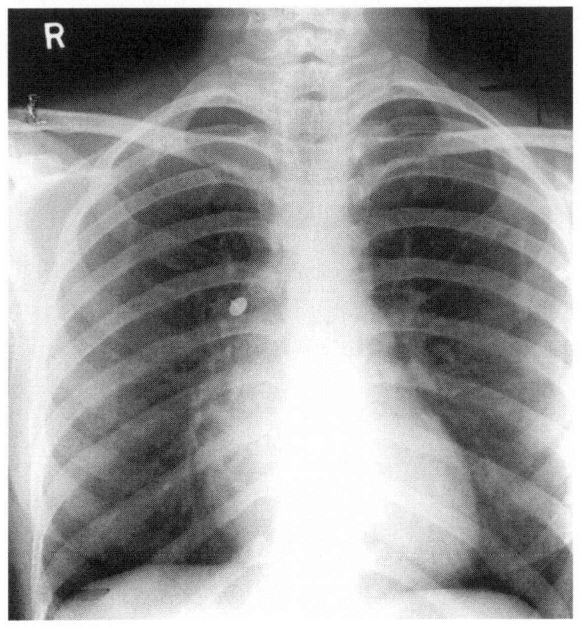

Arterial blood gases on air	pH	7.34	PCO_2	3.6
	PO_2	9.4		

The reason for her breathlessness is:

- A hysterical hyperventilation
- B inhaled foreign body
- C inspissated mucus plug blocking small airways
- D pneumothorax
- E pulmonary embolism

4.42 A 49-year-old man presented with progressive shortness of breath and dysphagia.

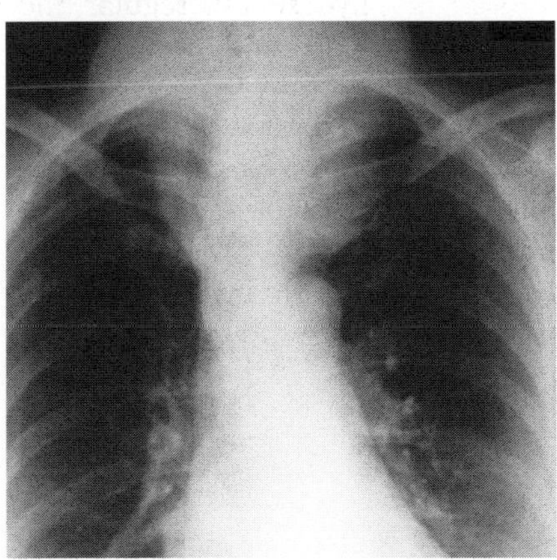

The chest X-ray findings are most consistent with:

A Hodgkin's lymphoma
B retrosternal goitre
C teratoma
D thoracic aortic aneurysm
E thymoma

4.43 A 13-year-old boy was referred by social services because of bruises and scars on his body. Other than generalised bruising, he had epicanthal folds and a flat nasal bridge. (Figure 4.43, page 389.)

The most likely diagnosis is:

A Ehlers–Danlos syndrome
B Marfan's syndrome
C Noonan's syndrome
D osteogenesis imperfecta
E pseudoxanthoma elasticum

4.44 A 45-year-old woman was brought to Accident & Emergency with pyrexia and dysuria for the past 2 days. Over the past month she had been complaining of increased lethargy. She had a previous medical history of rheumatoid arthritis affecting her hands and upper limbs for which she was receiving gold injections. She was not on any other medications.

On examination her temperature was 38.7°C, pulse 88 regular and blood pressure 130/78. Respiratory and abdominal examinations were normal with no organomegaly detected.

Bloods	Hb	6.4	MCV	95.4
	WCC	2.1	Platelets	42
	Neutrophils	1.1	Lymphocytes	0.5
	Reticulocytes	0.5%		
Urine	Blood +, protein ++, nitrites ++			
Chest X-ray	Normal			

Bone marrow aspirate and trephine (Figure 4.44, page 390.)

Regarding this patient's haematological diagnosis:

A rheumatoid arthritis per se can predispose to this condition
B severe disease is classed as marrow containing <50% cellularity and <50% of the cells are haemopoietic
C the condition can be caused by Epstein–Barr virus
D it is a type of Fanconi's anaemia
E it is myelodysplastic syndrome

4.45 A 25-year-old man with a history of Crohn's disease was referred with abdominal pain. There was no nausea or vomiting, his appetite was normal and he had not lost weight. He opened his bowels once a day and his stools were solid with some mucus but no blood. He was only on mesalazine tablets. He had a colonoscopy a year ago when he was diagnosed with Crohn's disease, which showed areas of quiescent disease up to the caecum.

On examination he was apyrexial. There was generalised abdominal tenderness but no masses and rectal examination was normal.

The next most appropriate investigation would be:

A barium enema
B capsule endoscopy
C CT abdomen
D repeat colonoscopy
E small bowel follow-through

4.46 A 16-year-old girl was referred because of 2-month history of seizures. They began with her seeing flashing lights and continued with jerking of the left upper limb for up to 5 min. Occasionally she had bitten her tongue but had never lost control of her bowels or bladder. She did not lose consciousness when fitting and had no post-seizure amnesia. She had no previous medical history; she was not on any medication and there was no family history of epilepsy.

On examination she looked well and no abnormalities were found on physical examination.

Full blood count	Normal
Urea & electrolytes	Normal

The most likely diagnosis is:

A absence seizures
B complex partial seizures
C myoclonic seizures
D simple partial seizures
E tonic-clonic seizures

4.47 A breathless 45-year-old man was referred for lung function tests.

	Absolute	Predicted (%)
FEV_1	1.2	33
FVC	2.6	55
TLC	5.5	112
DLCO	8.3	38
KCO	1.5	42

The results are most consistent with:

A atrial septal defect with left to right shunt
B emphysema
C extrinsic allergic alveolitis
D pulmonary embolus
E sarcoidosis

4.48 A 26-year-old Caucasian man was referred because of progressively worsening pain in his spine, hips and knees over the past 4 months. He also complained of skin darkening, especially on his ears. In addition to this his urine darkened markedly if it was allowed to stand. His father also suffered a similar problem.

On examination his skin was hyperpigmented and his ears were blue–black in colour. His pulse was 92 regular and blood pressure 110/82. His JVP was not elevated but there was an ejection systolic murmur. His chest was clear. There was loss of the lumbar lordosis and he had difficulty stooping forward. The knee joints were swollen and inflamed. There was no neurological deficit.

Lumbosacral X-ray	Calcification of the intervertebral discs
	Narrowing of the intervertebral spaces

The most likely diagnosis is:

A alkaptonuria
B ankylosing spondylitis
C homocystinuria
D maple syrup urine disease
E relapsing polychondritis

4.49 A 40-year-old man was admitted with worsening shortness of breath and cough productive of thick yellow sputum. This had been progressing over 2 years and it was his fourth admission this year. He was a smoker until he stopped last year.

On examination he was breathless and cyanosed. His temperature was 37.2°C, pulse 110 regular and blood pressure 120/78. His respiratory rate was 30 breaths/min and there were bilateral crackles in his lungs.

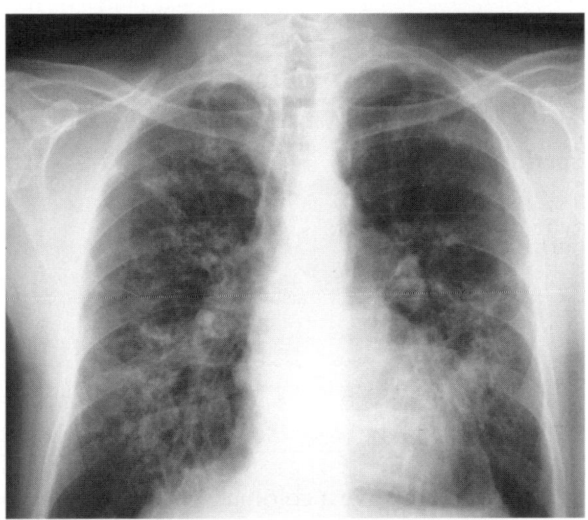

The condition that would be **LEAST** likely to have caused his chest X-ray appearances is:

A aspergillosis
B childhood pertussis infection
C chronic obstructive pulmonary disease
D cystic fibrosis
E tuberculosis

4.50 A 68-year-old man complained of a lump that had been growing on the top of his scalp for the past 2 months. (Figure 4.50, page 390.)

Of the following the **LEAST** likely cause of the scalp lesion is:

A arsenic exposure
B burn scars
C immunosuppressant treatment post-renal transplant
D pigmented naevi
E PUVA (psoralen + ultraviolet A light) treatment

4.51 A 22-year-old patient was referred with infertility. He has been married for 1 year but had so far failed to make his wife pregnant. He was very embarrassed, describing that he did have big breasts and that his genitalia were not very big. He had no previous medical history and did not smoke or drink alcohol.

On examination he was somewhat short but had a normal appearance. He was clinically euthyroid. There was gynaecomastia and both testes were present albeit very small.

Bloods	Testosterone	5.5	(normal 10–29 nmoL/L)
	FSH	40	(normal 1–7 U/L)
	LH	28	(normal 1–6 U/L)
Sperm count	Azoospermia		

The most likely karyotype of this patient is:

A 45,XO
B 46,XO
C 46,XY
D 47,XXY
E 47,XYY

4.52 A 35-year-old man was found to have a colonic tumour on colonoscopy. His father had developed carcinoma of the rectum aged 55 and his uncle had died from colonic carcinoma aged 60. He had a total colectomy and made an uneventful recovery.

The syndrome this patient is likely to have is:

A familial adenomatous polyposis
B Gardner's syndrome
C hereditary nonpolyposis colorectal cancer
D juvenile polyposis
E Peutz–Jegher's syndrome

4.53 A 35-year-old woman presented with worsening headaches and blurred vision. Over the past 3 months she had also noticed a 4 kg weight loss and an itchy rash on her legs. Her only previous medical history was of peptic ulcer disease that was diagnosed last year but responded to high dose proton pump inhibitors.

On examination she looked cachectic. There was a widespread erythematous rash on both lower limbs. There was no jaundice or lymphadenopathy. Epigastric tenderness was the only finding on examination of the abdomen. On testing the visual fields she had bitemporal hemianopia.

Bloods	Calcium	2.70	Phosphate	0.55
	Albumin	32	Glucose	13.4
	PTH	6.9	Prolactin	1000

The most likely diagnosis is:

A autoimmune polyglandular syndrome (APS) I
B APS 2
C multiple endocrine neoplasia (MEN) I syndrome
D MEN 2A syndrome
E MEN 2B syndrome

4.54 A 70-year-old woman was admitted with acute abdominal pain. She had had these symptoms on and off for the past 3 months. This time the pain was very severe and she had passed some fresh blood per rectum. She had no previous medical history and was not on any medication.

On examination she had a temperature of 38.0°C, pulse 95 regular and blood pressure 110/60. There was tenderness in the left iliac fossa, no organomegaly and rectal examination revealed some blood but no masses.

Bloods	Hb	10.5	WCC	13.5
	Neutrophils	11.7	Platelets	345
	Na	140	K	4.5
	Urea	7.8	Creatinine	96
	Albumin	30	Protein	60
	Bilirubin	10	ALT	20
	ALP	70	GGT	35
	Amylase	50	CRP	120
	ESR	55		
Chest X-ray	Normal			
Abdominal X-ray	No evidence of obstruction			

The most likely diagnosis is:

A acute diverticulitis
B Crohn's disease
C ischaemic colitis
D ovarian carcinoma
E pseudomembranous colitis

4.55 A 70-year-old woman was brought in drowsy and confused. Her daughter said that she had been off her food and had vomited several times that day.

She had decreased skin turgor and a furred tongue. Her temperature was 38.2°C, pulse 105, blood pressure 100/55 and JVP was not elevated. Heart sounds and chest were normal. Respiratory rate was 16 breaths/min. There was vague lower abdominal tenderness. She was unable to walk independently.

Bloods	Hb	12.5	WCC	13.4
	Platelets	200	Na	158
	K	4.0	Urea	19.0
	Creatinine	184	Glucose	58
Blood gases	pH	7.37	PCO_2	4.6
on air	PO_2	10.5	Bicarbonate	28
Urine osmolality	300 mosmol/kg			
Urinalysis	Protein 2+, glucose 3+, ketones 1+			

Of the following statements concerning this patient's management the one which is **FALSE** is:

A bring down her blood glucose as quickly as possible
B if she becomes drowsier, insert a nasogastric tube
C she may not need to be put on any long-term antidiabetic medication
D give 0.45% saline
E give prophylactic heparin

4.56 A 49-year-old man with chronic renal failure was referred with left loin pain and haematuria. He had a long history of renal stones. He had no other medical problems and was not on any medication.

On examination his temperature was 36.5°C, pulse 88 regular and blood pressure 148/92. There was tenderness in the left loin region but no organomegaly and rectal examination was normal.

Bloods	Hb	10.9	MCV	6.4
	WCC	8.6	Platelets	200
	Na	138	K	3.1
	Urea	18.3	Creatinine	220
	Protein	68	Albumin	38
	Bicarbonate	10	Chloride	114
	Calcium	2.42	Phosphate	0.98
	Renin (upright)	3.4		
	Aldosterone (upright)	420		
Urinalysis	pH 6.4, protein 2+, blood 1+, white cells 1+			
Abdominal X-ray	Nephrocalcinosis			
Intravenous pyelogram	Dilated medullary collecting ducts, 1cm stone in left ureter			

The most likely diagnosis is:

- A Bartter's syndrome
- B Conn's syndrome
- C renal tubular acidosis I
- D renal tubular acidosis II
- E renal tubular acidosis IV

4.57 A 27-year-old man presented with pyrexia for the past 7 days. He had just returned back from a holiday in the Gambia. (Figure 4.57, page 390.)

The organism seen in the blood film is:

- A *Leishmania donovani*
- B Loa loa
- C *Plasmodium falciparum*
- D *Schistosoma haematobium*
- E *Trypanosoma brucei gambiense*

4.58 A 28-year-old woman was referred with jaundice, neck stiffness and headache. She also complained of red, gritty eyes. Her symptoms had started 7 days ago as a flu-like illness and had got progressively worse. She had just returned from a camping holiday in the USA. There was no previous medical history and she was not on any medication. She did not drink alcohol or smoke.

On examination she was jaundiced and had bilateral conjunctivitis. Her temperature was 38.2°C, pulse 100 regular and blood pressure 120/90. Her JVP was not elevated and heart sounds were normal. Chest was clear. There was some right upper quadrant tenderness but no organomegaly. She was not encephalopathic. Kernig's sign was positive but the rest of the neurological examination was normal. There was no skin rash.

Bloods	Hb	11.9	MCV	93.0
	WCC	12.4	Platelets	259
	Na	138	K	4.4
	Urea	5.5	Creatinine	80
	Protein	70	Albumin	35
	Bilirubin	65	ALT	145
	ALP	135	CRP	189
Chest X-ray	Normal			

The most likely diagnosis is:

A hepatitis A
B histoplasmosis
C leptospirosis
D Lyme disease
E Rocky Mountain spotted fever

4.59 A 45-year-old woman was referred with widespread cervical and inguinal lymphadenopathy that was diagnosed as Hodgkin's lymphoma. She felt otherwise well.

Physical examination was normal apart from the lymphadenopathy.

Of the following which one is associated with a **BETTER** prognosis:

A lymphocyte-predominant disease
B mediastinal disease
C night sweats
D splenic involvement
E subdiaphragmatic disease

4.60 A 13-year-old boy was referred because of painless haematuria. He had no cough or shortness of breath. He was diagnosed with sensorineural deafness at the age of 5. His mother also had renal impairment. He was not on any medication.

On examination his pulse was 80 and blood pressure 90/50. Abdominal examination was normal.

Bloods	Hb	12.4	WCC	4.5
	Platelets	250	Na	138
	K	4.0	Urea	4.8
	Creatinine	79	Protein	70
	Albumin	39	Calcium	2.33
	Glucose	4.5		
Urinalysis	pH 6.4, blood 2+			
Retrograde pyelography	Normal			
Cystography	Normal			

The most likely diagnosis is:

A Alport's syndrome
B autosomal dominant polycystic kidney disease
C Fabry's disease
D juvenile nephronophthisis
E thin basement membrane nephritis

4.61 A 45-year-old man with persistent abdominal pain underwent a capsule endoscopy. On review of the pictures an abnormality was seen. (Figure 4.61, page 391.)

Regarding the diagnosis and management of this organism it is correct that:

A a full blood count will reveal a peripheral eosinophilia
B once treated re-infection rarely occurs
C praziquantel is the drug treatment of choice
D it is an important cause of occult anaemia
E it is most commonly found in the appendix and caecum

4.62 A 53-year-old man was referred because of deranged liver function tests and a distended abdomen. The abdominal distension had occurred over the past 6 months. In that time he had put on 10 kg. He had a normal appetite. He had no risk factors for viral hepatitis. He drank two glasses of wine a day and had smoked 15 cigarettes a day for over 35 years. He worked in an office. He had no other medical problems and was not on any medication.

On examination he was obese with weight 105 kg and BMI 32 kg/m^2. There was no jaundice, oedema or lymphadenopathy. His abdomen was not tender and there was no organomegaly or shifting dullness. There were no signs of chronic liver disease or encephalopathy.

Bloods	Hb	13.5	Platelets	170
	INR	1.2	Ferritin	250
	Albumin	38	Bilirubin	13
	ALT	90	ALP	120
	Glucose	6.4	IgA	1.4
	IgG	7.8	IgM	1.9
	AFP	12	Cholesterol	5.3
	Triglycerides	1.7		
Hepatitis A, B, C serology	Negative			
Liver ultrasound	Generalised bright echo texture No focal liver lesions No ascites with normal portal flow			

The **NEXT** step in the management of this patient is:

- A CT abdomen
- B liver biopsy
- C lose weight
- D start statin
- E start ursodeoxycholic acid

4.63 A 59-year-old man was admitted to the coronary care unit after suffering an acute myocardial infarction and was treated with thrombolysis. Three days later while sitting on his bed he suddenly collapsed. A cardiac monitor revealed ventricular fibrillation and he was successfully resuscitated by the cardiac arrest team. The rest of his inpatient stay was uneventful. It was felt he should have an implantable cardiovertor-defibrillator (ICD) fitted.

Regarding ICDs it is correct that:

- A it can be used for primary prophylaxis against life-threatening arrhythmia in patients with New York Heart Association (NYHA) grade 4 heart failure who are not considered heart transplant candidates
- B it can be used in asymptomatic hypertrophic cardiomyopathy patients
- C it is contraindicated in Brugada syndrome
- D it must not be used in patients already on amiodarone
- E the generator battery needs to be replaced every 2 years

4.64 A 56-year-old woman presented to Accident & Emergency with a 2-month history of increasing shortness of breath on exertion, dry cough and weight loss but no night sweats. She had smoked 20 cigarettes a day for >35 years. She did not drink alcohol. She had not travelled abroad recently.

On examination she was thin. Her temperature was 37.0°C, pulse 98 regular and blood pressure 115/75. Her JVP was not elevated and heart sounds were normal. The trachea was central, there was decreased chest expansion on the right and percussion note on this side was dull. Respiratory rate was 24 breaths/min. O_2 saturation on air was 93%. Abdominal examination was normal. A diagnostic pleural tap was performed and 50 ml of blood-stained fluid was aspirated.

Bloods	Hb	12.3	WCC	10.9
	Neutrophils	7.4	Platelets	130
	Protein	56	Albumin	35
	LDH	300	Glucose	6.0
Pleural fluid	pH	7.38	Protein	30
	Glucose	3.3	LDH	200
	Red cells	400	White cells	150
	Lymphocytes	70%		
Chest X-ray	Uniform shadowing of right middle and lower zones			

Of the following statements concerning the diagnosis it is correct that:

A CT chest should be performed after complete drainage of the effusion
B only 20% of malignant effusions can be diagnosed from fluid cytology
C pleural fluid lymphocytosis is consistent with malignant disease
D the effusion is likely to be due to an empyema
E the pleural effusion is a transudate

4.65 A 20-year-old woman was referred with amenorrhoea for the past 6 months. She denied being pregnant. She had had irregular menses since she underwent menarche aged 12 but had normal pubertal development. She had been putting on weight. She had also noticed a rash in both axillae. She did not smoke or drink alcohol. There was no relevant family history.

On examination she was obese and looked hirsute; height was 1.55 cm, waist 96 cm, weight 75 kg and BMI 31. Pulse was 100 and blood pressure 145/90. In her axillae there was a black, velvety, thickened hyperpigmentation of the skin. Breast, abdominal, rectal and vaginal examinations were normal.

Bloods	FSH	4.0	(normal 2.5–10 U/L)
	LH	12.0	(normal 2.5–10 U/L)
	Oestradiol	230	(normal 121–590 pmol/L)
	Testosterone	5.5	(normal: 0.5–3.0 nmol/L)
	Prolactin	350	
	Fasting glucose	6.5	

The following statement regarding her diagnosis is correct:

- A if she had late onset congenital adrenal hyperplasia there would be decreased levels of 17-hydroxyprogesterone
- B if she had polycystic ovarian syndrome (PCOS) she would be expected to have increased serum levels of sex hormone binding globulin
- C she fits the criteria for metabolic syndrome
- D she is likely to have primary ovarian failure
- E to diagnose PCOS she would have to have more than five cysts in both ovaries on ultrasound

4.66 A 55-year-old man presented to his local hospital on a Sunday night feeling unwell and complaining of acute right-sided abdominal pain. He had been discharged 2 days ago after receiving a renal transplant for diabetic nephropathy. He had made good progress postoperatively with his creatinine steadily improving. His creatinine at hospital discharge was 100. He had no cough or dysuria and had been taking his immunosuppressive medication as prescribed.

On examination he appeared in discomfort. His temperature was 37.4°C, pulse was 88 regular and blood pressure was 140/82. Heart sounds and respiratory examination were normal. There was tenderness over the right iliac fossa where his new graft was sited but the wound looked clean and bowel sounds were present. Neurological examination was normal.

Bloods	Hb	11.1	WCC	7.6
	Platelets	210	INR	1.1
	Na	134	K	4.8
	Urea	12.8	Creatinine	156
	Albumin	35	Bilirubin	12
	ALT	35	ALP	119
Chest X-ray	Normal			
Urine	Normal			

The next step in his management would be:

- A DMSA scan
- B MAG3 scan
- C renal biopsy
- D renal ultrasound with Doppler blood flow measurements
- E start intravenous methyl prednisolone

4.67 A 73-year-old man was reviewed in the clinic. Over the past 3 years there had been a progressive deterioration in his memory and mental state, so much so that it was now affecting his activities of daily living such as dressing and washing. His wife found it difficult to cope as he had recently been having aggressive mood swings. He was able to walk without a stick but tended not to go out very much. Until now he had no other medical problems and was on no medication. He did not smoke or drink.

On examination he did not appear distressed and there was no tremor. Pulse was 88 regular, blood pressure was 138/92 and there were no murmurs or bruits. Neurological examination was unremarkable with normal tone, power and reflexes. His mini-mental state examination was 15/30. Full blood count, urea & electrolytes, liver function tests, vitamin B_{12} and thyroid function tests were normal.

CT head Generalised cortical atrophy

The drug treatment of choice for this patient is:

A amantadine
B donepezil
C levodopa
D pyridostigmine
E reserpine

4.68 A 20-year-old woman on the postnatal ward was referred with confusion, rash and pyrexia. Two days ago she had an emergency Caesarean section. She had some abdominal pain and had vomited twice but there was no wound dehiscence. She had a headache, dizziness and upper and lower limb myalgia. She had no cough or urinary symptoms. She had previously been fit and well and her new baby was well.

On examination GCS was 15/15 and her temperature was 38.9°C. There was a diffuse, non-blanching, non-tender, macular rash around the wound site which extended to her thighs and up to her costal margin. Her pulse was 110 regular and blood pressure was 90/55. JVP was not elevated and heart sounds and chest examination were normal. There was generalized abdominal tenderness, worse over the wound scar, and bowel sounds were present. Neurological examination revealed no focal deficit, with Kernig's sign negative, and plantar responses were flexor.

Bloods	Hb	9.7	WCC	13.5
	Neutrophils	10.8	Platelets	98
	INR	1.4	Na	134
	K	5.8	Urea	14.8
	Creatinine	180	Albumin	34
	Bilirubin	30	ALT	50
	ALP	130	CRP	70
	Amylase	57	Creatine kinase	1200
Chest X-ray	Normal			

The most likely cause for this patient's deterioration is:

A haemolytic uraemic syndrome
B meningococcal septicaemia
C necrotising fasciitis
D toxic epidermal necrolyis
E toxic shock syndrome

4.69 A 33-year-old man was referred to the HIV clinic for treatment. He was on no treatment and had stopped injecting 'recreational' drugs 3 months ago. He did not drink alcohol. There was no history of foreign travel.

Physical examination was normal.

Bloods	Hb	11.4	WCC	9.8
	Platelets	110	INR	1.4
	Albumin	33	Bilirubin	12
	ALT	80	ALP	130
	GGT	60		
CMV IgG	Positive			
Toxoplasma IgG	Positive			
Cryptococcal antigen	Negative			
Varicella zoster virus IgG	Positive			
Hepatitis B serology	HBsAg positive, HBeAg negative			
Hep C IgG	Negative			
CD_4 count	400			
HIV viral load	4000			

The **NEXT** investigation in this patient should be:

A early morning urine for tuberculosis
B hepatitis B virus DNA
C liver biopsy
D *Mycobacterium avium intracellulare* culture
E *Strongyloides* serology

4.70 A 72-year-old man presented to Accident & Emergency with active haematemesis. He had a previous medical history of ischaemic heart disease and was on aspirin and clopidogrel.

He looked pale and was shocked with a pulse of 110 and blood pressure of 65/40.

Bloods				
	Hb	5.5	HCT	20%
	WCC	10.5	Platelets	200
	INR	1.0		

He was resuscitated with crystalloid and then rapidly transfused with 8 units of packed cells before having emergency endoscopy.

The complication that is **MOST** likely to follow transfusion is:

A hypercalcaemia
B hyperthermia
C metabolic acidosis
D thrombocytopaenia
E venous thromboembolism

4.71 A 63-year-old man presented to Accident & Emergency with a non-productive cough, lethargy and pyrexia. His symptoms had started 3 weeks ago and were getting worse. He had no previous medical problems. He did not smoke or drink alcohol.

On examination his temperature was 38.7°C and he had bilateral cervical lymphadenopathy. Respiratory and abdominal examination was normal. There was a petechial rash on both lower limbs.

Blood film (Figure 4.71, page 391.)

The condition that this patient **MOST** likely has is:

A acute lymphoblastic leukaemia
B acute myeloid leukaemia
C chronic lymphocytic leukaemia
D chronic myeloid leukaemia
E infectious mononucleosis

4.72 A 14-year-old boy was referred by his GP with a 3-month history of right-sided abdominal pain. He also complained of lethargy and decreased appetite. He had lost 2 kg in weight. There was no nausea or vomiting. He had no urinary or bowel symptoms. He had no previous medical history or family history of note.

On examination he looked pale. There was no jaundice, oedema or lymphadenopathy. He was apyrexial with a pulse of 65 and blood pressure 93/66. Cardiovascular and respiratory systems were normal. On palpation of the abdomen there was a mass in the right upper quadrant which was bimanually palpable and did not move with respiration. Neurological examination was normal.

Bloods	Hb	9.5	WCC	7.5
	Platelets	200	MCV	84.5
	Na	138	K	3.9
	Urea	4.3	Creatinine	78
	Protein	65	Albumin	35
	Bilirubin	10	ALT	25
	ALP	345	Calcium	2.20
Urinary VMA	90 mmol/24 h			
Urinary 5-HIAA	45 mmol/24 h			
Abdominal ultrasound	Right suprarenal mass			
	Normal liver, spleen and pancreas and left kidney			

The most likely diagnosis is:

A carcinoid tumour
B hepatoblastoma
C neuroblastoma
D phaeochromocytoma
E Wilm's tumour

4.73 A 63-year-old man had been admitted to ITU immediately following an elective abdominal aortic aneurysm repair. Unfortunately, he had developed a chest infection and remained on the ventilator. His treatment for the chest infection and a wound infection was cefotaxime, metronidazole and teicoplanin. He required a tracheostomy because he was unable to breathe spontaneously.

He had been on the ITU for over 2 weeks but over the past 5 days he had become anuric and was now on continuous venous–venous haemofiltration. His abdomen had become more distended. He was now off antibiotics and inotropic agents but had spiked a temperature of 38.5°C.

His pulse was 105 regular, blood pressure 100/55, CVP +8 and heart sounds normal. He was on pressure support ventilation with a respiratory rate of 20 breaths/min. There were decreased breath sounds in both bases. His abdomen was soft but distended. His wound site looked clean and there were no abdominal drains. He still had a urinary catheter in situ along with a right internal jugular CVP line, right forearm arterial line and right femoral vascular catheter; these had all been in situ for 10 days.

Bloods	Hb	10.6	WCC	14.5
	Neutrophils	11.4	Platelets	160
ECG	Normal sinus rhythm with a rate of 105			
Chest X-ray	Bilateral basal atelectasis			
Abdominal ultrasound	Normal liver, spleen and kidneys Large amount of ascites but no loculated collection seen			

Concerning the diagnosis and management of this patient is correct that:

A chest infection is the most likely cause for his pyrexia
B he is unlikely to have spontaneous bacterial peritonitis if there is no history of liver disease.
C he should be treated with intravenous meropenem and amikacin
D the source of sepsis is unlikely to his vascular access catheters if there is no surrounding erythema
E the urinary catheter should be removed

4.74 A 61-year-old man presented with abdominal pain to Accident & Emergency.

A CT abdomen was performed.

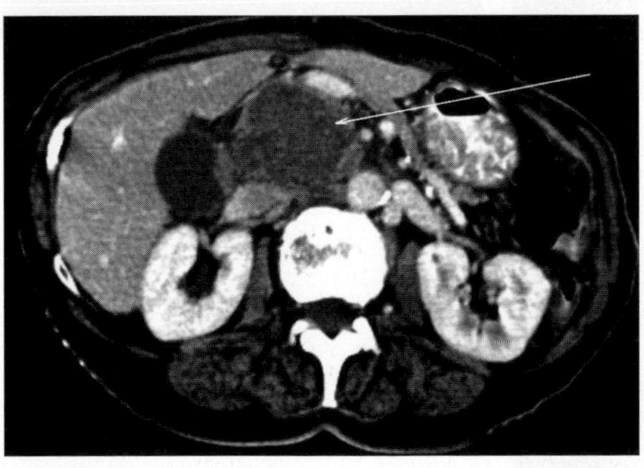

The lesion shown by the arrow is:

A abdominal aortic aneurysm
B acute cholecystitis
C carcinoid of the small intestine
D carcinoma of the head of pancreas
E portal vein thrombosis

4.75 A 42-year-old woman was referred to the clinic with altered sensation in her upper limbs. An MRI spine was performed.

The correct diagnosis is:

A Arnold–Chiari malformation
B Paraspinal abscess
C Spinal cord compression
D Syringomyelia
E Vertebral body fracture

(A) (B)

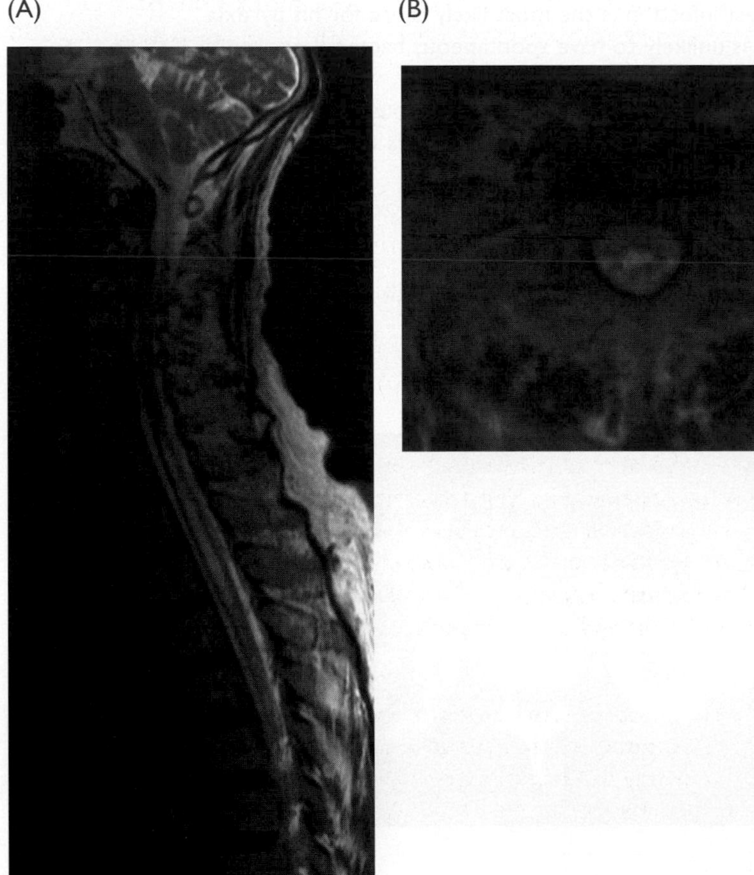

Paper 4

Answers

4.1 **B**** This patient has lone atrial fibrillation (AF). He has no other medical conditions so he would be considered a low risk for cerebrovascular disease. From the Stroke Prevention in Atrial Fibrillation Study, patients under 65 with lone AF would benefit from aspirin, not warfarin.

Warfarin versus aspirin for prevention of thromboembolism in atrial fibrillation: Stroke Prevention in Atrial Fibrillation II Study. *Lancet* 1994; **343**: 687–91

4.2 **D***** The PR interval is prolonged and there are two P waves for each QRS complex. This is fixed 2:1 atrioventricular block.

4.3 **B***** This patient has bradycardia, hypotension and dilated pupils suggestive of a β-blocker overdose. Tricyclic antidepressant overdose would typically cause a tachyarrhythmia. Digoxin would be expected to cause heart block but should not cause mydriasis. Codeine phosphate, as an opiate, would be expected to cause constricted pupils.

4.4 **A**** Impetigo is a superficial skin infection caused by staphylococci and streptococci. It starts with small, red macules that give way to small, fluid-filled vesicles. On top of these form honey-yellow crusting exudates, which may coalesce and enlarge. There may be associated pyrexia and painful lymphadenopathy.

4.5 **A**** The symptoms of cough, weight loss and abdominal pain, which he may have contracted abroad, are suggestive of tuberculosis. There is hyponatraemia, hyperkalaemia and hypoglycaemia. Hyponatraemia is possibly due to the adrenal glands failing to produce aldosterone and the hyperkalaemia is due to the relative deficiency of aldosterone, which helps excrete potassium. Postural hypotension is associated with Addison's disease and is due to relative hypovolaemia and hyponatraemia.

4.6 **A**** Of all the proposals, the only one that would be appropriate as a RCT would be investigating whether atenolol could prevent recurrence of stroke. RCTs are primarily used to test the efficacy of a treatment or intervention and not for diagnosis, determining causality or predicting prognosis.

4.7 **B***** This patient has all the features of Charcot's triad (fever, abdominal pain and jaundice) and so ascending cholangitis is the diagnosis until proven otherwise. Ultrasound should always be performed in the jaundiced patient to see if there is dilatation of the common bile duct and if there are residual stones. Blood cultures would identify the organism and hence confirm the diagnosis. *E. coli,* enterococci and *Pseudomonas* spp are the most likely organisms. ERCP may be necessary to remove a stone in the common bile duct that is acting as the source of infection; but as there is no mention of an ultrasound report, ERCP should not be the first-line investigation and may not give the diagnosis. The patient has a temperature of >39°C, so taking blood cultures is mandatory.

4.8 **C**** To diagnose polycythaemia rubra vera (PRV) secondary causes of erythrocytosis need to be excluded. These include Gaisbock's syndrome where there is polycythaemia secondary to hypoxia and renal tumours. With PRV, there is usually leucocytosis and increased neutrophil alkaline phosphatase score in the absence of infection. There may be an iron deficiency anaemia but there is increased vitamin B_{12} due to increased binding protein transcobalamin I; serum folate is normal. In PRV the serum erythropoietin level would be low, indicating an autonomic proliferative disorder.

4.9 **A**** The slide shows *Aspergillus fumigatus* with the characteristic septated hyphae. The chest X-ray shows two lesions on the right side of the chest, which could represent an aspergilloma. This represents the growth within previously damaged lung tissue of *A. fumigatus.*

4.10 **D**** Patients with HCV are at high risk of developing cirrhosis and hepatocellular carcinoma. As treatment may be curative and prevent both complications from occurring, patients should be encouraged to seek treatment. Continued drug use may reduce his chances of a successful cure but in reality most intravenous drug users do not seek help. Those that do should be treated if they are prepared to see out the course. There are at least six genotypes of which genotype 1 is the most resistant to treatment. The cure rate of genotype 1 is about 50% but can be as high as 80–90% with genotypes 2 and 3. With all genotypes, treatment with ribavirin and pegylated interferon is given for 6 months. Only patients with genotype 1, who have shown clinical improvement with treatment, are given a further 6 months of antiviral treatment. Interferon can cause bone marrow suppression and ribavirin can cause haemolysis, so it is important to monitor the full blood count; thrombocytopaenia is a reason to alter or stop treatment but not at this level.

4.11 **E***** This woman has myasthenia gravis with the characteristic fatigability of neuromuscular junction disease. Myasthenia gravis is an autoimmune disease involving antibodies targeted against the acetylcholine receptors of the neuromuscular junction. It can affect limb muscles as well as the ocular and bulbar muscles. It does not affect the heart and so there are no cardiac abnormalities, but the shortness of breath is due to respiratory muscle involvement. Eaton–Lambert syndrome is also a disorder of neuromuscular transmission but is due to antibodies targeting the presynaptic voltage-gated calcium channels. Unlike myasthenia gravis, muscle strength may improve for a short while after exercise. Also, this condition tends to affect the proximal limb muscles, not involve the bulbar muscles and can be associated with hyporeflexia. Over 60% of cases are associated with small cell carcinoma of the lung. A peripheral neuropathy could not account for all these symptoms.

4.12 B** The picture shows a segment of a white fluffy area radiating out from the disc. The rest of the disc looks normal. This is characteristic of myelinated fibres and does not affect vision.

4.13 A** This patient has a right lobar pneumonia, most probably due to *Streptococcus pneumoniae* acquired in the community. The vast majority of these are still sensitive to penicillin and so amoxicillin would be a sensible choice. There is nothing in the history to suggest that this is tuberculosis or legionnaire's disease.

British Thoracic Society (2001) Guidelines for the Management of Community Acquired Pneumonia in Adults. *Thorax* **56** (Suppl IV).

4.14 C, F, K*** A patient with arthritis, a rash affecting the face and alopecia is most likely to have systemic lupus erythematosus (SLE). To fully diagnose the condition, four of the following criteria need to be fulfilled: discoid rash, non-erosive arthritis, ANA-positive, positive anti-Sm (Smith) antibodies, evidence of haematological disorder (leucopaenia, thrombocytopaenia, normocytic anaemia or Coombs' positive haemolytic anaemia), evidence of renal disorder and serositis. Unlike other arthritides, SLE often has persistently high ESR and a normal CRP. Low C_3 and C_4 can be associated with SLE-induced nephritis. Anti-Ro and Anti-La antibodies may be positive in SLE patients with Sjögren's overlap syndrome.

4.15 D*** This patient has a puffy, thickened myxoedematous face with dry, pale skin and a slight malar flush.

4.16 A** The CT shows a low density area in the middle cerebral artery territory extending to the cortex, with some mass effect in the left fronto-parietal region. This is an acute infarct because the lesion appears hypodense/low attenuation (dark).

4.17 **C**** This barium swallow shows a long stricture with irregular shouldering. This is most likely to be an oesophageal neoplasm.

4.18 **B***** Normally with cardiac catheterisation there should not be large pressure differences as blood crosses between chambers. In this case there is a large pressure drop between the left ventricle and the aorta. This would suggest a stenotic lesion. If there were aortic regurgitation, there would be a large pulse pressure in the aorta.

4.19 **E**** This patient has Wolff–Parkinson–White syndrome with a short PR interval and the slurring upstroke of the delta wave. The treatment of choice is radiofrequency ablation of the accessory pathway.

4.20 **D**** This patient has developed acute liver failure following a paracetamol overdose. Normally the INR will peak at day 3 but even in this case it has reached dangerous limits. The King's College criteria for urgent referral to a specialist unit following paracetamol ingestion include: (1) arterial pH <7.3 following rehydration and at >24 h post overdose; (2) presence of encephalopathy; (3) creatinine >200 or oliguria; (4) PT >50 or INR >3.0 on day 2, PT >75 or INR >4.5 on day 3 and PT >100 or INR >6 on day 4; and (5) severe thrombocytopaenia (the current case is not low enough). Note the importance of the PT/INR, and it is for this reason that, unless a patient is bleeding, fresh frozen plasma should *not* be given to correct the coagulopathy; vitamin K is acceptable, however.

O'Grady JG, Alexander GJM, Hayllar KM, Williams R (1989) Early indicators of prognosis in fulminant hepatic failure. *Gastroenterology* **97**: 439–45

4.21 **C***** This patient has dermatitis artefacta. The lesions are multiple, bear no resemblance to any dermatological disease and are in easy reach of the patient's hands, and physical discomfort is minimal. She needs psychiatric assessment.

4.22 **C***** A man presents with progressive, painless obstructive jaundice and weight loss, as confirmed by dark urine, pale stools and cholestatic liver function tests. The ultrasound report shows dilated intrahepatic ducts in the absence of common bile duct dilatation; this suggests a stricture/obstruction more proximal in the biliary tree. The only two responses compatible with that diagnosis are obstruction at the porta hepatis or sclerosing cholangitis. This is less likely to be primary sclerosing cholangitis (PSC) because there is no previous medical history, particularly no history of inflammatory bowel disease. The cachexia would be in keeping with underlying malignancy, although PSC can be associated with cholangiocarcinoma.

4.23 B*** The sensitivity is the proportion of patients who have the condition that are detected by the test.

	Colon cancer +	**Colon cancer -**	
FOB +	80 (a)	65 (b)	145
FOB -	15 (c)	840 (d)	855
	95	905	1000

Sensitivity = a/a + c = 80/95 = 0.84

4.24 D** This is most likely to be cholestasis induced by flucloxacillin started for his cellulitis. Decompensated liver disease can occur especially after major operations but there is nothing to suggest he had this in the first place. Gallstones, likewise, may cause cholangitis but he is not pyrexial and does not complain of abdominal pain. The low globulin and raised ALP and GGT go against a picture of autoimmune hepatitis.

4.25 A* This slide shows periportal hepatocytes; the portal venule is to the extreme left-hand side. The purple globules are the α_1-antitrypsin, which accumulates and cannot be exported. PAS-D is the stain used to diagnose α_1-antitrypsin deficiency.

4.26 C** Motor neurone disease is a progressive disease of upper and lower motor neurones and can be classified as amyotrophic lateral sclerosis, progressive multiple atrophy and progressive bulbar palsy. There are no sensory signs, or evidence of cerebellar, extrapyramidal or dementia disease. With progressive bulbar palsy patients may present with nasal speech, wasted fasciculating tongue and palatal paralysis. Cervical myelopathy would need to be excluded. Some sensory involvement would be expected. Polio may resemble progressive muscular atrophy but exclusively affects the lower motor neurones. Sensory abnormalities would be expected in syringomyelia and Charcot–Marie–Tooth disease (HSMN).

4.27 B** This patient has respiratory acidosis, as evidenced by a low pH and raised PCO_2. There is also decreased bicarbonate and negative base excess, suggesting a metabolic acidosis as well. The PO_2 is above 8 and so there is no evidence of respiratory failure. These results would be consistent with chronic obstructive airways disease and intra-abdominal perforation. For an explanation of arterial blood gas interpretation, see **1.30**.

4.28 D** Takayasu's arteritis is a large vessel vasculitis and is associated with bruits, claudication, decreased pulses, hypertension, arthralgias and neurological symptoms. There are no specific tests but it is more common in young Asian women, although all racial groups are affected. Antiphospholipid syndrome would be unlikely given her lack of rash, normal platelet count, normal APTT and negative ANA.

4.29 **D**** The ascitic tap reveals chylous ascites, which is associated with obstruction of the thoracic duct and other major lymphatics. Acute pancreatitis does not usually result in ascites but when it does it may be haemorrhagic. The other causes are usually straw-coloured ascites.

4.30 **B**** The X-ray shows subperiosteal bone resorption, bony erosions and some soft tissue and arterial calcification. These are all the hallmarks of hyperparathyroidism.

4.31 **E***** This refugee's chest X-ray and his history of haemoptysis suggest that he has miliary tuberculosis. He should be isolated whilst infectious and started on quadruple anti-TB therapy: rifampicin, isoniazid, pyrazinamide and ethambutol.

4.32 **E**** This patient has signs of aortic stenosis. The intensity of the murmur is related more to the cardiac output than the severity of his condition. The decision to replace the valve depends on whether the patient is symptomatic: syncope, angina or heart failure; has an aortic valve gradient >50 mmHg; or has a surface area <0.8 cm^2 (normal area is 2.5–3.0 cm^2). There is no difference in prognosis between bioprosthetic valves and mechanical valves, even though the former avoid the need for life-long anticoagulation. Aortic valves are easy to replace; mitral valves are more likely to be repaired because of the difficulty in cutting the chordae tendinae in replacing the valve.

4.33 **E***** The cardiac monitor shows asystole. According to the universal treatment algorithm for non-VT/VF, cardiopulmonary resuscitation should be attempted with 30 chest compression to 2 breaths until the airway is secured. Once intravenous access is achieved, 1 mg intravenous adrenaline is given and this is repeated every 3–5 min. The rhythm should be rechecked every 2 min.

4.34 **B*** Circinate balanitis is characterised by small flesh-red erosions, with well-defined margins, which may coalesce. They may cause itching or burning but are often painless. Circinate balanitis and keratoderma blennorrhagicum are characteristic of Reiter's disease. Herpes simplex is associated with painful small ulcers that become vesicles which may burst to leave crusting erosions. Chancres are associated with primary syphilis and usually present as painless, indurated ulcers. Chancroid is a disease caused by *Haemophilus ducreyi* and often presents as one or more painful ulcers with a raised and undermined margin. There may also be associated lymphadenopathy. Condyloma accuminata is due to human papilloma virus and results in cauliflower-like genital warts.

4.35 **B**** This patient has increased prolactin secretion due to a prolactinoma. To diagnose prolactinoma, thyroid and renal disease have to be excluded as well as drug causes. The main regulatory factor in the release of prolactin is tonic inhibition of dopamine secretion by the hypothalamus. MRI pituitary would show the difference between a (non-functioning) macroadenoma and a microadenoma (i.e. differentiate between a tumour invading the pituitary stalk and a prolactin-secreting tumour). The treatment of a prolactinoma involves bromocriptine, a dopamine agonist, with surgery reserved for tumours that do not respond to medical treatment or non-functioning macroadenomas. The other drugs listed can cause high prolactin levels.

4.36 **D**** According to the GMC's guidelines on consent, if a child is under age 16, he/she may give consent if he/she is deemed to have the capacity to understand what the procedure involves, and does not require parental permission. Where a competent child refuses treatment, a person with parental responsibility or a court may authorise treatment or investigation if it is in the child's best interest.

4.37 **B**** The most likely diagnosis is Budd–Chiari syndrome, which is due to thrombosis of the three hepatic veins (right, middle and left). The caudate lobe of the liver drains directly into the inferior vena cava; if a block occurs to the hepatic veins, then there is compensatory hypertrophy of the caudate lobe, making it look enlarged on ultrasound or CT. There are a number of causes of Budd–Chiari syndrome: abdominal trauma; myeloproliferative disease; hepatocellular carcinoma; paroxysmal nocturnal haemoglobinuria; certain tumours like adrenal, pancreas and kidney; and pro-coagulative states like pregnancy, protein S and C deficiency, antithrombin III deficiency and contraceptive pills. In this case, liver failure looks imminent and so prompt referral to a liver unit should be undertaken. Ecstasy overdose can cause acute liver failure but not after 3 weeks.

4.38 **D***** This patient has a radiculopathy at S1, possibly due to a prolapsed intervertebral disc. The hallmark of nerve root disease is pain that may start in the back and radiate down the buttock and leg. Myopathy usually presents as a bilateral symmetrical (proximal) weakness without sensory loss. Peripheral neuropathy typically presents as distal and asymmetrical weakness with fasciculation and sensory loss. Myelopathy/spinal cord disease presents with spastic paraperesis causing symmetrical distal muscle weakness. There may also be a sensory level below which there is a decrease in sensation. Similarly there may be bowel and bladder symptoms. Subcortical lesions would cause a complete hemiparesis affecting the face, arm and leg.

4.39 **C***** Only 10–35% of patients with lung carcinoma have tumours that are surgically resectable. Contraindications include distant metastases involving the liver, brain and spine. Mediastinal spread includes: left recurrent laryngeal nerve involvement (which may result in hoarse voice), oesophagus (dysphagia), pericardium, phrenic nerve (causing high hemidiaphragm) and Horner's syndrome. Hypercalcaemia, if not due to metastases, is not a contraindication to surgery. Lung function tests are performed to assess the patient's ability to withstand thoracotomy pre- and post-operatively. Preoperatively the FEV_1 and FVC should be >50% of predicted; however, patients may survive the operation if the predicted postoperative FEV_1 is >0.8l.

4.40 **C**** This man presents with urethritis, migratory arthritis, skin rash and tenosynovitis. He has multiple sexual partners, which would make him at risk of getting gonorrhoea. Gonococcal arthritis is more common in females than males. Failure to identify the organism in the joint fluid (up to 80%) does not exclude the diagnosis. Secondary syphilis, not primary, can be associated with arthritis. It should be suspected in a patient with a primary chancre, maculopapular rash on the hands and feet, and generalized lymphadenopathy. Behçet's syndrome (see **3.42**) and Reiter's syndrome (see **5.41**) are discussed elsewhere in this book. Ankylosing spondylitis is not associated with genital lesions.

4.41 **B**** The chest X-ray shows a drawing pin in the right lung as the cause of her condition, ruling out the other plausible options.

4.42 **B**** The chest X-ray shows a mass that extends into the neck. Teratoma and thymoma do not extend into the neck. This cannot be a thoracic aortic aneurysm as there is a normal aortic knuckle. Hodgkin's lymphoma would be unlikely as there is no hilar involvement.

4.43 **A**** The photograph of this young boy shows a scar with poor healing, which could be confused for keloid but the associated features are characteristic of Ehlers–Danlos syndrome (EDS). EDS is an inherited disorder of elastic tissue and is associated with increased joint mobility, skin fragility and hyperextensibility. Pseudoxanthoma elasticum involves degeneration and calcification of the elastic fibres of the eyes, skin and arteries. It is associated with cutis laxa, where the skin appears wrinkled and sagging rather than breaking easily.

4.44 C Aplastic anaemia is the most likely diagnosis in a patient with evidence of bone marrow failure, pancytopaenia and no splenomegaly. The trephine shows a hypocellular bone marrow with a lot of fat. In the bone marrow the residual haemopoietic cells are morphologically normal. In her case, the aplasia is most likely due to gold; other drugs that have been implicated include chloramphenicol, phenylbutazone, sulphonamides and nifedipine. Other causes include viruses such as hepatitis, Epstein–Barr virus and human parvovirus B19, interferon-γ and external radiation. Paroxysmal nocturnal haemoglobinuria is closely associated with aplastic anaemia and part of the investigation would be to exclude CD59/PIG-related antigens. Fanconi's anaemia is a congenital form of aplastic anaemia with most patients diagnosed in childhood. Bleeding and infection are the most common presenting conditions. Myelodysplastic syndrome comprises a group of stem cell disorders characterised by dysplasia and recurrent anaemia, which may ultimately transform into an acute leukaemia. Symptoms are non-specific and are often related to underlying anaemia. Hepatosplenomegaly and lymphadenopathy are not characteristic and patients may present only with petechiae secondary to thrombocyto paenia. Bone marrow is characterised by the presence of immature and abnormal precursors.

4.45 E** This patient with Crohn's disease presents with abdominal pain rather than diarrhoea. A colonoscopy shows extensive large bowel involvement. He may have subacute small bowel obstruction due to small bowel involvement or stricture formation. The best test that would show this would be a small bowel enema or follow-through. Capsule endoscopy can look for areas of inflammation and is useful in the investigation of occult bleeding in anaemic patients, but there is the risk of causing bowel obstruction if this patient has strictures.

4.46 D** Seizures are classified as partial if they are confined to one cerebral hemisphere, or generalised if they involve both hemispheres. Partial seizures can be further subdivided into simple if consciousness is not impaired, or complex if there is loss of consciousness. This patient has simple partial seizures associated with an aura. Absence seizures, myoclonic and tonic-clonic seizures are generalised seizures.

4.47 B** This patient has an obstructive lung function picture as the FEV_1:FVC ratio is 46%. All the other options would result in a restrictive pattern. The large TLC makes emphysema much more likely than chronic bronchitis.

4.48 A** Alkaptonuria or ochronosis is a rare defect in tyrosine catabolism due to deficiency of homogentisic acid oxidase. Patients present with degenerative arthritis, aortic stenosis, abnormal pigmentation and deposition of homogentisic acid in the sclera, ear and cochlea, leading to deafness. The arthritis may resemble ankylosing spondylitis but the X-ray findings do not show the annular ossification or sacroiliac joint fusion.

4.49 C** The X-ray appearances are those of bilateral bronchiectasis with dilated bronchi seen end on and longitudinally. There are many causes of bronchiectasis, including respiratory infections in childhood (particularly whooping cough, measles and tuberculosis), cystic fibrosis, hypogammaglobulinaemia states, bronchial obstruction conditions, fibrosis complicating lung infections and allergic bronchopulmonary aspergillosis. Chronic obstructive pulmonary disease does not cause bronchiectasis.

4.50 D* This patient has a squamous cell carcinoma on top of his head. Recognised causes include sunlight and ultraviolet light exposure; radiation; chronic skin injury including burns and ulcers; chemical exposure like arsenic; immunosuppression; and human papilloma virus. Pigmented naevi are associated with the development of melanoma.

4.51 D** This patient has all the classical features of Klinefelter's syndrome: gynaecomastia, small testes and azoospermia. It is caused by an abnormal chromosome complement.

4.52 C* To diagnose hereditary non-polyposis colorectal cancer three criteria have to be satisfied: at least three relatives who have suffered from colorectal cancer; involvement of two generations; and one of the individuals should be aged under 50. Familial adenomatous polyposis and Gardner's syndrome are associated with the development of multiple colonic adenomas.

Vasen HF, Watson P, Mecklin JP, Lynch HT (1999) New clinical criteria for hereditary nonpolyposis colorectal cancer (HNPCC, Lynch syndrome) proposed by the International Collaborative group on HNPCC. *Gastroenterology* **116**: 1453–6.

4.53 C* MEN I syndrome is associated with hyperplasia or neoplastic transformation of the parathyroids, pancreatic islets and pituitary gland. This patient has a prolactinoma, hyperparathyroidism, causing the peptic ulcer, and a probable glucagonoma suggested by the necrolytic migratory erythema and diabetes.

4.54 A** A neoplasm may be a possibility and, if she had a change in bowel habit, anaemia and loss of weight, this would have to be excluded. However, she appears to have acute inflammation with some bleeding rectally, so acute diverticulitis is the most likely diagnosis. Inflammatory bowel disease would be unusual in this age group. Pseudomembranous colitis may be considered if there was a history of antibiotic use.

4.55 A** This patient has a hyperosmolar non-ketotic (HONK) state (see **2.5**). The principles of treatment differ slightly from that of diabetic ketoacidosis (DKA). In DKA the main aim is to rehydrate, correct acidosis and prevent further ketosis. In HONK it is important to treat the underlying cause as well as to rehydrate. Big shifts in the osmolality caused by large doses of insulin to bring down the blood glucose can lead to central pontine myelinolysis; far safer would be to have a small but constant infusion of intravenous insulin and then to use a 'sliding scale' insulin regimen when the blood glucose has come down gradually. Because of the high osmolality there is increased blood viscosity and so thromboembolism is a risk. Gastroparesis can also occur and so nasogastric intubation may be necessary to prevent aspiration. As such patients are not insulin dependent, they will remain diabetic but may not need tablets or insulin once recovered.

4.56 C* This patient with long-standing renal calculi has medullary sponge kidney, as shown by the intravenous pyelogram demonstrating a dilated medullary collecting duct system. In this autosomal recessive condition the flow of urine is slowed from the tubules into the renal pelvis, leading to supersaturation of the urine and stone formation. RTA I is characterised by a defect in urinary acidification and renal ammoniagenesis, which results in a net accumulation of acids within body fluids. Unlike RTA II, where there is a failure to reabsorb bicarbonate ions in the proximal tubule, RTA I results in an inability to excrete H^+ ions in the distal tubule and so urinary pH is never <5.3. Other features of RTA I include association with renal parenchymal disease, normal anion gap and profound hypokalaemia due to increased exchange between Na and K ions at the distal tubule. Feature of RTA II include variable urine pH, serum bicarbonate between 14 and 20, Fanconi's syndrome (hypophosphataemia, hyperuricaemia, glycosuria and volume depletion) and osteomalacia. RTA IV is associated with hyporeninaemic hypoaldosteronism, hyperkalaemia and diabetic nephropathy. Conn's syndrome is a cause of hypokalaemia associated with primary hyperaldosteronism. Bartter's syndrome is a salt-losing state due to defective chloride reabsorption at the loop of Henle and is associated with hypokalaemia and hyperreninaemia.

4.57 B** The blood film shows a long nematode worm between blood cells. They may present with swellings on the limbs known as Calabar swellings.

4.58 C* This patient presents with symptoms of jaundice, conjunctivitis, anaemia and meningism following the onset of a flu-like illness after a camping trip. During that time she may have come into contact with contaminated water and contracted leptospirosis. If allowed to progress it may lead to hepatic failure, meningitis and renal failure. There may occasionally be a rash but this is non-specific. Rocky Mountain spotted fever and Lyme disease are both associated with a characteristic rash and do not cause liver dysfunction.

Histoplasmosis may mimic tuberculosis but she has no chest signs and a clear chest X-ray. Hepatitis A does not usually cause conjunctivitis or meningitis.

4.59 A** The poor prognostic factors for Hodgkin's lymphoma include: male sex, lymphocyte-depleted disease, bulky mediastinal disease, older age and development of B symptoms. B symptoms include unexplained fever, drenching night sweats and weight loss of >10% over 6 months. Subdiaphragmatic disease is associated with wider disseminated disease; in this case, the patient has disease on both sides of the diaphragm, making her stage III disease according to the Ann Arbor staging system.

4.60 A* Alport's syndrome is an X-linked dominant disease where sensorineural deafness presents by age 7 and microscopic haematuria is usually present by age 10. Proteinuria and renal failure tend to develop well into adulthood. Ocular abnormalities can also occur and include myopia, retinitis pigmentosa, anterior lenticonus and cataracts. Urogenital investigations reveal no evidence of structural abnormalities. Juvenile nephronophthisis is an inherited tubulointerstitial nephropathy, which eventually leads to renal failure, and patients present with polyuria, polydipsia and weight loss, progressive loss of vision (secondary to retinal degeneration) and small, cystic, hyperechoic kidneys on ultrasound. Fabry's disease is an X-linked recessive deficiency of α-galactosidase A, which leads to progressive haematuria, proteinuria, renal failure, skin lesions and peripheral neuropathy. Thin basement membrane disease is an autosomal dominant condition characterised by persistent microscopic haematuria but normal renal function. Autosomal dominant polycystic kidney disease tends to present with loin pain, haematuria, renal dysfunction, hypertension, nephrolithiasis and recurrent urinary tract infections; there may also be extrarenal complications, including liver cysts and fibrosis, intracranial and aortic aneurysms, colonic diverticula and pancreatic cysts.

4.61 E** Wireless capsule endoscopy is a method of visualizing the gastrointestinal tract from the oesophagus down to the caecum. The patient swallows the 'pill' containing a camera while wearing a sensor attached to the abdomen. The camera records two images per second over an 8 h period before the pill is excreted with normal bowel movements. The picture shows multiple, small, slender pinworms or *Enterobius vermicularis*. They are often an incidental finding and are usually found in the caecum, appendix and right side of the colon. Unlike hookworms, which may be associated with anaemia, pinworms can be associated with diarrhoea and pruritus ani. Pinworms do not penetrate the intestinal wall and so are not associated with an eosinophilia. The treatment of choice is mebendazole; praziquantel is used to treat other helminth infections such as schistosomiasis and *Taenia solium* infections. Reinfection after treatment is common.

4.62 C*** This patient has elevated ALT, most likely secondary to fatty liver/non-alcoholic steatohepatitis. In a proportion of patients this can progress to fibrosis and cirrhosis. However, in this case the patient needs to be encouraged to lose weight, eat less and exercise more as he is at risk of developing the metabolic syndrome. The most sensible measure would be to review his liver function tests in 4–6 months and, assuming he has lost some weight, only then make a decision on a liver biopsy if these have worsened. Statins are useful in patients with metabolic syndrome and hypercholesterolaemia but can cause deterioration of liver function tests. These need to be carefully monitored once started.

4.63 B* ICD generator batteries typically last 7 years but this depends on the number of shocks delivered. ICDs can be inserted as primary prophylaxis in patients who have had a MI and are NYHA heart failure grade 3. Patients with grade 4 heart failure have a very high mortality from progressive pump failure. ICDs are indicated for primary prophylaxis, including familial conditions such as Brugada syndrome, arrhythmogenic right ventricular dysplasia, hypertrophic cardiomyopathy, and in patients who have had surgery for congenital heart disease. Brugada syndrome is a rare inherited condition which can cause sudden death due to the development of life-threatening ventricular arrhythmias. It is characterised on the ECG by a 'pseudo' right bundle branch block with ST elevation in V_{1-3}. It can be unmasked in patients given a sodium channel blocker, like flecainide or procainamide. ICDs should avoid the need for having to be on antiarrhythmic agents but in some cases additional treatment with amiodarone can be given. If that is the case, an electrophysiological study should be done after loading the drug as there may be interactions and an increase in the defibrillation threshold.

4.64 C*** The first step in evaluating a pleural effusion is to determine whether it is a transudate or an exudate. Transudate effusions are due to systemic factors which alter the balance of production and absorption of pleural fluid, although capillary permeability is normal, i.e. heart failure, hypoalbuminaemia, nephrotic syndrome and cirrhosis. Exudative effusions occur as a result of local factors affecting the pleural surface and/or capillary permeability, i.e. neoplastic disease, parapneumonic effusions and rheumatoid arthritis. Transudate effusions usually respond to treatment of the underlying disease, while exudate effusions require further investigation. Transudates have a pleural protein content <30 g/L and exudates have pleural protein content greater than this. A more accurate diagnostic method, however, is to use Light's criteria. Pleural fluid is exudative if one or more of the following criteria are met: (1) pleural fluid protein divided by serum protein is >0.5; (2) pleural fluid LDH divided by serum LDH is >0.6; and (3) pleural fluid LDH is more than two-thirds the upper limit of normal of serum LDH. Normal fluid pH is 7.60 (due to the high bicarbonate concentration) while a pH ≤7.20 is consistent with empyema. Infective pleural effusions are associated with low pH ≤ low glucose, high protein and high LDH. Pleural fluid white cell count and differential can give an indication of the cause: predominant neutrophilia is associated with parapneumonic effusions and pulmonary embolism; lymphocytosis is consistent with tuberculosis and malignancy. The lung cancer detection rate from fluid cytology is approximately 60%, but greater for adenocarcinoma than squamous cell carcinoma. CT chest should be performed prior to drainage of the effusion as pleural abnormalities will be better visualized by CT.

Light RW (2001) *Pleural Diseases*, 4th ed. New York: Lippincott Williams & Wilkins. Maskell NA, Butland RJA (2003) BTS guidelines for the investigation of a unilateral pleural effusion in adults. *Thorax* **58** (Suppl II): ii8–ii17

4.65 C** A young woman with oligomenorrhoea, now developing into secondary amenorrhoea, but normal sexual development, raised LH and testosterone, hirsutism, obesity and acanthosis nigricans is suggestive of polycystic ovary syndrome (PCOS). According to the modified Rotterdam criteria to diagnose PCOS, patients need to have two of the following three criteria: (1) oligomenorrhoea $\pm$ anovulation; (2) clinical and/or biochemical signs of hyperandrogenism: raised testosterone and dehydroepiandrosterone-sulphate DHEA and decreased sex hormone binding globulin; and (3) 12 or more follicles in each ovary measuring 2–9 mm in diameter and/or increased ovarian volume (>10 ml). Imaging is not necessary to make a diagnosis of PCOS. A differential diagnosis for PCOS is late-onset 21-hydroxylase deficiency congenital adrenal hyperplasia but there would be increased levels of 17-hydroxyprogesterone, especially in response to ACTH stimulation. A normal FSH goes against a diagnosis of primary ovarian failure. There are a number of definitions of the metabolic syndrome but a commonly used set of criteria is that of the International Diabetes Federation: central obesity/increased waist circumference (>94 cm) *plus* any two of the following: (1) raised triglyceride level (>1.7 mmol/L); (2) reduced high density lipoprotein cholesterol (HDL-C) (<1.03 mmol/L in males and <1.29 mmol/L in females); (3) raised blood pressure ≥130/85 mmHg or the need to be on antihypertensives; and (4) raised fasting plasma glucose (≥5.6 mmol/L) or previously diagnosed type 2 diabetes.

Rotterdam Consensus Working Group (2004) Revised 2003 consensus on diagnostic criteria and long-term health risks related to polycystic ovary syndrome (PCOS). *Hum Reprod* **19**: 41–7

Alberti KG; Zimmet P; Shaw J (2005) The metabolic syndrome – a new worldwide definition. *Lancet* **366**: 1059–62

4.66 D** This patient is acutely unwell post renal transplant. The main possibilities are urinary tract infection, arterial or venous thrombosis, drug toxicity or acute cellular rejection. The most important initial test is a renal ultrasound with Doppler to exclude any arterial or venous thrombosis. Other tests that should be done include MSU, tacrolimus level, CMV and BK virus serology. If the tacrolimus level were high, this would need to be reduced and then observe what effect this has on renal function. If the tacrolimus level were low and the ultrasound were normal, a MAG 3 scan should be done to look at perfusion of the graft. Following this, a renal biopsy may be performed to look for rejection and, if present, steroids started.

4.67 B* This patient with progressive memory loss and cognitive deterioration with no metabolic or other neurological cause for his dementia most likely has Alzheimer's disease (AD). The diagnosis is usually made on clinical grounds; while the brains of patients are characterized by the deposition of amyloid-beta protein, neurofibrillary tangles and senile plaques, there are no specific laboratory or imaging diagnostic tests. In AD, there is a decrease in acetylcholine production and this worsens with disease progression. Anti-cholinesterase drugs like donepezil, rivastigmine and galantamine have been shown to slow the progression of the disease. Pyridostigmine is an anti-cholinesterase which works at the neuromuscular junction but it is used in the treatment of myasthenia gravis. There is no evidence of parkinsonism and so levodopa and amantadine are not indicated. Reserpine is a dopamine antagonist used in treating psychosis.

4.68 E*** Toxic shock syndrome (TSS) is an inflammatory response to a particular exotoxin produced by *Staphylococcus aureus* or group A β-haemolytic streptococci. The exotoxin can act as a superantigen and lead to the activation of multiple T cells, resulting in massive cytokine response. Staphylococcal TSS is characterized by fever, hypotension and diffuse macular erythematous rash *plus* involvement of three or more organ systems. Streptococcal TSS is also characterized by hypotension, fever and rash *plus* isolation of group A streptococcus from a sterile (i.e. CSF) or non-sterile (i.e. throat) site *plus* involvement of two or more organ systems. TSS is most prevalent in menstruating females, especially with the use of super absorbent tampons, but can also occur following operations and post partum. The mainstay of treatment is aggressive fluid replacement with or without pressor agents, a search for the source of infection and broad-spectrum antibiotics that will cover both organisms. As she has contracted the infection in hospital there is a risk of this infection being MRSA.

4.69 B* This patient has hepatitis B. In a significant proportion of patients the virus is active but a mutation prevents them from producing HBeAg; these have been referred to as pre-core mutants. If HBV DNA level was performed and it was positive and very elevated, this patient may need treatment for his hepatitis B. Percutaneous liver biopsy is an important investigation but should be delayed until an ultrasound of the liver is performed to ensure there is no focal liver lesion or ascites.

4.70 D* Massive transfusion is defined as replacement of >50% of blood volume in 12–24 h, and is associated with a number of homeostatic and metabolic complications. Packed cells are devoid of platelets and clotting factors which are removed soon after collection. This transfusion dilutes the patient's own platelets and coagulation proteins and can result in thrombocytopaenia and disseminated intravascular coagulation. To help store the blood, sodium citrate is added. This can bind to ionized calcium and lead to a significant fall in the plasma free calcium concentration. Citrate also generates bicarbonate so that metabolic alkalosis can occur if the kidneys fail to excrete bicarbonate in the urine. Blood is typically stored at 1–6 °C and rapid transfusion can lead to an abrupt cooling of core temperature, which may result in arrhythmias developing: a blood warmer should be used whenever >3 units of blood are transfused.

4.71 B* ** The blood film shows a myeloblast with a number of Auer rods in the cytoplasm. This is characteristic of acute myeloid leukaemia.

4.72 C* Hepatoblastoma, neuroblastoma and Wilm's tumour (nephroblastoma) may all present as abdominal masses in children. Wilm's tumour arises from the kidney and can be associated with haematuria and hypertension. Hepatoblastoma is excluded by a normal liver on ultrasound. Neuroblastomas arise from neural crest tissue with the most common sites being the adrenal medulla retroperitoneal sympathetic nervous tissue, although a number of other primary sites occur and present with different signs and symptoms ranging from back pain, cord compression and loss of bladder control to Horner's syndrome and myoclonus. Though urinalysis shows increased homovanillic acid (HVA) and vanillylmandelic acid (VMA), unlike phaeochromocytoma, neuroblastomas rarely present with sweating, hypertension and diarrhoea.

4.73 E** This patient probably has developed sepsis but the source is not clear. The bilateral basal atelectasis on the X-ray could be due to his previous chest infection and does not conclusively point to a chest source. He has not passed any urine for 5 days and therefore a urinary catheter is only acting as a source of infection in a patient who is being filtered; it can be re-introduced when his kidney function recovers. Line sepsis is a possibility and the risk of this occurring is increased when lines have been in for longer than 7 days even if there is no evidence of local cellulitis. Any patient with ascites could potentially develop spontaneous bacterial peritonitis. The ascites is more likely due to his acute inflammatory condition and hypoalbuminaemic state rather than liver dysfunction. Antibiotic treatment should be guided by the patient's clinical state and likely source of infection.

4.74 D** The large central mass, which is slightly irregular in shape and appears to be squashing the duodenum, is highly suspicious of a pancreatic head neoplasm. The gallbladder is to the right of this structure. The aorta is posterior and to the left of the mass; an aortic aneurysm would have to encompass the true lumen and would typically have a calcified rim, whereas this lesion is separate from the aorta. Carcinoid of the small intestine would appear as a small lesion with serpiginous lines fanning out into the surrounding fat.

4.75 **D******* The coronal MRI shows the syrinx in the centre of the spinal cord. The sagittal section shows a white line within the spinal cord beginning at C7 and extending to T3. There is no Arnold–Chiari formation because there is no herniation of the cerebellar tonsils through the foramen magnum.

Paper 5

Questions

5.1 A 67-year-old male patient on the ward developed severe central chest pain that did not respond to glyceryl trinitrate. He had been admitted 2 days ago with progressive shortness of breath on exertion but no chest pain. The pain radiated up to the neck and he felt nauseous. He had a previous medical history of hypertension and chronic renal failure. His only medication was furosemide and enalapril. He smoked 20 cigarettes a day and drank 2 units of alcohol a week. There was a family history of myocardial infarction.

On examination he was in pain, looked unwell and was sweating. His temperature was 36.6°C, pulse 100 regular and blood pressure 150/88. His JVP was not elevated and heart sounds were normal with no murmurs, but he did have bilateral crackles in his chest. Abdominal examination was normal.

Bloods	Hb	12.0	WCC	9.3
	Platelets	400	Na	143
	K	4.1	Urea	15.4
	Creatinine	220	Glucose	4.2
	Magnesium	0.86		
Chest X-ray	Some upper lobe blood diversion			
	No pulmonary oedema			
ECG	T wave inversion V_{4-6} present on admission			

The patient was suspected of having an acute coronary syndrome/non Q-wave MI.

The most important diagnostic test to enable urgent further treatment would be:

- A development of right bundle branch block on further ECG
- B plasma BNP (B-type natriuretic peptide)
- C serum CK-MB (creatine kinase)
- D serum LDH
- E serum troponin T and I

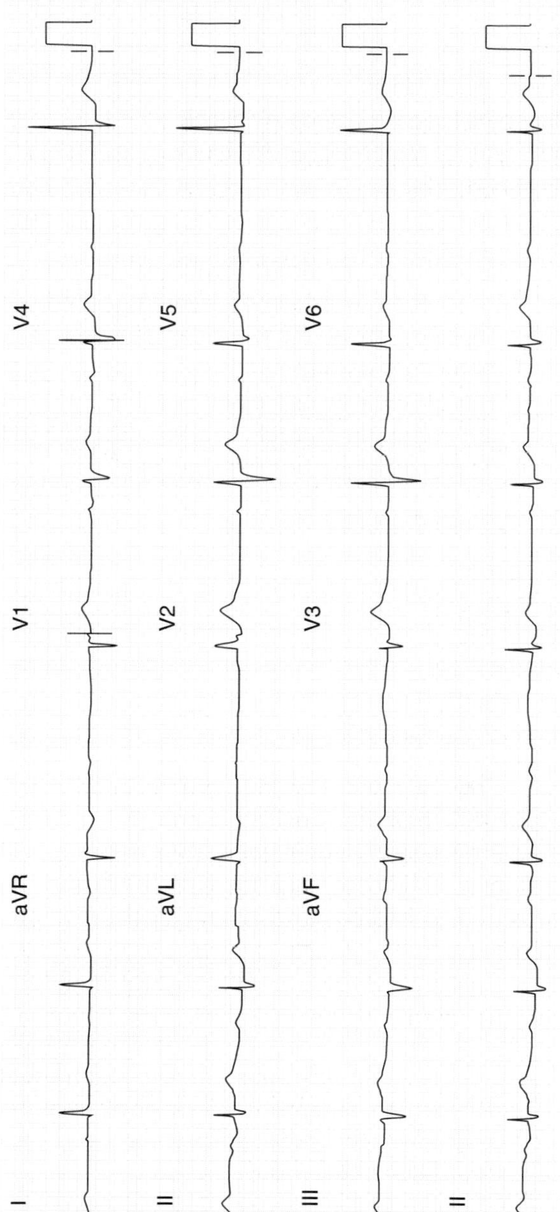
I
aVR
V1
V4
II
aVL
V2
V5
III
aVF
V3
V6
II

5.2 A 73-year-old man was referred with collapse.

His ECG shows:

A first-degree AV block
B complete heart block
C Mobitz type I second-degree AV block
D Mobitz type II second-degree AV block
E sinus bradycardia

5.3 A 19-year-old girl was admitted with difficulty in swallowing; 36 h previously she took an overdose of metoclopramide. Over the last 3 h she had developed progressively worse dysphagia and drooling. She also complained of blurred vision.

On examination she was distressed but alert. There was drooping of the left side of her mouth. Her left eye was deviated to the left. The rest of her cranial nerve examination was normal.

The treatment of choice for this patient is:

A adrenaline
B chlorphenamine
C hydrocortisone
D prochlorperazine
E procyclidine

5.4 A 37-year-old woman was admitted with headache, fever, neck stiffness and malaise. She had also noticed a non-pruritic rash on her left leg, which had progressively got bigger. Two weeks ago she had returned from a camping holiday in the USA with her family. No one else in her family was ill. She had no previous medical problems and was not on any medication.

On examination she had a temperature of 38.3°C and bilateral, tender, cervical lymphadenopathy. Her pulse was 92 regular and blood pressure 135/78. There was some tenderness in her lower limb joints but no swelling, erythema or effusions, and she had normal range of movements. Cranial nerve examination was normal. (Figure 5.4, page 392.)

The skin rash is most likely to be:

A erythema chronicum migrans
B erythema gyratum repens
C erythema marginatum
D erythema nodosum
E granuloma annulare

5.5 A 45-year-old man presented with worsening chest pain that came on with exertion. He was a smoker and drank 5 units of alcohol a day. He had no other medical problems and was not on any medication.

He was rather obese on examination. His pulse was 80 regular and his blood pressure was 130/80.

Bloods	Glucose	12.0	TSH	2.5
	Free T_4	20.5	Cholesterol	3.5
	Triglycerides	35	LDL cholesterol	2.7
	HDL cholesterol	0.8		

Aside from lifestyle changes, the drug treatment of choice is:

A bezafibrate
B cholestyramine
C nicotinic acid
D simvastatin
E thyroxine

5.6 A large randomised controlled trial (RCT) comparing aspirin to warfarin in preventing recurrence of ischaemic stroke was published. All 2000 patients had a previous history of ischaemic stroke, of whom 1000 patients were male. The age ranges for the two groups were similar. Randomisation was determined by the toss of a coin. All patients received the same care apart from the drug being investigated. There were equal numbers of withdrawals from both groups. Both groups' data were analysed in exactly the same way and on an intention to treat basis. A significant reduction in recurrence of stroke in the warfarin group (absolute risk reduction 10%; 95% confidence interval 120–443) was found.

The Type of flaw that occurred in this study is:

A detection bias
B exclusion bias
C performance bias
D recall bias
E selection bias

5.7 A 66-year-old man was referred for PEG (percutaneous endoscopic gastrostomy) tube insertion. A stroke 4 weeks ago had affected his swallowing and he was currently fed via a nasogastric tube which he kept pulling out.

Endoscopic placement of a PEG can safely and successfully be undertaken in:

A achalasia
B ascites
C morbid obesity
D partial gastrectomy
E small bowel obstruction

5.8 A 14-year-old Afro-Caribbean boy presented with severe abdominal pain and shortness of breath for 1 day. He was known to suffer from sickle cell anaemia and had had similar attacks before but could not remember how they had been treated. He was not on any medication and had no other medical problems.

On examination he was in pain and jaundiced. His temperature was 37.5°C, pulse 100 regular and blood pressure 98/60. His respiratory rate was 22 breaths/min and his chest was clear. He had tender hepatomegaly with no lymphadenopathy or ascites. There was no pain in his limbs. Neurological examination was normal.

Bloods	Hb	3.5	MCV	60.2
	WCC	4.0	Platelets	320
	Reticulocytes	18%	Na	135
	K	4.0	Urea	3.3
	Creatinine	70	Protein	65
	Albumin	35	Bilirubin	80
	ALT	25	ALP	345
Chest X-ray	Normal			

The type of flow that occurred in this study is:

A acute chest syndrome
B aplastic
C haemolytic
D infarctive
E sequestration

5.9 A 49-year-old man was referred with a shortness of breath on exertion associated with a non-productive cough. He had normal exercise tolerance and no cardiac history. He had a normal appetite and no loss of weight. He had smoked 15 cigarettes a day for over 20 years. He had no other medical problems, was not on any medication and had not travelled abroad recently.

On examination he was apyrexial, pulse 79 regular and blood pressure 138/88. His respiratory rate was 18 breaths/min and his chest sounded clear.

Chest X-ray	Right hilar lymphadenopathy
Lymph node biopsy	(Figure 5.9, page 392.)

The most likely diagnosis is:

- A lipoma
- B lung carcinoma
- C lymphoma
- D reactive lymphadenopathy
- E sarcoidosis

5.10 A 36-year-old male nurse had a pre-employment health screen. He was originally from Mozambique and had no history to suggest high risk behaviour. He felt well and had a normal appetite with no weight loss. He was married with one son.

Physical examination was normal.

Bloods	Albumin	38	Bilirubin	12
	ALT	78	ALP	110
	INR	1.0		
HBsAg	Positive			
HBeAg	Positive			
Total anti-HBc	Positive			
IgM anti-HBc	Positive			
Anti-HBe	Negative			
HBV DNA	1 x 10^7 IU/ml			

Concerning his diagnosis and management it is correct that:

- A he has evidence of recently acquired hepatitis B
- B he should be screened for HIV and hepatitis D
- C he should be treated with interferon and ribavirin
- D hepatocellular carcinoma is a risk only if there is evidence of cirrhosis
- E his wife and son should be treated with hepatitis B immunoglobulin

5.11 A 60-year-old woman presented with progressive fatigue and weakness. She found writing a real struggle and had to stop often. However, there were no paraesthesiae and her symptoms improved with rest. She also complained of some double vision, dysphagia and shortness of breath on exertion. She had had no recent illnesses.

On examination she had bilateral ptosis and strabismus. Her face lacked expression and her voice was weak and nasal. The rest of her cranial nerve examination was normal. Her pulse was 72 regular and blood pressure was 120/80. Respiratory examination was normal. There was no limb muscle wasting or weakness. Tone, power, reflexes and sensation in upper and lower limbs were normal.

The test that would give the definitive diagnosis is:

A anti-Jo I antibodies
B edrophonium (tensilon) test
C muscle biopsy
D nerve conduction studies
E temporal artery biopsy

5.12 A 55-year-old woman was referred with blurred vision. Fundoscopy was performed. (Figure 5.12, page 393.)

The fundoscopic appearance is most likely due to:

A choroidoretinitis
B hypertensive retinopathy
C optic atrophy
D retinal artery occlusion
E retinitis pigmentosa

5.13 A 22-year-old known asthmatic man presented very wheezy to Accident & Emergency. Three days previously he had developed a cough productive of white sputum. Since then he had become increasingly short of breath and was using his inhalers much more frequently. His asthma had been well controlled and he had never been admitted to hospital because of it. He did not have a nebuliser at home. The ambulance crew had put him on high flow oxygen and given him two nebules of salbutamol. He had now been treated for over an hour with another nebule of 5 mg salbutamol and 100 mg of hydrocortisone, but there was no improvement in his clinical state.

On examination, he was panting and sitting forward. He was unable to complete a sentence or perform a peak flow. His temperature was 37.8°C, pulse 120 regular and blood pressure 95/60. Respiratory examination revealed central trachea, intercostal recession, respiratory rate 32 breaths/min and soft bilateral wheeze.

Bloods	Hb	14.6	WCC	9.0
	Platelets	368	Neutrophils	5.5
	Na	140	K	3.9
	Urea	3.9	Creatinine	65
	O_2 saturation	93%		

Concerning his immediate management, it is correct that:

A aminophylline has no role in the management of acute asthma
B a chest X-ray should be done as soon as possible
C he should be treated with intravenous benzyl penicillin and clarithromycin
D he should be treated with intravenous magnesium sulphate regularly
E he should be treated with nebulised ipratropium bromide using oxygen

5.14 A 67-year-old woman was admitted with melaena having passed 500 ml of black stools. She had no abdominal pain, was not on NSAIDs or anti-coagulants and did not drink alcohol. She suffered with intermittent dysphagia and arthritis affecting her hands. She also complained that her hands changed colour if she put them in cold water. She no longer smoked cigarettes.

On examination she looked pale. She had telangiectasia on her face, lips and neck. Her pulse was 98 and blood pressure 135/90 with no postural drop on standing. Respiratory examination was normal. Her abdomen was soft and tender. Rectal examination confirmed melaena. The skin of her hands was thickened and rough and her fingers were thin and spindly. The wrist and finger joints were tender but not obviously inflamed and she had normal range of movements.

Bloods				
	Hb	9.8	MCV	73.6
	WCC	7.9	Platelets	450
	Na	145	K	4.2
	Urea	8.7	Creatinine	99
	Protein	70	Albumin	35
	Bilirubin	12	ALT	16
	ALP	56	ESR	35
	CRP	28		

The most likely diagnosis is:

A amyloidosis
B CREST syndrome
C hereditary haemorrhagic telangiectasia
D Sjögren's syndrome
E systemic sclerosis

5.15 A 45-year-old man was referred for endoscopy because of indigestion. (Figure 5.15, page 393.)

The endoscopic findings are consistent with:

A Barrett's oesophagus
B benign oesophageal stricture
C oesophageal candidiasis
D oesophageal varices
E Schatzki ring

5.16 A 62-year-old man presented with collapse. His GCS at the time of presentation was 14/15.

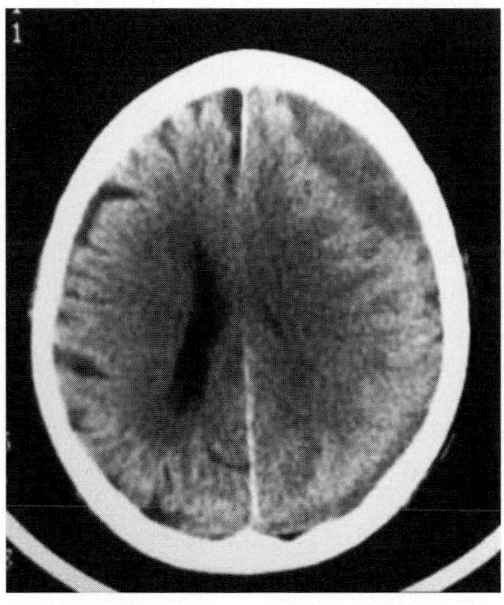

The CT scan shows:

A extradural haematoma
B hydrocephalus
C intracerebral haemorrhage
D subarachnoid haemorrhage
E subdural haematoma

5.17 A 35-year-old HIV-positive man presented with headaches. He had no neck stiffness or personality change.

On examination he had a temperature of 38.1°C and cervical lymphadenopathy. There was no rash. His pulse was 88 regular and blood pressure 120/78. Chest examination was normal. Fundoscopy and cranial nerve examination were normal.

Chest X-ray Normal
CT head

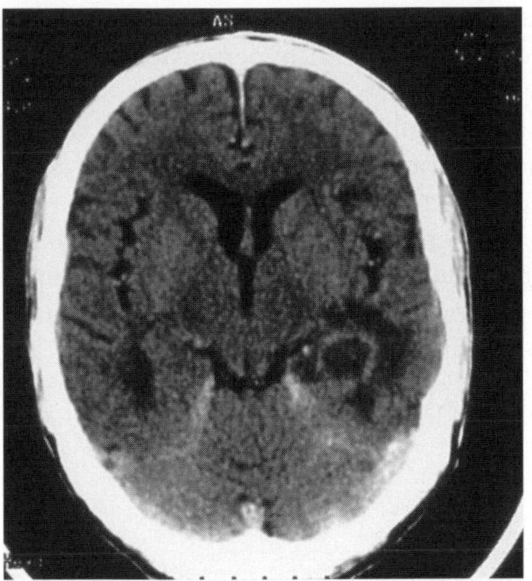

This patient should be started on:

- A aciclovir
- B cefotaxime
- C co-trimoxazole
- D dexamethasone
- E pyrimethamine and sulphadiazine

5.18 A 15-year-old boy was referred because he found that he became short of breath when he tried to play football with his friends. He had to stop after only a few minutes and this was progressively getting worse. He had no previous medical problems and was not on any medication.

On examination he looked well and was not cyanosed. His pulse was 75 regular and blood pressure 120/72. His JVP was just visible and he had a fixed split second heart sound. There was a systolic murmur, loudest at the left upper sternal edge. The apex was not displaced. Respiratory examination was normal.

ECG Right bundle branch block
Right axis deviation
No ischaemic changes

The most likely diagnosis is:

- A Fallot's tetralogy
- B ostium primum atrial septal defect
- C ostium secundum atrial septal defect
- D patent ductus arteriosus
- E ventricular septal defect

5.19 A 64-year-old man presented with acute diplopia, dysphagia and dysarthria. He suffered from diabetes and hypertension. He had never had these symptoms before.

On examination he had a right Horner's syndrome. There was decreased temperature and pinprick sensation on the right side of the face. There was right-sided palatal paralysis with absent gag reflex. He had right-sided ataxia and nystagmus. There was no dysphasia but some dysarthria. There was normal tone, power and reflexes in the upper and lower limbs but decreased pinprick sensation on the left upper and lower limbs.

The blood vessel most likely to be occluded is:

A basilar artery
B middle cerebral artery
C posterior cerebral artery
D posterior inferior cerebellar artery
E superior cerebellar artery

5.20 A 45-year-old man was referred because of a 3-day history of severe pain in his right middle finger. (Figure 5.20, page 393.)

The most likely diagnosis is:

A Heberden's node
B rheumatoid nodule
C septic arthritis
D tophaceous gout
E tuberous xanthoma

5.21 A 75-year-old Caucasian woman suffered a fall at home. Her daughter was concerned she had osteoporosis. A DEXA scan was performed and the patient has returned wanting to know the result.

DEXA scan of total hip	T score	–0.8
	Z score	–0.5

The interpretation of the DEXA scan result is:

A normal bone mass
B osteopaenia appropriate for her age
C osteopaenia inappropriate for her age
D osteoporosis appropriate for her age
E osteoporosis inappropriate for her age

5.22 A 35-year-old woman who was 27 weeks pregnant was admitted with severe headache and blurred vision. She reported no neck stiffness or photophobia. She had no previous medical problems. This was her first pregnancy and up until now she had had no complications. She was not on any medication.

On examination she had a temperature of 38.1°C, pulse 100 regular and blood pressure 100/68. Chest and heart sounds were clear. Her abdomen was distended consistent with pregnancy. There was no focal neurological defect and plantar responses were flexor. She had widespread purpuric lesions on her back and lower limbs. There was no peripheral oedema.

Bloods	Hb	8.0	MCV	106.2
	WCC	23.2	Neutrophils	19.1
	Platelets	35	Reticulocytes	13%
	INR	1.0	Na	137
	K	4.4	Urea	35.3
	Creatinine	300	Protein	68
	Albumin	37	Bilirubin	35
	ALT	20	ALP	96
	GGT	50		
Blood film	Red cell fragments			
Chest X-ray	Normal			

The most likely diagnosis is:

A disseminated intravascular coagulopathy
B fatty liver of pregnancy
C pre-eclampsia
D thrombotic thrombocytopaenic purpura
E toxic shock syndrome

5.23 It had been proposed that helical CT chest could be used to screen for lung carcinoma. A trial in 500 patients was carried out and 140 cases of carcinoma developed. CT detected 60 cases and 25 false-positives.

The specificity of CT as a screening test is:

A 60/85
B 60/140
C 335/360
D 335/415
E 395/500

5.24 A 64-year-old woman with osteoarthritis presented with a several month history of lethargy and itching, which kept her awake at night. She had decreased appetite but had been putting on weight, which she attributed to her abdomen becoming larger.

On examination there were scratch marks over her forearms and legs. She had moderate ascites and 3 cm hepatomegaly.

Bloods	Hb	12.4	WCC	5.7
	Platelets	100	Bilirubin	38
	Albumin	32	Protein	69
	ALT	40	ALP	170
	GGT	120		

This patient should be treated with:

A azathioprine
B chlorphenamine
C cholestyramine
D penicillamine
E prednisolone

5.25 A 16-year-old boy presented with a 3-day history of bleeding gums and generalised purpura.

On examination he had a temperature of 39.1°C. He had bilateral cervical lymphadenopathy and palpable splenomegaly.

Bloods	Hb	13.1	WCC	2.9
	Platelets	30		
Blood film	Atypical lymphocytes			

The most likely diagnosis is:

A acute lymphoblastic leukaemia
B acute myeloid leukaemia
C aplastic anaemia
D Henoch-Schönlein purpura
E infectious mononucleosis

5.26 A 25-year-old HIV-positive man was admitted with bloody diarrhoea that had been going on for 3 weeks. He had a decreased appetite and some weight loss. He was not on any medication. He contracted HIV from an infected needle but was hepatitis B and C negative. He did not drink alcohol but did smoke.

On examination he looked thin. His temperature was 37.3°C, pulse 88 regular and blood pressure 130/89. His chest was clear. His abdomen was generally tender with no organomegaly. Rectal examination revealed no masses.

Chest X-ray Normal

Colonoscopy was performed and biopsies were taken. (Figure 5.26, page 394.)

The most likely diagnosis is:

A cytomegalovirus colitis
B giardiasis
C Kaposi's sarcoma
D *Mycobacterium avium intracellulare* complex
E *Mycobacterium tuberculosis*

5.27 A 36-year-old woman was admitted from Accident & Emergency with a provisional diagnosis of deliberate self-harm because she kept burning herself with cigarettes. She denied any suicidal ideation but felt depressed that she had no pain sensation in her hands, which were ugly and deformed. She had no previous medical history and no family history of note. She was a heavy smoker.

On examination she had right Horner's syndrome and mild kyphosis of her spine. There was no cyanosis or lymphadenopathy. There was wasting of the small muscles of her hands but tone, power and reflexes in her upper limbs was decreased. There was loss of pinprick sensation but intact light touch and vibration sense. In her legs there was increased tone, some muscle weakness, increased reflexes and extensor plantars but she was able to walk. Cranial nerve examination was normal. Examination of the cardiovascular and respiratory systems revealed no abnormality.

The most likely diagnosis is:

A cervical myelopathy
B Charcot–Marie–Tooth disease (HSMN)
C motor neurone disease
D Pancoast's tumour
E syringomyelia

5.28 A 68-year-old woman who was known to have chronic obstructive pulmonary disease was admitted with shortness of breath. She was on home nebulisers of salbutamol and ipratropium bromide but not home oxygen. Her last admission with the same problem was 6 months ago and she had never required ventilation. Today she had used her nebuliser four times without relief. The ambulance crew had given her another two nebules plus oxygen.

On examination in Accident & Emergency she was on 40% oxygen. She was drowsy. Her temperature was 36.9°C, pulse 120 regular and blood pressure 130/80. Respiratory rate was 26 breaths/min but she was unable to talk in full sentences. She had bilateral wheeze in her chest.

Arterial blood gases on 40% O_2	pH	7.25	PCO_2	10.5
	PO_2	9.5	Bicarbonate	34
	Base excess	6.2	O_2 saturation	90%
Chest X-ray	No pneumothorax or consolidation			
	Hyperinflated lungs			

The next most appropriate immediate management step would be to:

A increase the oxygen to 60% with a rebreathing bag and repeat arterial blood gases in 30 min
B reduce the oxygen to 28% and repeat arterial blood gases in 30 min
C start a doxapram infusion
D start non-invasive partial pressure ventilation
E start on oral prednisolone and oral antibiotics

5.29 A 45-year-old man was referred with bilateral paraesthesia up to mid-shin that had been present for 3 months. He also complained of pain in his hips and knees and had a purpuric rash on his legs. He used to be an intravenous drug abuser and 6 months ago had become jaundiced, which had resolved spontaneously.

On examination he was not in pain. His temperature was 36.5°C, pulse 78 regular and blood pressure 147/76. Respiratory examination was normal. He had mild abdominal tenderness but no organomegaly. He had decreased sensation to light touch and pinprick up to the level of mid-shin. There was normal lower limb tone and power but absent ankle and plantar reflexes.

Bloods	Hb	11.9	MCV	92.4
	WCC	7.6	Platelets	459
	Na	138	K	4.8
	Urea	10.8	Creatinine	130
	Protein	74	Albumin	38
	Bilirubin	15	ALT	55
	ALP	100	ESR	65
	CRP	58	C_3	70
	C_4	30		
Antinuclear antibody	Negative			
ANCA	Negative			
Hepatitis A, C serology	Negative			
Hepatitis B serology	HBsAg positive, HBeAg positive			
Chest X-ray	Normal			

The most likely diagnosis is:

A microscopic polyangiitis
B mixed cryoglobulinaemia
C polyarteritis nodosa
D systemic lupus erythematosus
E Wegener's granulomatosis

5.30 A 45-year-old man was referred because of a pruritic rash that had developed on his right forearm 2 weeks after cleaning out his aquarium. On examination he was apyrexial. (Figure 5.30, page 394.)

The most likely diagnosis is:

A anthrax
B Herpes simplex
C molluscum contagiosum
D *Mycobacterium marinuum*
E orf

5.31 A 59-year-old man presented with a 5-month history of frontal headaches.

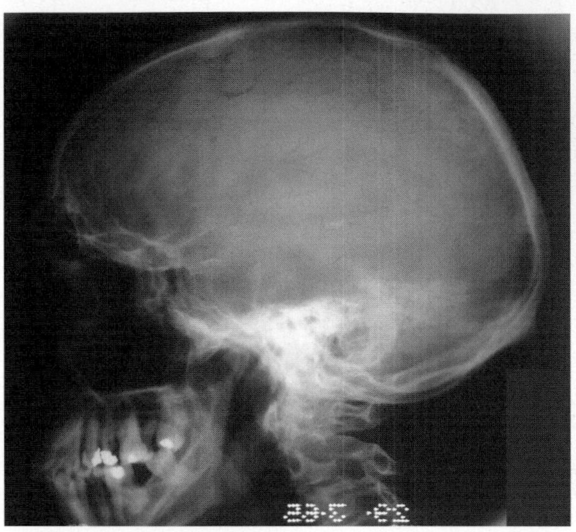

The most likely diagnosis is:

A acromegaly
B hyperparathyroidism
C hypophysis tumour
D multiple myeloma
E Paget's disease of bone

5.32. A 76-year-old woman was referred with shortness of breath and acute abdominal pain. She has no previous medical history of note.

Cardiovascular and respiratory examinations were normal but she had diffuse abdominal tenderness. Bowel sounds were infrequent.

An abdominal x-ray was performed (see plate section)

The MOST likely diagnosis is

A caecal volvulus
B diverticular abscess
C large bowel obstruction
D sigmoid volvulus
E toxic megacolon

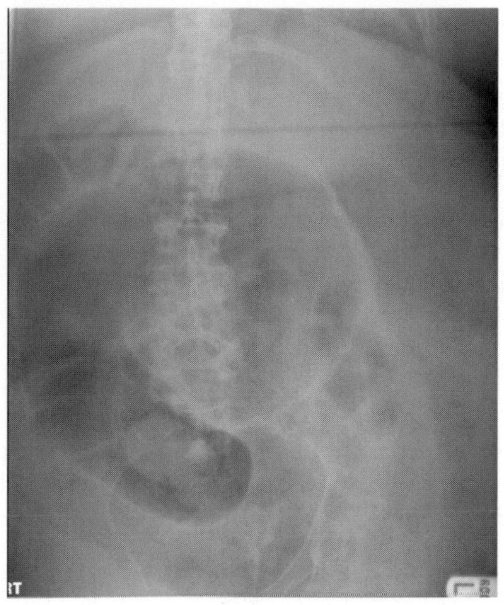

5.33 A 14-year-old boy was referred with worsening syncopal episodes. He had a heart murmur at birth and an operation soon afterwards. He became very short of breath with exercise.

On examination there was finger clubbing and central cyanosis. There was a thoracotomy scar. His pulse was 88 regular and blood pressure 100/76. The left radial pulse was weaker than the right radial pulse. There was a left parasternal heave and a systolic thrill at the left upper sternal edge accompanied by a loud ejection systolic murmur. His chest was clear.

Concerning this patient's condition it is likely to be true that:

- A β-blockers are the drug treatment of choice
- B he has pulmonary hypertension due to development of Eisenmenger's syndrome
- C squatting would make his symptoms worse
- D syncope is due to left to right intracardiac shunting of blood
- E syncope is likely to be due to dislodged vegetations from infective endocarditis

5.34 A 56-year-old woman had an emergency operation for a ruptured aortic aneurysm; 4 h postoperatively she became tachycardic and hypotensive. While talking to the doctor who had been asked to see her she lost consciousness. He could not feel a pulse or hear any breath sounds. The cardiac monitor showed the following trace.

The next step in the immediate management of this patient would be:

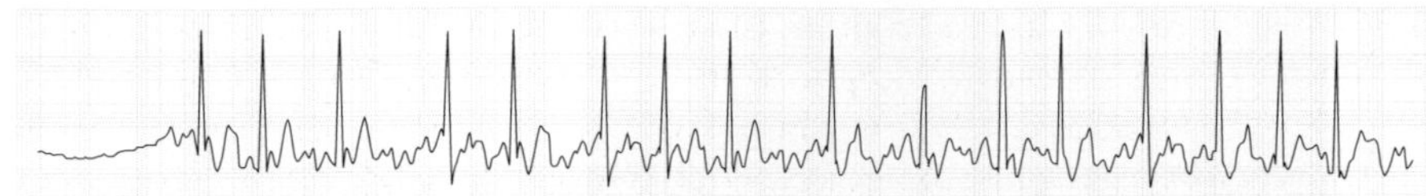

A adrenaline (epinephrine) 1 mg intravenously
B defibrillate 200 J
C lignocaine 100 mg intravenously
D precordial thump
E start cardiopulmonary chest compressions

5.35 A 63-year-old man had just returned from a holiday in India. His previous medical history included non-insulin dependent diabetes mellitus, hypertension and atrial fibrillation for which he was on a number of medications.

He had a rash on the back of his neck. (Figure 5.35, page 395.)

The most likely cause of his rash is:

A atenolol
B digoxin
C gliclazide
D hydrochlorthiazide
E metformin

5.36 A 65-year-old woman presented with a 2-month history of a painless swelling in her neck. It was getting bigger but not causing problems with swallowing or breathing. She had a normal appetite and no weight loss. She had no previous medical history and was not on any medication.

On examination there was a 3 cm firm, non-tender single nodule in her thyroid gland. There was no associated lymphadenopathy or goitre. She was clinically euthyroid.

Bloods TSH 1.6 Free T_4 20

The next most appropriate investigation in this patient would be:

A CT thoracic inlet
B fine needle aspiration of the nodule
C flow volume loop
D radioisotope scan
E ultrasound of the thyroid

5.37 You have been asked to sit on the research and development committee to consider a research application for a screening test for Creutzfeldt–Jakob disease (CJD). It is claimed that CJD patients who present with myoclonic jerks have abnormally high levels of enzyme *x* in their blood. The prevalence of CJD is estimated to be 1 in 20 000 and the test has a specificity of 90% and a sensitivity of 92%.

The major flaw with this screening test is:

- A too harmful to the patient
- B disease is too rare
- C too difficult to measure
- D too expensive
- E will not alter management

5.38 A 45-year-old man presented with a 2-day history of worsening severe central abdominal pain. He had vomited four times but had no haematemesis. The pain was like a knife and radiated to the back; movement made his symptoms worse. He had not opened his bowels today. He also suffered from ulcerative colitis. His inflammatory bowel disease was difficult to control and he was on azathioprine, mesalazine and a course of prednisolone. He drank 4 units of alcohol a day and smoked 10 cigarettes a day.

On examination he was in severe pain. He had a temperature of 38.2°C and he looked pale. His pulse was 110 regular and blood pressure 98/59. His abdomen was distended and there was rebound tenderness and generalised guarding. Bowel sounds were absent.

Bloods	Hb	11.5	WCC	25.4
	Neutrophils	22.8	Platelets	345
	Na	135	K	4.0
	Urea	7.8	Creatinine	150
	Bilirubin	25	ALT	35
	ALP	95	GGT	130
	Albumin	33	Calcium	2.82
	Phosphate	0.7		
Chest X-ray	Free air under the right hemidiaphragm			
Abdominal X-ray	No obstruction			

The following statements concerning this patient's condition is true:

- A ERCP should be performed as soon as possible
- B fall in the haematocrit >10% after 48 h carries a worse prognosis
- C hypocalcaemia is a cause of this patient's symptoms
- D serum amylase >2000 has a poor prognosis
- E urgent laparotomy should be performed if he fails to improve within the first 72 h

5.39 A 69-year-old woman was admitted with dysarthria and dysphagia of sudden onset. She was known to suffer from atrial fibrillation. There was a family history of stroke and she smoked 20 cigarettes a day.

On examination she had no facial abnormalities. She was able to name objects and follow commands. Her speech was slow and indistinct. She was unable to protrude her tongue, which was small and tight. Saliva dribbled persistently from her mouth. The corneal reflex was intact. The jaw jerk appeared brisk. The gag reflex was intact.

The patient is most likely to have:

- A bulbar palsy
- B cerebellopontine angle lesion
- C jugular foramen syndrome
- D medial medullary syndrome
- E pseudobulbar palsy

5.40 A 55-year-old man was referred for lung function tests because of shortness of breath and chronic cough.

- Flow Volume Loop

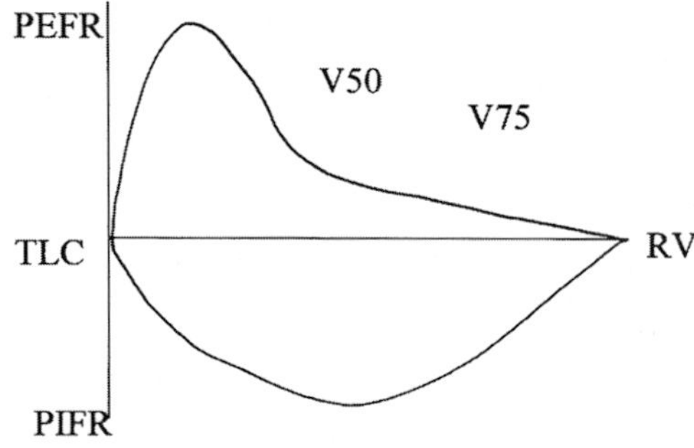

His flow–volume loop is most consistent with:

A chronic bronchitis
B emphysema
C fibrosing alveolitis
D normal
E retrosternal goitre

5.41 A 28-year-old man presented with a 3-week history of pain and stiffness in his right ankle; no other joints were affected. A month ago he had had conjunctivitis involving the right eye, which had resolved spontaneously. He also had a painless ulcer on his penis and some discomfort when he passed urine. He was heterosexual and had multiple sexual partners.

On examination his temperature was 37.2°C, pulse 88 regular and blood pressure 130/74. Respiratory and abdominal systems were normal. The right ankle was swollen and tender. There was also some thickening and tenderness of the Achilles' tendon. His other leg and hands were normal and there was no skin rash.

The most likely diagnosis is:

A ankylosing spondylitis
B Behçet's syndrome
C gonococcal arthritis
D Reiter's syndrome
E rheumatoid arthritis

5.42 A 50-year-old woman was referred with a 3-month history of burning in both ears that came and went, and was associated with deafness and vertigo. She also had a deformity of her nose and in the past had suffered from episcleritis and arthritis of the shoulder and hip. (Figure 5.42, page 395.)

The most likely diagnosis is:

A Reiter's syndrome
B relapsing polychondritis
C syphilis
D systemic lupus erythematosus
E Wegener's granulomatosis

5.43 A 45-year-old woman presented with collapse. Her GCS at the time of presentation was 14/15.

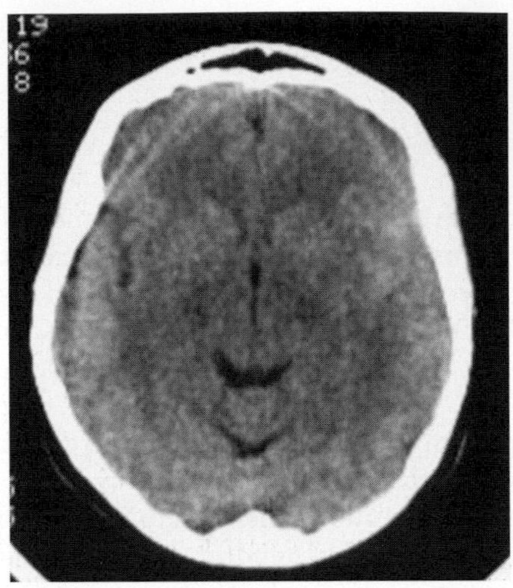

The CT scan shows:

A cerebral infarct
B extradural haematoma
C intracerebral haemorrhage
D subarachnoid haemorrhage
E subdural haematoma

5.44 A 16-year-old boy was admitted with a 3-day history of malaise, abdominal pain and microscopic haematuria. He was not on any medication. Further to this he had now developed a non-pruritic rash affecting his lower limbs.

His temperature was 37.4°C, pulse 88 regular and blood pressure 110/88. He had generalized abdominal tenderness and urine dipstick was positive for red cells and protein. (Figure 5.44, page 395.)

Concerning the patient's condition it is true that:

A he is at risk of developing haemolytic uraemic syndrome
B he is likely to have a low platelet count
C he should be started on high dose intravenous antibiotics immediately
D he should be given intravenous hydrocortisone
E skin biopsy would provide the definitive diagnosis

5.45 A 40-year-old woman was admitted with weakness, paraesthesia, muscle cramps, headaches and palpitations. Her symptoms had been getting worse over the past month. She had no previous medical history. She did not smoke or drink alcohol.

On examination her pulse was 90 regular and blood pressure 190/105. Her JVP was not elevated and heart sounds and chest examination were normal. Abdominal examination was normal.

Bloods				
	Na	137	K	2.9
	Urea	5.5	Creatinine	98
	Glucose	5.9	Magnesium	0.69
	Bicarbonate	37		

The most appropriate treatment for her hypertension is:

A methyldopa
B nifedipine
C phenoxybenzamine
D propanolol
E spironolactone

5.46 A 29-year-old man presented with a 4-week history of abdominal pain and bloody diarrhoea. He opened his bowels up to five times per day and his stools were liquid, containing fresh blood. He had not eaten anything unusual nor been abroad recently. He had a decreased appetite and had lost over 3 kg in weight. He had no previous medical history and there was no relevant family history.

On examination he looked ill and had a temperature of 38.0°C. His pulse was 110 regular and blood pressure 95/60. Chest examination was normal. His abdomen was very tender and distended. Rectal examination revealed bloody stool.

Bloods				
	Hb	10.4	WCC	13.5
	Platelets	450	INR	1.0
	Na	138	K	3.9
	Urea	7.5	Creatinine	100
	Albumin	28	Bilirubin	12
	Protein	60	ALT	20
	ALP	65	Amylase	30
	Calcium	2.20	Phosphate	0.8
	ESR	65	CRP	250

The next most appropriate investigation of this patient would be:

A abdominal ultrasound
B abdominal X-ray
C barium enema
D CT abdomen
E flexible sigmoidoscopy

5.47 A 33-year-old man was brought to Accident & Emergency with generalised fits. They had started 20 min ago and had continued despite the patient being given 2 x 10 mg of diazepam intravenously. He had associated tongue biting and jerking of all limbs. He was not conscious and did not respond to commands. He had no previous medical history of epilepsy.

On examination he had a temperature of 38.5°C, pulse 110 regular and blood pressure 150/90 when he briefly stopped fitting. His chest sounded clear. Pupils responded to light and his plantar responses were bilaterally extensor.

Bloods				
	Hb	14.4	WCC	12.3
	Platelets	160	Na	138
	K	4.0	Urea	4.9
	Creatinine	89	Glucose	5.6
	Calcium	2.1	Magnesium	0.8
	Protein	70	Albumin	40

Concerning the diagnosis and management of this patient it is correct that:

A bilateral extensor plantars are consistent with a permanent intracranial event
B he should be restrained as he is at risk of hurting himself and other patients
C intravenous sodium valproate should be considered next in his immediate management
D lorazepam could be used just as effectively as diazepam
E pyrexia, urine dipstick and microscopy showing blood but not haemoglobin are suggestive of an underlying urinary tract infection

5.48 A 69-year-old woman presented to her GP with low back pain that had been getting progressively worse over the past 3 months.

The symptom that would suggest her condition was due to an infiltrative, non-inflammatory cause is:

- A activity makes back pain worse
- B back pain is only felt down one side
- C symptoms are unaffected by change in position and not improved by supine position with hips flexed
- D associated morning stiffness lasting >1 h
- E nocturnal pain

5.49 A 61-year-old woman presented with bloody diarrhoea that had been going on for 4 weeks. She had decreased appetite and had lost 3 kg in weight. She opened her bowels five times per day and twice at night, and the stools were liquid with blood. She was not on any medication.

A barium enema was performed.

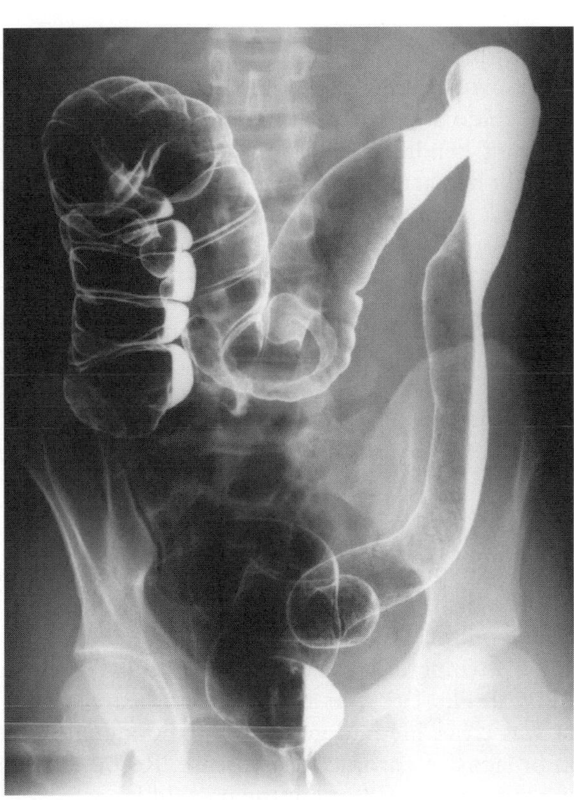

The barium enema shows:

A Crohn's disease
B diverticulitis
C ischaemic colitis
D normal colon
E ulcerative colitis

5.50 A 32-year-old woman presented with a facial rash that had worsened over 6 weeks and was limited to the chin, cheeks and nose. (Figure 5.50, page 395.)

The most likely diagnosis is:

A acne vulgaris
B erysipelas
C gingivostomatitis
D impetigo contagiosa
E rosacea

5.51 A 52-year-old woman presented with increasing tiredness, irritability and sweating that was worse at night. Her husband had complained that she had a decreased libido and was rather more forgetful. Recently she had been experiencing headaches and dizziness. She had a normal appetite and her weight had actually increased. She smoked 15 cigarettes a day. She did not drink alcohol or take any medication.

There were no abnormal findings on examination.

The next most appropriate test would be:

A 24-h ECG
B CT head
C serum gonadotrophins
D serum prolactin
E thyroid function tests

5.52 A 55-year-old Nepalese man presented with abdominal pain. Unfortunately he spoke no English, having arrived just 3 days ago from his native Nepal claiming political asylum.

On examination his temperature was 37.2°C, pulse 100 regular and blood pressure 120/70. His JVP was not elevated, heart sounds were normal and chest was clear. He had generalised abdominal tenderness but no distension or signs of chronic liver disease. Rectal examination was normal. Urine output was 500 ml in the past 24 h.

Bloods	Hb	12.5	WCC	4.8
	Platelets	45	INR	3.5
	Na	140	K	4.2
	Urea	8.2	Creatinine	215
	Bilirubin	55	Albumin	33
	Protein	64	ALT	4800
	ALP	240	GGT	150
	Amylase	80	Glucose	3.5
Hepatitis A, B, C serology	Negative			
Malaria films	Negative			
Blood cultures	No growth			
Chest X-ray	Normal			
Abdominal ultrasound	No abnormality found in liver, gallbladder, spleen, kidneys Normal portal vein flow			

The next most appropriate test would be:

- A dengue fever serology
- B hepatitis E serology
- C HIV test
- D paracetamol level
- E yellow fever serology

5.53 A 28-year-old man was referred with difficult to control hypertension. The GP had tried bendrofluazide and amlodopine without success. The patient also complained of palpitations, feeling sweaty and a swelling in his neck that appeared to be getting bigger. Two years ago renal stones were diagnosed and since then he had been told to drink plenty of fluids.

On examination he was anxious. He had an obvious goitre but was clinically euthyroid. His pulse was 90 regular and blood pressure 170/86. His JVP was not elevated and heart sounds were normal. His chest was clear and there were no abnormal findings on abdominal examination.

Bloods	Calcium	2.75	Phosphate	0.65
	Albumin	38	PTH	1.9
	TSH	1.5	Free T_4	22
	Calcitonin	50		
24-h urinary adrenaline	330			
24-h urinary noradrenaline	750			

The most likely diagnosis is:

A autoimmune polyglandular syndrome (APS) I
B APS 2
C MEN (multiple endocrine neoplasia) I syndrome
D MEN 2A syndrome
E MEN 2B syndrome

5.54 A 45-year-old man presented with gross ascites. A diagnostic tap was performed on the fluid.

Serum albumin	32
Ascitic fluid albumin	20

These results are most consistent with:

A intra-abdominal malignancy with peritoneal seeding
B large bowel obstruction
C nephrotic syndrome
D portal vein thrombosis
E tuberculous peritonitis

5.55 A 19-year-old man was referred because of a 3-day history of increased thirst and polyuria. Random blood glucose was 15.8. He had no other symptoms. He had no other medical problems and was not on any medication. He did not drink alcohol or smoke.

On examination his temperature was 37.0°C, pulse 78 regular and blood pressure 115/78. The rest of the physical examination was normal. His body mass index was 23.2.

Arterial blood gases on air	pH	7.34	PCO_2	3.8
	PO_2	12.7	Bicarbonate	23.1
	Base excess	0.5		
Urinalysis	Glucose 2+, ketones 1			

The best management plan for this patient would be:

A acarbose
B diabetic diet
C gliclazide
D insulin
E metformin

5.56 A 30-year-old man was referred with ankle and facial swelling, lethargy and proteinuria. He had no previous medical history and was not on any medication.

On examination his face was puffy. He was apyrexial, pulse 88 regular and blood pressure 160/98. His JVP was not elevated and chest and heart sounds were normal. His abdomen was soft and non-tender. He had pitting oedema up to his thighs.

Bloods	Hb	13.7	WCC	4.8
	Platelets	190	INR	1.0
	Na	138	K	4.7
	Urea	12.9	Creatinine	160
	Protein	54	Albumin	25
	LDL cholesterol	8.9		
24-h urinary protein collection	14.8 g/L			
Renal biopsy	Focal segmental glomerulosclerosis			

Regarding this patient's management:

A first-line treatment of his oedema should be with spironolactone
B he is likely to go into and stay in remission with steroids
C he should be anticoagulated if his albumin drops below 25
D he would benefit from a low protein diet
E his blood pressure should be treated with bendroflumethiazide (bendrofluazide)

5.57 A 32-year-old woman presented to Accident & Emergency with pyrexia and splenomegaly. Two weeks ago she had returned from holiday in West Africa.

A blood film was performed. (Figure 5.57, page 396.)

The film shows:

A *Plasmodium falciparum*
B Loa loa
C *Leishmania donovani*
D *Trypanosoma brucei gambiense*
E *Schistosoma haematobium*

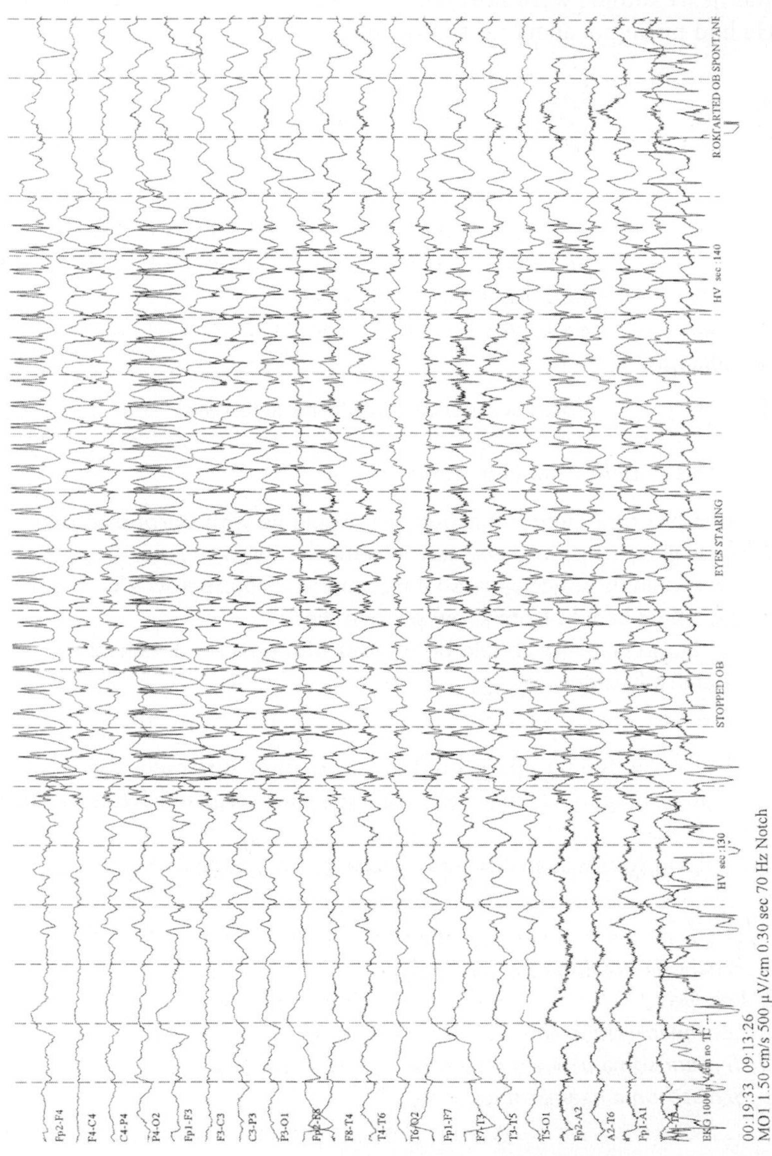
Fp2-F4
F4-C4
C4-P4
P4-O2
Fp1-F3
F3-C3
C3-P3
P3-O1
Fp2-F8
F8-T4
T4-T6
T6-O2
Fp1-F7
F7-T3
T3-T5
T5-O1
Fp2-A2
A2-T6
Fp1-A1
A1-T3
HV sec:130
STOPPED OB
EYES STARING
HV sec:140
00:19:33 09:13:26
MO1 1.50 cm/s 500 μV/cm 0.30 sec 70 Hz Notch

5.58 A 15-year-old boy was referred for an EEG because of fits associated with loss of consciousness. He was not on any medication. While he was having another attack an EEG was performed. His EEG showed the following trace with 3 Hz spikes:

The most likely diagnosis is:

A absence seizures
B complex partial seizures
C Creutzfeld–Jakob disease
D subacute sclerosing panencephalitis
E tonic-clonic seizures

5.59 A 37-year-old HIV-positive man was referred because of difficulty swallowing. He was not on any medication and had no other medical problems. He did not smoke or drink alcohol.

Apart from oropharyngeal candidiasis the rest of the physical examination was normal.

Bloods	Hb	12.4	WCC	3.9
	Platelets	150		
CD_4	250			
Viral load	16 000			

The treatment of choice for this patient is:

A intravenous aciclovir
B intravenous amphotericin
C intravenous ganciclovir
D oral fluconazole
E oral nystatin

5.60 A 62-year-old man was admitted with unstable angina and shortness of breath. He was treated with aspirin, diltiazem, furosemide, glyceryl trinitrate infusion, intravenous heparin and simvastatin. As the chest pain continued coronary angiography was undertaken. This showed 75% occlusion of the left anterior descending artery and he was treated with a coronary stent. Two days later he complained of painful, discoloured toes. His renal function was noted to have deteriorated. Prior to the procedure his creatinine was 120.

On examination there were no splinter haemorrhages in his fingernails. His temperature was 37.6°C, pulse 110 regular and blood pressure 150/90. His JVP was not elevated and chest and heart sounds were normal. Abdominal examination was normal. Toes from both feet were blue and mottled. Foot pulses and sensation were normal.

Bloods	Hb	13.8	WCC	8.9
	Neutrophils	5.8	Lymphocytes	2.1
	Eosinophils	1.0	Platelets	200
	Na	139	K	4.0
	Urea	13.8	Creatinine	250

Urinalysis Protein 2+, blood 1+, WCC 2+, eosinophiluria, no red cell casts

Chest X-ray Normal

The most likely diagnosis is:

A acute interstitial nephritis secondary to aspirin
B acute vasculitis
C cholesterol embolus
D contrast-induced nephropathy
E over diuresis with furosemide

5.61 A 40-year-old man presented to Accident & Emergency with dysuria, lethargy, muscle cramps and increased thirst. Two weeks ago he had been discharged from hospital following small bowel resection and formation of a jejunostomy. For many years he had suffered with Crohn's disease that was difficult to control and had necessitated numerous operations, leading to loss of colon and ileum and leaving him with 180 cm of small bowel. There was no abdominal pain or vomiting. He was on a normal oral diet at home. His stoma output had increased from 1.5 to 3 L but contained no blood.

On examination he looked dehydrated with a dry tongue and reduced skin turgor. His temperature was 37.2°C, pulse 100 regular and blood pressure 108/68. His abdomen was soft and non-tender and his stoma site looked healthy.

Bloods	Hb	15.2	WCC	10.4
	Platelets	250	Na	130
	K	4.0	Urea	7.0
	Creatinine	90	Calcium	2.10
	Magnesium	0.40	Albumin	32

Urine dipstick Nitrites ++

Concerning his management:

A he should be encouraged to increase oral intake of food and fluids
B intravenous dextrose and K+ supplements will correct the hypomagnesaemia
C loperamide is contraindicated
D metoclopramide should be given to reduce his stoma output
E omeprazole should be given

5.62 A 40-year-old man with known hepatitis C (HCV) genotype 1 was referred for treatment. He had factor VIII haemophilia and had contracted HCV from an infected blood transfusion in the 1980s. He did not drink alcohol or smoke cigarettes but did smoke cannabis on a regular basis.

Examination of his abdomen was normal and there was no evidence of encephalopathy.

Bloods	Albumin	32	Bilirubin	14
	ALT	70	ALP	138
Viral load	1.2×10^5 IU/ml			
Liver ultrasound	Normal with no focal lesions or ascites			

Regarding treatment of this patient:

A before treatment can start he must have a liver biopsy
B continued cannabis use is a contraindication to starting anti-HCV treatment
C if by 12 weeks of combination treatment the viral load has not dropped to 1.2×10^4, treatment should be terminated
D patients with depression should be first assessed by a psychiatrist
E ribavirin can predispose to venous thromboembolism

5.63 A 36-year-old woman was referred to the cardiology clinic with a 6-month history of worsening dyspnoea, now experienced with minimal exertion. Episodes of angina were also occurring with exertion. Over the last year she had noticed increased leg oedema. She had no other medical problems and did not smoke or drink alcohol.

On examination she was cyanosed. Her pulse was 74 regular and blood pressure was 140/90. Her JVP was elevated to +10 cm and heart sounds were normal. Respiratory and abdominal examination was normal except that she was moderately obese with a BMI of 27. A provisional diagnosis of idiopathic pulmonary arterial hypertension (IPAH) was made.

The following finding would be consistent with a diagnosis of IPAH:

- A echocardiogram showing left ventricular dilatation and hypertrophy
- B enlarged aortic knuckle on chest X-ray
- C increased transfer factor (DLCO) on lung function tests
- D mean pulmonary artery pressure > 20 mmHg after exercise
- E normal sleep study test

5.64 A 34-year-old female nurse was referred to the occupational health department prior to starting employment. She was asymptomatic. She had had BCG vaccination as a child in her native Kenya. Her husband and son were fit and healthy. She had no previous medical history, was on no medication and did not smoke or drink alcohol.

Physical examination was normal.

Mantoux skin test	25 mm induration at 72 h
Chest X-ray	Normal

Concerning this patient's condition:

- A a whole blood interferon-γ assay would most likely be negative
- B all patients she has come into contact with in the last 2 months should be contact traced and screened for tuberculosis
- C her husband and son should receive BCG vaccination if their Mantoux tests are negative
- D she should receive treatment with rifampicin, isoniazid and pyrazinamide for 6 months
- E the Mantoux test result is as expected in someone who has had BCG vaccination

5.65 A 45-year-old man with primary hyperparathyroidism underwent surgery. At operation he was found to have a parathyroid adenoma and this was removed. His immediate postoperative progress was unremarkable and he was discharged from hospital. Two months later he was seen in clinic and complained of nausea, vomiting abdominal pain and lethargy.

Examination findings were normal and he was haemodynamically stable.

Bloods	Calcium	3.25	Phosphate	0.8
	Albumin	38	ALP	127
	PTH	7.9		

Despite being treated with intravenous fluids and pamidronate his serum calcium remained above 3.3 mmol/L.

Regarding this patient's diagnosis and management it is **NOT** true that

A he could be treated with cinacalcet
B he is likely to have a high PTH related protein if he has a parathyroid carcinoma
C he is likely to need a total parathyroidectomy and autotransplantation of parathyroid tissue
D he may have ectopic/accessory PTH glands missed at initial operation
E he should have a ^{99m}technetium-sestamibi scan

5.66 A 73-year-old woman was admitted to hospital with a fractured neck of femur. She underwent a dynamic hip screw operation. She had a previous medical history of congestive cardiac failure. Two days postoperatively she developed a chest infection that was complicated by hypotension, tachycardia and renal impairment resulting in oliguria. She was treated with fluids and antibiotics and appeared to be improving with some cough but no chest or abdominal pain.

On examination she was apyrexial but mildly icteric with peripheral oedema up to her thighs. Her pulse was 95 regular and her blood pressure was 90/55. Her JVP was elevated +6 cm and heart sounds were normal. She had some crackles in her right lung base and 2 cm tender hepatomegaly. Neurological examination was normal.

Bloods	Hb	10.0	WCC	10.9
	Platelets	190	PT	16
	INR	1.4	Na	133
	K	3.9	Urea	13.4
	Creatinine	149	Albumin	35
	Bilirubin	40	ALT	2400
	ALP	130	GGT	100
	LDH	1600		
Chest X-ray	Some patchy consolidation in the right lower zone			
ECG	Normal sinus rhythm with no ischaemic changes			

Concerning the diagnosis it is true that:

A her acute deterioration is most likely to be due to non-steroidal anti-inflammatory drugs and antibiotics
B she is in acute liver failure
C she needs an urgent liver biopsy to establish the diagnosis
D the most likely diagnosis is portal vein thrombosis
E the severity of her condition is related to her underlying heart failure

5.67 A 15-year-old boy was referred to the clinic because of weakness, worse after exercise or running at school. This problem had been going on for a number of months. Sometimes he would be weak for 1-2 days post exercise. If he did not exercise he had no problems. There was no altered sensation. He had no problems with his bowels or bladder. He had no other medical problems and he was not on any medication.

On examination he looked well with no signs of muscle wasting, and normal tone, power, reflexes and sensation. After being made to run up and down stairs a number of times there was decreased muscle tone and marked upper and lower limb weakness. Cranial nerves, cardiovascular, respiratory and abdominal examination was normal.

Bloods (post exercise)	Na	138	K	2.7
	Urea	3.2	Creatinine	55
	Glucose	4.0	Calcium	2.2
	Phosphate	0.65	TSH	2.0
	Free T_4	20	Creatine kinase	430

The most likely diagnosis is:

- A chronic inflammatory demyelinating polyradiculoneuropathy
- B McArdle's syndrome
- C myasthenia gravis
- D myopathic carnitine deficiency
- E periodic paralysis

5.68 A 60-year-old man presented to Accident & Emergency with a 2-month history of cough, shortness of breath at rest and haemoptysis. He also complained of headache and right arm swelling. He had smoked 20 cigarettes a day for over 45 years but did not drink alcohol.

On examination he looked plethoric and had facial, neck and right upper limb oedema, but no cervical or axillary lymphadenopathy. His temperature was 37.3°C, pulse 100 regular and blood pressure 105/75. His JVP was elevated +8 cm and heart sounds were normal. The trachea was central but there were decreased breath sounds in the right upper zone; respiratory rate was 24 breaths/min. Abdominal examination was normal.

O_2 saturation on air	93%
Chest X-ray	Opacity in right middle zone

The **BEST** first step in his management would be:

- A emergency radiotherapy
- B anticoagulation until tissue biopsy can be performed
- C thrombolysis with tissue plasminogen activator
- D immediate intravenous dexamethasone
- E symptomatic relief from intravenous diuretics

5.69 A 26-year-old heterosexual African man was seen in the outpatient clinic complaining of painful inguinal lymphadenopathy. He had multiple sexual partners. Four weeks ago he had returned from Ghana where he had his last sexual contact. Last week he had noticed a painless ulcer on his penis but that had now disappeared. He was not on any medication and was HIV-negative when tested 6 months ago.

On examination his external genitalia looked normal. There were large, tender, fluctuant inguinal lymph nodes on the right side. Rectal examination was unrevealing. He was apyrexial and there was no axillary or cervical lymphadenopathy.

Regarding his diagnosis and management it is **FALSE** that:

A a positive *Chlamydia* test will not be helpful in diagnosing the condition
B if untreated, long-term sequelae include distortion to the architecture of curvature of the penis
C rectal involvement can lead to proctitis
D surgical incision of buboes is contraindicated
E this condition can be adequately treated with a prolonged course of doxycycline

5.70 A 56-year-old woman was admitted with right upper quadrant pain which started a week ago.

A CT abdomen was performed.

The **MOST** significant abnormality on the CT is:

A ascites
B gallbladder sludge
C hepatocellular carcinoma
D lung abscess
E subcapsular haematoma

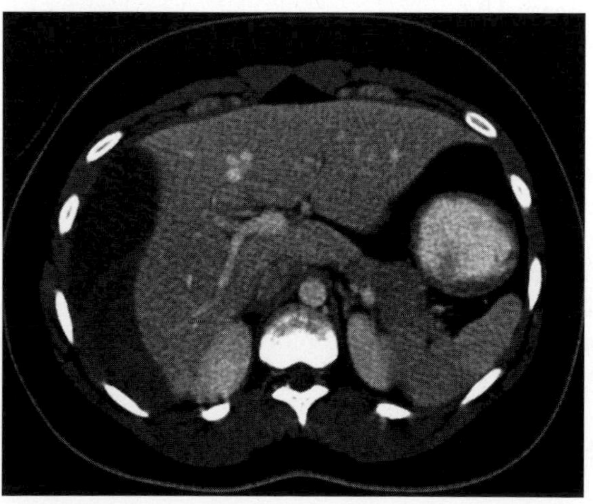

5.71 A 63-year-old woman diagnosed with chronic lymphocytic leukaemia 18 months ago was reviewed in the clinic. She was asymptomatic and was not on any medication. She had no other medical problems.

Physical examination was normal except for some bruising on her forearm following a fall.

Bloods	Hb	9.1	MCV	95.3
	Platelets	88	WCC	24.9
	Neutrophils	2.5	Lymphocytes	20.7
	INR	1.0	Reticulocytes	3.5%
Direct antibody test	Positive			

The next step in her management is to:

A observe and review in 3 months' time
B prescribe cyclophosphamide
C prescribe prednisolone
D prescribe rituximab
E splenectomy

5.72 A 55-year-old man was referred to the oncology clinic for consideration for radiotherapy. He had been diagnosed with squamous cell oesophageal carcinoma that showed evidence of vascular invasion. He had a previous medical history of HIV, hepatitis B and pulmonary TB but was now not on any medication. He still drank 5 units of alcohol a day.

His upper GI endoscopy had revealed a 5 cm tumour at 25 cm, oesophageal varices, gastritis and duodenitis.

Palliative radiotherapy would be contraindicated by:

A AIDS
B oesophageal varices
C previous pulmonary TB
D squamous cell carcinoma in middle third of oesophagus
E tracheobronchial fistula

5.73 A 77-year-old man had been admitted to the ward with acute left ventricular failure. He had a history of ischaemic heart disease and used to be a heavy smoker. Despite being on intravenous furosemide and glyceryl trinitrate infusion, his shortness of breath was getting worse.

On examination his GCS was 14/15 and he had a temperature of 37.8°C. His pulse was 106 regular and blood pressure was 108/70. His JVP was elevated +10 cm and both heart sounds were normal. His respiratory rate was 32 breaths/min and he had bilateral crackles throughout his lungs. Abdominal examination was normal.

Arterial blood gases on 10 L O_2	pH	7.29	PCO_2	6.3
	PO_2	8.4	Bicarbonate	33
	Base excess	3.5	O_2 saturation	90%
Chest X-ray	Bilateral pulmonary oedema with added suspicion of consolidation in the right lower zone			

A decision was taken to start the patient on non-invasive positive pressure ventilation (NIPPV).

Concerning the use of NIPPV in this patient it is true that:

A concomitant pneumonia is a contraindication to starting NIPPV
B decreased conscious level is a contraindication to using NIPPV
C he should be treated with CPAP (continuous positive airways pressure) rather than BiPAP (bilevel positive airways pressure)
D NIPPV is associated with increased risk of barotrauma compared to endotracheal intubation
E NIPPV results in decreased intrathoracic pressure, resulting in increased venous return

5.74 A 45-year-old man was admitted with generalised abdominal pain for over 1 week. He had had similar attacks of abdominal pain in the past but now it was getting worse.

A CT abdomen was performed:

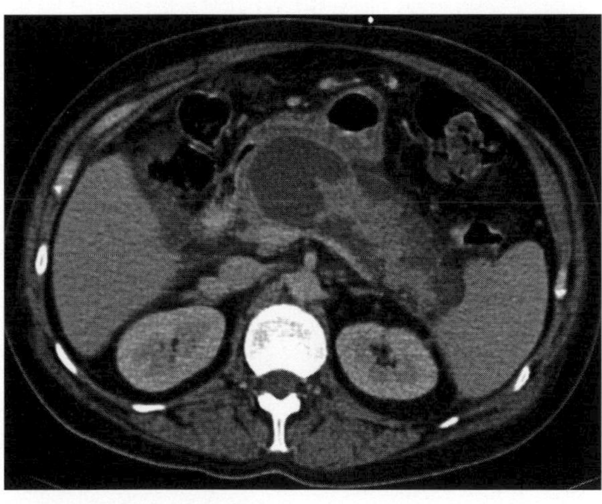

The **MOST** likely diagnosis is:

A acute cholecystitis
B acute pancreatitis
C acute pyelonephritis
D chronic pancreatitis
E gastric carcinoma

5.75 A 32-year-old woman presented to Accident & Emergency with shortness of breath and chest pain.

A CT chest was performed.

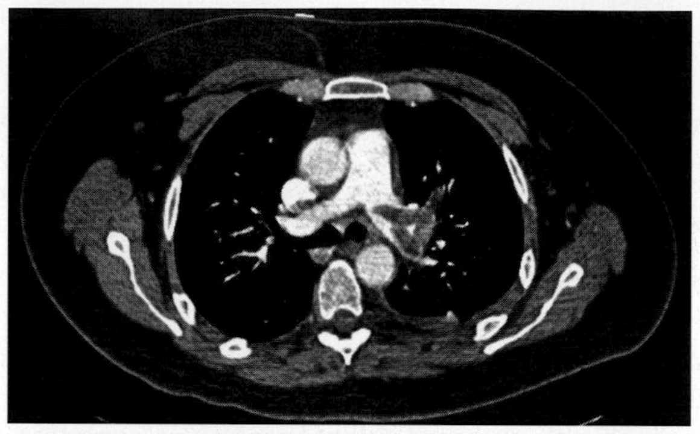

The **MOST** likely diagnosis is

- A lung carcinoma
- B pneumothorax
- C pulmonary embolus
- D sarcoidosis
- E thoracic aortic dissection

Paper 5

Answers

5.1 **E**** This patient has a history suggesting an acute coronary event but no ECG evidence. Blood tests could confirm the diagnosis and would be important for determining future prognosis. Serum LDH peaks at 72 h and lasts for 7–10 days. Creatinine kinase peaks at 24 h but normalizes by 48–96 h. It may give a false-positive result in patients with chronic renal failure. Serum troponins would be most appropriate at this stage in this patient. An echocardiogram may show new wall-motion abnormalities but in the absence of a new murmur will not affect management in the present scenario. New onset left bundle branch block with a history suggestive of MI is an indication to thrombolyse. Plasma BNP is released by the ventricles during pressure and volume overload; it is used in the diagnosis and monitoring of patients with heart failure.

5.2 **C**** The PR interval is getting progressively longer until after the third QRS complex the P wave is not followed by a QRS complex. This is characteristic of Wenckebach second-degree AV block.

5.3 **E**** This patient presents with an oculogyric crisis, a form of drug-induced dystonia. Dopamine antagonists are well known to cause such effects. Prochloperazine will make it worse. The correct treatment is procyclidine or benzatropine.

5.4 **A**** The patient has symptoms of headache, meningitis and fever consistent with Lyme disease. The rash is caused by the spirochaete bacterium *Borrelia burgdorferi* and starts off as an inflamed red papule, which then develops into a red, oedematous plaque with central livid regression. It may remain for many months. Erythema marginatum is associated with rheumatic fever, has a predilection for the trunk and is transient in nature. Erythema gyratum repens is a figurate erythema that is a paraneoplastic syndrome.

5.5 **A**** The patient has hypertriglyceridaemia but he is also diabetic. Before starting drug treatment this patient should try to lose weight, start a diabetic diet and reduce his alcohol intake. Metformin may be started before antilipid treatment as he is overweight and diabetic. The treatment of choice is a fibrate like gemfibrozil or bezafibrate if the triglyceride level is persistently >10.

5.6 **E**** The study is flawed by the way the patients were randomised. Tossing a coin is not a true randomisation procedure because, although the outcome is either 'heads' or 'tails', there may still be a disproportionate number in one group. A better method would involve a random number generator where each subject was given a number that, once chosen, would allocate him/her to a particular treatment arm.

5.7 **A**** PEG insertion involves passing the endoscope into the body of the stomach and shining a light (transillumination) through the anterior abdominal wall. The abdominal wall is indented with a finger and this should be seen by the endoscopist. Using aseptic technique and local anaesthetic, a small incision is made at this point on the abdominal wall and a needle catheter is inserted. A guidewire is fed through the catheter and is snared by the endoscopist and brought out through the mouth. The PEG tube is attached to this guidewire, which is now pulled through the anterior abdominal wall. There is a significant risk of bleeding and misplacement of feeding tubes so transillumination must ensure apposition of the anterior gastric wall to the abdominal wall. Conditions like gastric resection, ascites and morbid obesity prevent transillumination from occurring. Bowel obstruction is associated with abdominal distension and increased risk of perforation. Oesophageal and pharyngeal obstruction will prevent insertion of an endoscope into the stomach but achalasia per se is not a contraindication to PEG insertion. As there is the possibility of recovery of swallowing within the first 4 weeks in patients who have suffered a stroke, a PEG should not be considered for feeding until this time period has elapsed.

5.8 **E**** This is a sequestration crisis as there is sudden drop in haemoglobin with the red blood cells being trapped in the liver, which enlarges rapidly; in a younger child this may also occur in the spleen. These can occur repeatedly, over a very short period of time and may be life-threatening. Treatment involves transfusion, hydration, preventing hypoxia, opioid analgesia and possibly splenectomy if there is splenic sequestration. Chest syndrome is characterised by pleuritic chest pain, anoxia and anaemia from pulmonary vessel blockage. Aplastic crises can occur secondary to parvovirus infection and result in a rapid fall in haemoglobin levels without other clinical findings; the reticulocyte count is low, which differentiates it from haemolytic crises where there is marked haemolysis complicating a painful/infarctive crisis. Infarctive crises are characterised by bone pain.

5.9 **E**** The slide shows a lymph node, which stains blue. The large pink lesion represents granuloma, which would be consistent with sarcoidosis. If this were lymphoma, the whole slide would appear blue with lymphoid cells. Lung carcinoma consists of large pleiomorphic cells with big nucleoli. Reactive lymphadenopathy is associated with an exaggerated normal architecture with large germinal centres. Lipomas consist of lots of fat.

5.10 **B**** This patient has acute hepatitis B (HBV) as he is HBsAg positive and IgM anti-HBc positive. This may not necessarily represent a recent infection as the patient may have had chronic HBV which has now acutely reactivated. Unlike hepatitis C (HCV), HBV can cause hepatocellular carcinoma even without the development of cirrhosis. The aim of therapy is to develop anti-HBs antibodies and lose HBsAg; if this is not possible then the next goal is seroconversion with the development of anti-HBe antibodies and loss of anti-HBeAg, histological improvement and normalisation of the liver function tests. Treatment would be with interferon alone; interferon and ribavirin are used in combination for the treatment of HCV. Before starting treatment it is important to exclude HIV, as lamivudine is used as an antiretroviral and should not be given as monotherapy. Superinfection with hepatitis D (HDV) is a possibility and this needs to be excluded. Any sexual intercourse should be protected and he should not share utensils with his family that may transmit blood, such as toothbrushes, forks, knives or razors. His family should be vaccinated against HBV using standard vaccine rather than HBIg (immunoglobulin), which is used for vaccinating the fetuses of HBV-positive mothers and people exposed to HBV through needlestick injuries.

Foster GR, Goldin RD (2005) *Management of chronic viral hepatitis*, 2nd edn. London: Taylor & Francis.

5.11 **B***** This woman has myasthenia gravis (see **4.11**), which can be confirmed by finding anti-acetylcholine receptor antibodies, single-muscle fibre electromyography or an edrophonium/tensilon test. Edrophonium is a short acting anticholinesterase, which will cause an improvement in muscle weakness and fatiguability if patients have myasthenia gravis.

5.12 **B*** This patient has malignant hypertensive retinopathy. There is swelling of the optic disc with definite blurring of the disc margin, severely attenuated arteries, cotton wool spots, scattered flame-shaped haemorrhages, dilated tortuous veins and a partial macular star. The fundus looks tessellated, which is a normal variant. Note this cannot be defined as papilloedema because papilloedema is bilateral optic disc swelling due to raised intraocular pressure only and is not secondary to malignant hypertension.

5.13 **E**** A young man presents to Accident & Emergency with status asthmaticus. He has features of life-threatening asthma: inability to perform peak flow; unable to complete sentences; using accessory muscles of respiration; hypotension; respiratory rate >30 breaths/min; acidosis; and increasing PCO_2. He has already had nebulised salbutamol and 100 mg of intravenous hydrocortisone with little improvement in his clinical state. He should be treated additionally with ipratropium bromide nebulisers using oxygen (not air) and these can be given every 15 min to improve bronchodilatation. A single dose of intravenous magnesium 1.2–2 g can be given in patients with severe asthma.

Intravenous aminophylline or intravenous salbutamol can be given to those patients who are not improving. Chest X-ray is not necessary in all patients and is done to exclude pneumothorax or pneumonia, which this patient does not have clinically. Similarly, arterial blood gases do not need to be done in patients who have oxygen saturation levels >92%. Antibiotics are not necessary unless there is evidence on chest X-ray of lobar consolidation. He may need to be assessed for mechanical ventilation if he continues to deteriorate.

BTS/SIGN 2003 British Guideline on the Management of Asthma. *Thorax* **58** (Suppl I).

5.14 B** This woman has thickened skin, Raynaud's phenomenon, oesophageal dysmotility symptoms and telangiectasia. All of these features, along with positive anticentromere antibodies, would be consistent with CREST syndrome, although calcinosis is absent. The upper gastrointestinal haemorrhage is due to bleeding from gastric telangiectasia. This is unlikely to be systemic sclerosis because she has normal blood pressure, renal function and skin involvement limited to the hands. Amyloidosis can affect the gastrointestinal system and can cause haemorrhage but is usually secondary to another chronic illness like rheumatoid arthritis if it is not associated with myeloma. Hereditary haemorrhagic telangiectasia is not associated with Raynaud's phenomenon or arthralgia. Raynaud's phenomenon may be the initial symptom of CREST syndrome.

5.15 A* Barrett's oesophagus is defined as metaplastic change in the squamous epithelial lining of the oesophagus. With chronic reflux this changes to a more reddish, gastric columnar epithelial lining. It produces no symptoms but may lead to adenocarcinoma.

5.16 E** The CT scan shows a chronic left subdural haematoma. It is due to tearing of the bridging veins and blood collects between the dura and the arachnoid. The lesion follows the shape of the brain to display a more 'semi-circular' appearance. Compare and contrast this with **1.17**.

5.17 E** This patient has a ring-enhancing lesion on his CT head. The differential diagnosis in a patient with HIV would be toxoplasmosis, lymphoma or abscess. The most sensible treatment option after taking all appropriate cultures would be to treat as though he had cerebral toxoplasmosis. There is no midline shift and so no need to start steroids.

5.18 C** The fixed, split second heart sound is the hallmark of atrial septal defect. There may be a systolic murmur heard loudest in the pulmonary area because of increased flow across the pulmonary valve. Patients may present with cyanosis, clubbing and a loud second heart sound when pulmonary hypertension and Eisenmenger's complex develop. On the ECG there may be incomplete or complete right bundle branch block. If there is a secundum lesion with a patent fossa ovalis, then there is right axis deviation. With ostium primum lesions, which occur just above the atrioventricular valves, there is left axis deviation.

5.19 **D**** This patient presents with signs and symptoms of Wallenberg's syndrome or lateral medullary syndrome. The vessel that is usually occluded is likely to be the posterior inferior cerebellar artery, a branch of the vertebral artery. The clinical effects are ipsilateral V, VI, VII and VIII cranial nerve lesions, ipsilateral bulbar palsy, ipsilateral Horner's syndrome and ipsilateral cerebellar lesion. The jerking nystagmus on turning the head may make the patient complain of diplopia. Damage to the lateral spinothalamic and, sometimes, pyramidal tracts will cause contralateral hemianaesthesiae and upper motor neurone signs in the arm and leg.

5.20 **D**** This patient has tophi, which appear as nodular structures usually around joints, especially in the foot, and ear lobes. If the overlying skin is eroded they may discharge a whitish, crumbing mass, which if analysed microscopically will often show sodium urate needles. Tophi may occur after an acute attack of gout and may be painless. Heberden's nodes affect the distal interphalangeal joints but the joint per se does not look inflamed. Rheumatoid nodules hardly ever affect the distal interphalangeal joints.

5.21 **A**** The answer is normal bone mass as both her T score and Z score are above –1. For an explanation of how to interpret DEXA scan results, see **1.7**.

5.22 **D*** This pregnant patient has fever, low platelet count with associated bruising, impaired renal function, neurological changes and evidence of microangiopathic haemolytic anaemia, which are all features of thrombotic thrombocytopaenic purpura. This can be differentiated from disseminated intravascular coagulopathy (DIC) because there is normal clotting. Pre-eclampsia is characterised by hypertension, proteinuria and oedema and can be associated with DIC and HELLP syndrome (haemolytic anaemia, elevated liver enzymes and low platelets). Acute fatty liver of pregnancy and HELLP would be associated with marked derangement of liver function tests. For a discussion of toxic shock syndrome, see **4.68**.

5.23 **E**** The specificity is the proportion of patients who do not have the disease, which the test excludes as not having the condition.

	Lung cancer +	Lung cancer -	
CT +	60 (a)	25 (b)	85
CT -	80 (c)	335 (d)	415
	140	360	500

Specificity = d/d + b = 335/360 = 0.93

5.24 C** A middle-aged woman with history of ascites, weakness and pruritus with cholestasis is very suggestive of primary biliary cirrhosis (PBC). In most cases of pruritus there is release of histamine and so antihistamines like chlorpheniramine would be very useful. However, in PBC, the main problem is cholestasis and so a bile acid sequestrant such as cholestyramine is used. The other treatment for primary biliary cirrhosis is ursodeoxycholic acid (UDCA). Steroids and azathioprine are used in autoimmune hepatitis. Penicillamine is used to treat Wilson's disease. There is no effective treatment to prevent the progression of PBC and ultimately a liver transplant may have to be considered.

5.25 E** A boy presents with bruising, pyrexia, lymphadenopathy and splenomegaly. Full blood count shows low platelet count, leucopaenia and normal haemoglobin. All these features would be consistent with infectious mononucleosis or glandular fever. It must always be a differential diagnosis for cervical lymphadenopathy. Acute myeloid leukaemia can be associated with gum hypertrophy. The fact that there are no blasts on the film goes against this being acute leukaemia. Although not always the case, infectious mononucleosis can be associated with atypical lymphocytes on the blood film.

5.26 A** In the centre of the slide is a capillary with infected endothelial cells. Cytomegalovirus is characterised by bloated endothelial cells with inclusion bodies and occasional nuclear 'Owl's eye inclusions'. With TB, there would be caseating granulomas. With *Mycobacterium avium intracellulare* complex there would be more cells out in the periphery with clear cytoplasm. Kaposi's sarcoma is associated with spindle cells with red cells in between.

5.27 E** Syringomyelia results from a longitudinal cystic cavity that develops within the spinal cord and which may extend over a number of segments or even into the medulla (syringobulbia). The clinical features are those of a myelopathy or disease affecting the spinal cord. At the level of the syrinx, the involvement of the anterior horn cells causes a lower motor neurone lesion that results in wasting of the upper limb muscles and decreased tone and reflexes. For some unknown reason fasciculation is uncommon. The dissociated sensory loss is due to involvement of the lateral spinothalamic tract but sparing of the dorsal columns.

Below the level of the syrinx, there can be involvement of the pyramidal tracts causing a spastic paraperesis. The Horner's syndrome is due to involvement of the cervical sympathetic nerves. A Pancoast's tumour could also produce wasting of the small muscles of the hand due to involvement of the lower brachial plexus and Horner's syndrome, but would not cause bilateral lower limb signs or kyphoscoliosis. Cervical myelopathy can produce the spastic paraparesis and wasting of the small muscles of the hand but not the Horner's syndrome. HSMN can present as wasting of the small muscles of the hand but could not explain the dissociated sensory loss and pyramidal signs.

5.28 **B**** This patient with COPD has a normal PO_2 but evidence of uncompensated respiratory acidosis. Her drowsiness may be due to carbon dioxide narcosis. She may have carbon dioxide retention, which could get worse on increasing her oxygen concentration. The safest option would be to reduce the oxygen concentration to see if there is an improvement in her acidosis. If there is worsening acidosis and the PCO_2 remains elevated, then NIPPV could be considered.

5.29 **C*** Presentation with peripheral neuropathy, vasculitic rash, arthralgia, mild renal impairment and a history of hepatitis B infection are features consistent with polyarteritis nodosa. This is a vasculitis of small and medium-sized blood vessels. When associated with hepatitis B (HBV) infection, patients tend to be e antigen- and HBV DNA-positive but ANCA antibodies are negative. Unlike cryoglobulinaemia there are normal complement levels. Microscopic polyangitis is more associated with alveolar haemorrhage, not associated with hepatitis B, and p-ANCA is positive in 50–80% of cases.

5.30 **D*** *M. marinuum* can produce 'fish tank granulomas', which are bluish-red inflammatory nodules that occur at the sites of injury and track up the arm or leg. They can ulcerate but are not infectious.

5.31 **C**** The X-ray shows enlargement of the sella turcica and erosion of the dorsum sella. This would be consistent with a hypophyseal/pituitary tumour.

5.32 **A***** Volvulus refers to torsion or twisting of a segment of alimentary canal along with its mesentery and blood supply. It is due to increased mobility of that segment as a result of anomalous fixation and can lead to bowel ischaemia and gangrene. It most commonly occurs in the sigmoid and caecum. In caecal volvulus, the caecum looks like a coffee bean or is kidney shaped with the apex pointing up towards the left hemidiaphragm. In sigmoid volvulus, the sigmoid has its apex under the right hemidiaphragm at about the level of the 10th rib.

5.33 A* This patient has Fallot's tetralogy and almost certainly has had a Blalock–Taussig shunt (brachial to pulmonary artery anastomosis) as an infant. The clinical features are: pulmonary stenosis, ventricular septal defect (with right-to-left shunt), right ventricular hypertrophy and overriding aorta. Squatting improves symptoms because it increases systemic vascular resistance and so reduces the amount of blood returning to the heart and hence through the right-to-left shunt. This can lead to pooling of blood in the legs. Eisenmenger's syndrome is when there is reversal of flow in conditions that produce left-to-right shunts. β-Blockers reduce right ventricular outflow obstruction.

5.34 E*** The cardiac monitor shows a trace that resembles atrial fibrillation; however, in the context of a patient with no pulse this is pulseless electrical activity or electromechanical dissociation. According to the universal treatment algorithm for non-VT/VF, cardiopulmonary resuscitation should be attempted with 30 chest compression to two breaths until the airway is secured. Once intravenous access is achieved, 1 mg intravenous adrenaline (epinephrine) is given and this is repeated every 3–5 min. The rhythm should be rechecked every 2 min. During resuscitation the aim should be to treat the cause of her cardiac arrest; in this case, this is most likely to be due to hypovolaemic shock.

5.35 D** This patient has a photosensitive dermatitis affecting the back of the neck. Amiodarone is associated with photosensitivity, digoxin is not.

5.36 B** This patient possibly has a cold nodule that may be malignant. The only way to be sure is to do a fine needle aspiration. Ultrasound would reveal whether the nodule was cystic or not. Isotope scanning would reveal whether it is a hot or cold nodule, depending on whether it takes up tracer. A significant proportion of cold nodules are malignant and hence fine needle aspiration is mandatory.

5.37 E** This test fits most of the criteria for a screening test: easy to administer, high sensitivity and specificity, inexpensive, not harmful to patients and the disease is not too rare. The only problem is that CJD is incurable and the screening test can only be used after the patient has presented with the clinical disease. Screening tests ideally should detect the disease before clinical problems develop so that future management can be altered.

5.38 B** A middle-aged man presents with acute pancreatitis. He is on a number of drugs that could have caused this, including steroids, mesalazine and azathioprine. Hypercalcaemia is another cause of acute pancreatitis. With time, saponification develops, which results in hypocalcaemia. Treatment is usually conservative because there is a very high mortality if operations are undertaken in the first 2 weeks. ERCP may be a cause of pancreatitis but if the condition is due to gallstones then endoscopic pancreatic duct decompression may be beneficial. Alcohol is the usual cause of acute pancreatitis. The serum amylase usually confirms the diagnosis of pancreatitis but adds nothing to predicting a patient's prognosis. For that, Ranson's criteria are used, taking measurements at admission (age >55; WCC >15; glucose >10; LDH >600; and AST >60) and at 48 h (haematocrit drop >10% ; urea >16; PO_2 <8; calcium <2; albumin <32; and base excess >–4).

5.39 **E**** Bulbar palsy is a syndrome of lower motor neurone paralysis that affects the muscles innervated by the cranial nerves that originate in the medulla/bulb. Unlike bulbar palsy, pseudobulbar palsy is an upper motor neurone lesion and does not originate in the brainstem. It affects the corticobulbar system above the brainstem bilaterally to produce similar clinical features. Dysarthria and dysphagia are common to both but the palate and pharynx are hyperactive in pseudobulbar palsy. Bulbar palsy speech has a more nasal twang and the tongue is flaccid and fasciculating. Jugular foramen syndrome affects IX, X and XI cranial nerves, and presents with palatal paralysis, uvula drawn up to the contralateral side, absent gag reflex and weakness and wasting of sternocleidomastoid. Medial medullary syndrome results in ipsilateral paresis of the tongue, contralateral hemiplegia and contralateral loss of joint position and vibration sense. Cerebellopontine angle lesions are discussed in 3.67.

5.40 **B*** The normal flow–volume should have a triangular expiratory loop (above the x-axis) and a semi-circular inspiratory loop (below the x-axis). With emphysema there is pressure dependent collapse of the airways soon after expiration occurs, which results in the early drop in the expiratory limb. With chronic bronchitis and asthma, there is a normal inspiratory loop but a more gradual flattening of the expiratory limb (volume dependent collapse). If there is a fixed intrathoracic or extrathoracic lesion, like goitre or lymph nodes, there is flattening of both inspiratory and expiratory limbs.

5.41 **D**** This young man presents with urethritis, conjunctivitis and arthritis, which may have followed a urogenital infection by *Chlamydia trachomatis.* The heel pain and thickening of the Achilles' tendon would be consistent with enthesitis, which is inflammation of the ligaments and tendons that is characteristic of 'reactive arthritides'. Gonococcal arthritis does not cause enthesitis or conjunctivitis and is associated with a migratory arthritis. Behçet's syndrome is associated with orogenital ulceration, arthritis and eye symptoms but not enthesitis, and usually presents with skin lesions.

5.42 **B**** The photograph shows a reddish-brown discoloration of the patient's ear. The disease affects the cartilaginous pinna with sparing of the inferior soft lobules. With progressive dissolution of the cartilage the ear becomes floppy ('cauliflower ear'). The nasal cartilage can also be affected, resulting in a 'saddle-shaped' deformity.

5.43 **D*** There is blood in the left Sylvian fissure consistent with a subarachnoid haemorrhage. Compare both sides of the CT head scan. On the right there appears to be a low attenuation (black) line, whereas on the left this line is high attenuation (white), signifying blood.

5.44 **E**** This patient has the rash and symptoms of Henoch–Schönlein purpura (HSP). HSP is a type of vasculitis and type III hypersensitivity. It may develop post-viral or -streptococcal infection and is associated with headache, malaise, abdominal pain, arthralgia, haematuria and possibly glomerulonephritis. The rash consists of sharply demarcated pink or red haemorrhagic patches, mainly on the lower limbs and buttocks. As it is a vasculitis there is no thrombocytopenia. Skin biopsy would show deposits of IgA about the dermal vessels. There is no effective treatment.

5.45 **E*** This patient has Conn's syndrome (see **3.58**). As she is most likely to have an aldosterone-secreting adenoma, the best drug would be an aldosterone antagonist: spironolactone. The definitive treatment would be to localize the tumour and perform an adrenalectomy.

5.46 **B**** This patient has a history and examination findings suggestive of acute colitis. Toxic megacolon needs to be excluded. The most appropriate investigation should be a plain abdominal X-ray. The other tests can be performed at a later date if necessary.

5.47 **D***** Status epilepticus is a medical emergency and should be managed aggressively as there is a risk of permanent neurological damage, coma and death. Pyrexia and urine that shows blood but not haemoglobin is a possible indicator that this patient may have rhabdomyolysis. The main aim of treatment is to stop the fits using a benzodiazepine. This can be with either diazepam or lorazepam. If this should fail to control them, intravenous phenytoin should be administered. Phenobarbitone can also be given but by this stage an anaesthetist ought to be assessing the patient for ventilation. Patients who continue to fit should be moved to a place where they will not harm themselves but only when their fits have stopped; no attempt should be made to move them while they are fitting.

5.48 **C**** Certain signs and symptoms suggest that low back pain is not due to a mechanical, inflammatory or soft tissue cause. These include the pain that does not respond to changes in position; pain associated with fever, rigours and weight loss; bilateral pain that is progressive; and abnormal neurological signs.

5.49 **E***** There is loss of the haustral folds and superficial ulceration from the rectum in continuity to the mid-transverse colon. This would be consistent with ulcerative colitis rather than the discontinuous lesions of Crohn's colitis or the predominant splenic flexure location of ischaemic colitis.

5.50 **E**** Rosacea is a disease characterised by papules and pustules on the central face against a livid erythematous background with telangiectasia, and is exacerbated by sunlight. Acne vulgaris would be an unusual presentation so late in adulthood and is characterised by pustules and comedones.

5.51 **C**** This patient presents with all the features of a woman going through the menopause. Other symptoms include amenorrhoea, depression, arthralgia and hot flushes. Such patients would be expected to have a high FSH and high LH.

5.52 **D*** A patient presents with acute liver failure. There is a possibility he may have a viral haemorrhagic fever, although he would be expected to be more jaundiced and show signs of bleeding. Hepatitis E has an incubation period of 3–9 weeks so it is possible that he may have been harbouring this virus. However, the test is only carried out in specialist centres where there is a high index of suspicion. HIV can cause very deranged liver function tests but testing for this should not be considered a first-line investigation. Paracetamol overdose is very common and must be excluded along with salicylate overdose in any patient with unexplained deranged liver function tests. He should be treated with intravenous vitamin K, adequately filled $\pm$ haemofiltration and started on N-acetylcysteine, and then urgently referred to a liver transplant centre.

5.53 **D*** The cause of this patient's hypertension is phaeochromocytoma, as shown by the high urinary catecholamines and the failure to respond to thiazide diuretics and calcium antagonists (see **1.53**). He also has hyperparathyroidism and this has caused renal calculi in the past. The goitre and high calcitonin level are associated with medullary carcinoma of the thyroid. These are all associated with MEN 2A syndromes. MEN 2B syndromes are associated with hyperplasia or neoplastic transformation of the thyroid parafollicular cells and adrenal medulla with concomitant development of mucosal neuromas and possibly a Marfanoid appearance.

5.54 **D*** The serum–ascites albumin gradient gives an indication of whether a patient has portal hypertension or not. If $\text{albumin}_{serum} - \text{albumin}_{ascites} \geq 11$ g/L, then the patient has portal hypertension. Causes of portal hypertension include: cirrhosis, portal vein thrombosis, Budd–Chiari syndrome; veno-occlusive disease, hepatic (not peritoneal) metastases, fatty liver of pregnancy and myxoedema. All the other causes in the question are associated with a low gradient.

Runyon B, et al 1992 The serum-ascites albumin gradient is superior to the exudates-transudate concept in the differential diagnosis of ascites. *Ann Intern Med* **117**: 215–220.

5.55 **D**** This young patient with new onset diabetes is likely to be an insulin dependent diabetic. At the moment he is becoming symptomatic of diabetes and unless he is started on insulin very soon he will develop ketoacidosis.

5.56 **C**** This patient has nephrotic syndrome secondary to focal segmental glomerulosclerosis (FSGS). FSGS is a type of glomerulonephritis characterised by focal mesangial collapse of some glomeruli and segmental scarring in part of the glomerular capillary tufts. Fifty per cent of patients with heavy proteinuria go onto develop end-stage renal failure. Blood pressure should be treated with ACE inhibitors and/or angiotensin II antagonists because these drugs have been shown to reduce glomerular causes of proteinuria. Hyperlipidaemia should be treated with statins, and oedema should be treated with loop diuretics, not spironolactone as first-line treatment. Another complication of nephrotic syndrome is an increased thrombotic tendency, which is believed to be due to a combination of a loss of anticoagulants and increased production of procoagulants. An albumin <25 is arbitrarily set as the point at which to start anticoagulation. Low protein diet is controversial as it may decrease the protein-losing state but may make the hypoalbuminaemia worse. Unlike minimal change glomerulonephritis or membranous nephropathy, FSGS patients often fail to remain in remission with steroids.

5.57 **D*** The blood film shows the characteristic 'S-shaped' trypomastigotes between blood cells. African trypanosomiasis or sleeping sickness is a disease caused by protozoa carried by tsetse flies. There are two types: *T. brucei gambiense* (West Africa) and *T. rhodesiense* (East Africa).

5.58 **A*** EEGs are difficult to interpret but absence seizures are associated with a characteristic waveform. The discharges appear and discharge suddenly but have a regular 3 spike per second frequency. CJD and subacute sclerosing panencephalitis also have characteristic waveforms but are a lot slower, lasting 1s and 4–14 s, respectively. Complex partial seizures are characterised by spikes followed by slow waves.

5.59 **D***** This patient has oropharyngeal candidiasis and so it would be safe to presume that the oesophageal candidiasis is the cause of his symptoms. The correct treatment is oral fluconazole. Only if his symptoms persist after treatment would upper GI endoscopy be indicated to look for another cause.

5.60 C* This patient has developed a cholesterol embolus, as suggested by the discoloration of the toes due to small vessel infarction, mild fever and eosinophilia and eosinophiluria. Such complications can occur after invasive procedures such as angioplasty. Acute interstitial nephritis can also cause fever and eosinophilia but does not give toe discoloration. Contrast-induced nephropathy and overdiuresis with furosemide are not associated with eosinophilia. Acute vasculitis would be unlikely, given the time frame and lack of active urinary sediment.

5.61 E* The normal small bowel length measured from the duodenaljejunal flexure varies between 275 and 800 cm; patients with <200 cm will have reduced intestinal absorptive ability for water and electrolytes and will require nutrient and fluid supplements. The amount of small bowel remaining, along with whether there is an intact colon or not, will determine whether these supplements can be given orally or parenterally. This patient's short bowel syndrome has been complicated by a urinary tract infection. He has increased stoma output which has led to him becoming dehydrated and hypomagnesaemic. Stoma output is often driven by oral intake, especially if the fluids taken in are hypotonic. In this case he should be kept nil by mouth and given intravenous saline. Over the next 2–3 days the intravenous fluids can be withdrawn and restricted and oral glucose–saline solutions containing ≥90 mmol/L can be re-introduced. Drugs like proton pump inhibitors (omeprazole) and H_2 antagonists (ranitidine) reduce gastric acid secretion but may also delay gastric emptying; this can reduce stomal output and increase water and sodium absorption. Octreotide has been shown to achieve similar results. Metoclopramide is a pro-kinetic agent which speeds up gastric emptying and will worsen stoma output. Loperamide and codeine phosphate can reduce intestinal motility and stoma output by 20–30%. Hypokalaemia may occur as a result of hypomagnesaemia but the converse is not true, and hypomagnesaemia does not respond to the addition of potassium supplements; hypokalaemia is unusual in patients with a jejunostomy, as is the case here.

Nightingale J, Woodward JM. (2006) Guidelines for management of patients with a short bowel. *Gut* **55** (Suppl IV): iv1–iv12.

5.62 D** Standard treatment for HCV is pegylated interferon-α and ribavirin. Both drugs have side effects but major ones include the development of bone marrow aplasia, thyroid abnormalities, alopecia, lethargy and asthenia. Ribavirin can also cause a haemolytic anaemia which may require erythropoietin treatment to maintain haemoglobin. Interferon can induce depression and can make an already severe depression even worse, including the development of suicidal ideation. A liver biopsy is useful prior to starting treatment to assess the degree of liver damage but is not a prerequisite and indeed may be hazardous in a patient with haemophilia. Inhaled or intravenous drug misuse is not a contraindication to starting treatment but probably would not help his chances of a cure. Treatment is terminated if there is no evidence of an early virological response at 12 weeks, defined as a 2 log drop, i.e. his viral load would have to be lower than 1.2×10^3.

5.63 E*** Idiopathic pulmonary arterial hypertension or primary pulmonary hypertension is a rare condition that is characterized by an elevated pulmonary arterial (PA) pressure in the absence of another demonstrable cause. The PA pressure is >25 mmHg at rest or >30 mmHg with exercise. Other causes such as parenchymal lung disease, chronic thromboembolic disease, left sided valvular or myocardial disease and connective tissue diseases need to be excluded first. Obstructive sleep apnoea is another cause of secondary pulmonary hypertension. The echocardiogram usually shows right heart enlargement, paradoxical motion of the interventricular septum and tricuspid regurgitation. An enlarged right heart and central pulmonary arteries may be seen on chest X-ray. Increased DLCO would be seen with pulmonary haemorrhage.

5.64 C *** The Mantoux skin test is used to screen for latent tuberculosis (TB). In patients who have not had BCG, an induration >6 mm would suggest active infection; in someone who has had BCG, a 25 mm induration is still larger than expected. If an interferon-γ blood test were performed, this would most likely be positive. When specific T lymphocytes encounter mycobacterial antigens they secrete interferon-γ; detection of this secretion appears to detect latent TB with a greater sensitivity and specificity than the tuberculin skin test. Its utility in active TB and in immunosuppressed individuals remains unclear. This patient needs to be treated with isoniazid for 6 months or isoniazid and rifampicin in combination for **3** months. If she had smear-positive sputum for acid fast bacilli, contact tracing of close contacts would be necessary; as it is, only her family need to be screened and if they are Mantoux negative they should be given BCG vaccination.

Richeldi L (2006) An update on the diagnosis of tuberculosis infection. *Am J Respir Crit Care Med* **174:** 736–742.

5.65 B** If a patient has never had neck surgery, localization studies prior to parathyroid surgery may not be necessary. If there is an adenoma, this is removed along with a normal parathyroid gland; subtotal parathyroidectomy is reserved for parathyroid hyperplasia. There is the possibility of ectopic parathyroid glands in the neck, thymus, thyroid or mediastinum. This patient needs accurate localization of the remaining parathyroid glands through a ^{99m}technetium-sestamibi scan and ultrasound. CT, MRI and venous sampling may also be used. Cinacalcet is a calcimimetic which acts by increasing the sensitivity of calcium sensing receptors in the parathyroid gland so as to reduce serum PTH and subsequently serum calcium. PTH related protein is released by various squamous cell and adenocarcinomas but not parathyroid cancer.

5.66 **E*** Patients with congestive cardiac failure have decreased hepatic blood flow; any event that can affect this blood supply, such as shock, can lead to an ischaemic hepatitis. With sepsis and hypotension there is an imbalance between oxygen supply and demand to the hepatocytes, which leads to liver injury. It is important to note that ischaemic hepatitis can occur without an obvious hypotensive event but that elevated right heart pressures also play a role (as in this case). The condition is related to the severity of the underlying disease. It can be diagnosed clinically by an acute rise in serum transaminases 25–250 times the upper limit of normal, a concomitant large rise in LDH and milder rises in bilirubin and ALP. The deranged blood results typically occur 1–3 days post insult. The synthetic function of the liver is not usually significantly affected but a coagulopathy can occur. Liver biopsy, while unnecessary to make the diagnosis, reveals a picture of congestive hepatopathy with zone 3 acinar damage. In the liver acinus, zone 1 hepatocytes are closest to the portal tract (periportal) and hence receive more oxygen and nutrients than zone 3 hepatocytes (perivenular) which are furthest away from the portal tract. If severe, then renal failure and altered mental state can occur due to decreased cerebral perfusion rather than hepatic encephalopathy. This patient is not in liver failure as there is no evidence of encephalopathy. Ultrasound of the liver should be done to exclude interruption of the liver blood flow but it is unlikely to show portal vein thrombosis. Acute portal vein thrombosis can be associated with deranged liver function tests but is often associated with abdominal pain and procoagulant conditions. Antibiotics can affect liver function, usually by causing intrahepatic cholestasis. NSAIDs can affect renal prostaglandin synthesis, which can lead to renal failure. With the resumption of haemodynamic stability there is resolution of the blood results within 7–10 days. There is no specific treatment but some evidence that N-acetylcysteine has a cytoprotective effect. Diuretics should be used judiciously because their overuse can lead to hepatic hypoperfusion and so worsen the problem.

5.67 **E*** This young man develops muscle weakness post exercise with no wasting and no change in sensation; this is consistent with a metabolic myopathy. Periodic paralysis can be classified according to its aetiology (primary or secondary) or according to the changes in serum potassium during the attack (hypo-, normo- or hyper-kalaemia). The pathogenesis of primary periodic paralysis is not fully understood but there is an hereditary component and there are abnormalities with various voltage-gated ion channels: sodium, calcium and potassium. Hypokalaemic periodic paralysis is associated with weakness of the limb muscles and sparing of the respiratory and cranial muscles; it can last a few days, is brought on by strenuous exercise and can be made worse by eating a high carbohydrate meal. During an attack patients may have low blood potassium and phosphate with a moderately elevated CK. With hyperkalaemic periodic paralysis, patients tend to present younger, and the weakness lasts for only a few hours and is more associated with myotonia. Thyrotoxicosis can be associated with a hypokalaemic periodic paralysis. McArdle's disease is a type V glycogen storage disorder in which there is deficiency of myophosphorylase, leading to abnormal accumulation of glycogen in affected tissues (like the liver) but fatigue and weakness when muscle glycogen supply is depleted. Patients tend to present in the second decade of life and often have a very elevated CK post exercise, dark urine due to myoglobinuria, and hypoglycaemia. Myopathic carnitine deficiency causes slow progressive weakness of limb, neck and trunk muscles and can be associated with cardiomyopathy and peripheral neuropathy. Sensation is normal which goes against radiculoneuropathy. For a discussion of myasthenia gravis, see **4.11**.

5.68 **B***** The superior vena cava (SVC) drains the head, neck, upper limbs and upper thorax, and so obstruction leads to engorgement of these vessels, resulting in facial and upper limb oedema. There may be dyspnoea, plethora and peripheral cyanosis. If the condition is chronic, collaterals can develop. The SVC can be easily compressed by any enlargement of the trachea, aorta, right main stem bronchus, pulmonary artery, sternum or surrounding pretracheal and perihilar lymph nodes. Tissue diagnosis is important and will affect treatment: small cell carcinoma, high-grade lymphoma and germ cell tumours respond well to chemotherapy, while non-small cell carcinoma responds better to radiotherapy. CT chest often shows decreased flow in the SVC and this may lead to the development of pulmonary embolus, so patients should be anticoagulated until diagnosis is confirmed. Eighty per cent of cases are due to underlying malignancy with small cell lung carcinoma far more common than non-small cell carcinoma. Empiric treatment with steroids and radiotherapy should be avoided until a diagnosis is established, unless the condition is life-threatening, such as the development of stridor suggesting central airway obstruction.

5.69 **A**** This patient has lymphogranuloma venereum (LGV) but there is a wide differential diagnosis and often the diagnosis cannot be made clinically. The disease is caused by serovars L_1, L_2 and L_3 of *Chlamydia trachomatis*. It is endemic in several tropical areas, including Africa, Southeast Asia, India and the Caribbean. The clinical course is divided into three stages. Primary disease is characterized by a genital ulcer that is transient and tends to heal spontaneously. The second stage involves extension of the infection to the regional lymph nodes (femoral and inguinal). These can become inflamed and enlarged (buboes). In 15–20% of cases these buboes can be separated by the inguinal ligament (the groove sign). Buboes can rupture and lead to sinus and fistula formation. A small number of patients, in particular homosexual men and heterosexual women, progress to the tertiary stage (genito-ano-rectal syndrome). These patients can develop proctocolitis (rectal discharge, tenesmus, proctitis), distortion of the penis known as saxophone penis, chronic infection and rarely systemic spread. Diagnosis can be made from isolation of the L_1–L_3 serovars of *C. trachomatis* from culture of ulcers, lymph node aspirates and nucleic acid amplification techniques like ligase chain reaction (LCR) and polymerase chain reaction (PCR) from genital samples. The treatment for LGV is doxycyline or erythromycin for 3 weeks. Aspiration of buboes can give symptomatic relief, but surgical incision is contraindicated because of the risk of sinus and fistula formation. The differential diagnosis includes chancroid, herpes simplex infection, primary syphilis and granuloma inguinale.

5.70 **E**** The CT shows a liver with an extensive haematoma with layering of the blood. There is no ascites, which would appear dark and low attenuated and usually surrounds the liver. There are no focal liver lesions.

5.71 **C*** Chronic lymphocytic leukaemia does not usually require treatment as there is controversy about whether it will improve long term prognosis, especially in asymptomatic patients. One indication for treatment to be started is the development of haemolytic anaemia and thrombocytopaenia, even if the patient is not symptomatic, because this is an autoimmune complication. The DAT/Coombs' test is positive along with a raised reticulocyte count, suggestive of a haemolytic anaemia. She should be started on oral steroids. If this fails, she could be considered for splenectomy. Cyclophosphamide and rituximab are drugs that can be used for more advanced disease, either alone or in combination with other chemotherapeutic agents.

5.72 **E***** The major contraindications to radiotherapy for oesophageal carcinoma are mediastinitis, acute upper gastrointestinal haemorrhage and tracheobronchial fistula.

5.73 **B**** NIPPV is a means of delivering mechanically assisted or generated breaths without the need for an endotracheal tube or tracheostomy. It can improve gas exchange by increasing alveolar ventilation and decrease the work of breathing. It has been shown to be of benefit in patients with COPD, cardiogenic pulmonary oedema and hypoxaemic respiratory failure. It increases intrathoracic pressure and leads to a reduction in preload and venous return. Both BiPAP and CPAP can be used to treat cardiogenic pulmonary oedema. CPAP utilises expiratory positive airways pressure while BiPAP also delivers inspiratory positive airways pressure. Contraindications to NIPPV include cardiac or respiratory arrest, severe non-respiratory organ failure, facial or neurosurgical surgery or trauma, and inability to protect the airway, i.e. decreased conscious level because of the high risk of aspiration. Pneumonia is not a contraindication provided the patient is able to clear secretions.

5.74 **B*** The CT abdomen shows an inflamed pancreas with a central pseudocyst around the head of the pancreas. The lack of calcification suggests that this is acute rather than chronic pancreatitis. The gallbladder is not seen on this CT scan. Pyelonephritis would show up as bright kidneys.

5.75 **C***** The CT scan shows dark filling defects in the left pulmonary trunk consistent with multiple large pulmonary emboli. It would be difficult to diagnose pneumothorax from a scan showing the mediastinal windows rather than the lung window. There is no dissection flap (see **2.63**).

Paper 6

Questions

6.1 A 49-year-old man was admitted with an inferior myocardial infarction. He was thrombolysed and appeared to make a good recovery, becoming pain free. He had no previous medical history. He was a heavy smoker. Twelve hours later he became acutely unwell, feeling cold, clammy and sweating. He had no shortness of breath or palpitations but had a recurrence of his chest pain.

On examination he was unwell and in pain. His temperature was 35.9°C, pulse 110 regular and blood pressure 80/45. His JVP was elevated +8 cm but his heart sounds were normal and there were no murmurs or added sounds. His chest was clear and his abdomen soft and non-tender.

Bloods	Hb	14.2	WCC	12.4
	Platelets	234	INR	1.1
	Na	138	K	4.8
	Urea	4.7	Creatinine	78
	Magnesium	0.90	Calcium	2.23
Chest X-ray	Normal			
ECG	ST elevation in II, III and aVF ST depression in V_{1-3} Normal sinus rhythm			
Arterial blood gases on air	pH	7.39	PCO_2	3.52
	PO_2	13.8	Bicarbonate	22.8
	Base excess	1.0		

The most likely complication this patient has suffered is:

A cardiac tamponade
B pulmonary embolism
C right ventricular infarction
D rupture of the interventricular septum
E rupture of the papillary muscles

6.2 A 53-year-old woman was admitted with central crushing chest pain while walking to work.

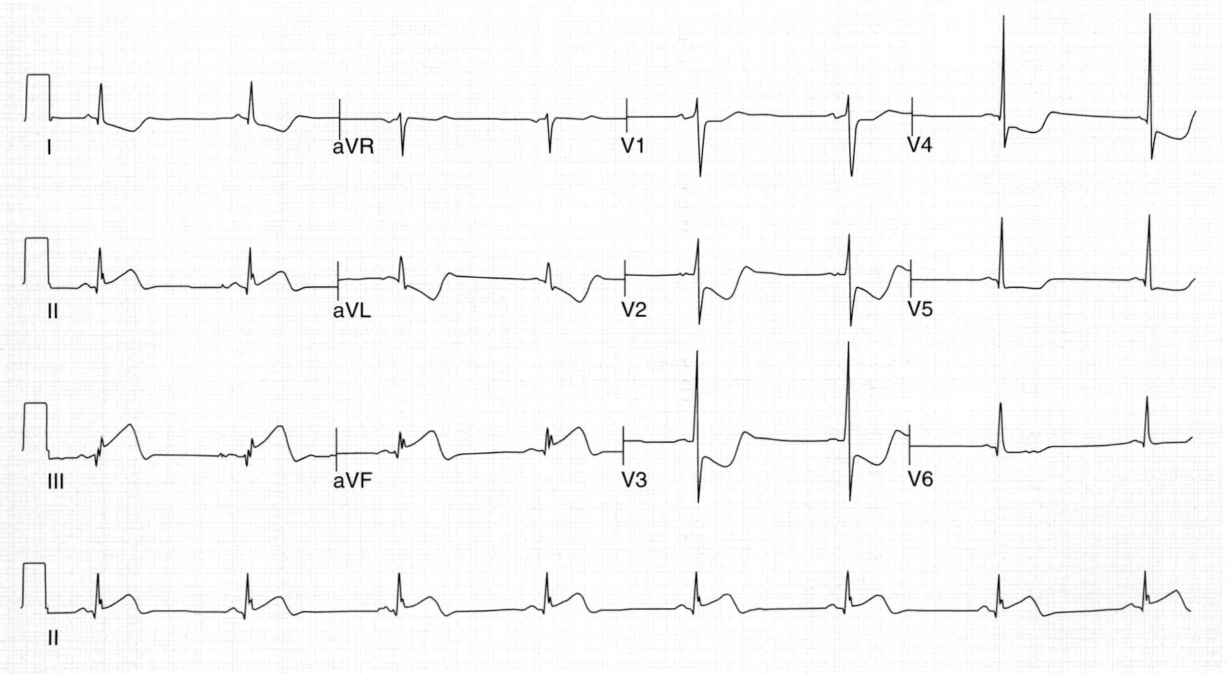
I
aVR
V1
V4
II
aVL
V2
V5
III
aVF
V3
V6
II

Her ECG shows:

A anterior MI
B anterolateral MI
C inferior MI
D inferolateral MI
E inferoposterior MI

6.3 A 16-year-old girl was brought to Accident & Emergency in a state of collapse. She had been at a nightclub and her friends thought she might have taken something there. Normally she was fit and well and not on any medication.

On examination, she was drowsy but responded to command. She was disorientated in time and place. Her temperature was 40.6°C, pulse 120 regular and blood pressure 195/114. Her JVP was not elevated and heart sounds were normal. Her chest was clear. Abdominal examination was normal. She was uncooperative on neurological examination but her pupils were dilated and her plantars were flexor. She had only passed 40 ml of urine over the preceding 4 h.

Bloods	Hb	10.8	WCC	5.4
	Platelets	100	INR	1.4
	Na	130	K	6.9
	Urea	22.3	Creatinine	328
	Protein	64	Albumin	37
	Bilirubin	15	ALT	350
	ALP	140	Calcium	1.81
	Phosphate	1.82		
Chest X-ray	Normal			
Arterial blood gases on air	pH	7.29	PCO_2	2.9
	PO_2	12.5	Bicarbonate	12.3
	Base excess	−13.1		

Concerning this patient's condition it is **FALSE that:**

A alkalinization of urine with bicarbonate is indicated
B dipstick and microscopy of her urine is likely to show blood and red blood cells.
C hypertension should be treated with labetalol infusion
D mannitol diuresis should be considered if oliguria persists in spite of intravenous fluid resuscitation
E she is at risk of compartment syndrome

6.4 A 58-year-old woman was referred with weight loss and anorexia. On examination she had a rash in her axilla. (Figure 6.4, page 396.)

The condition **LEAST** likely to be associated with this skin rash is:

A carcinoma of the breast
B carcinoma of the colon
C carcinoma of the kidney
D carcinoma of the pancreas
E carcinoma of the uterus

6.5 A 27-year-old woman presented with shortness of breath, tiredness and a swelling of her neck over the past 2 weeks.

Thyroid function	TSH	0.4	Total T_4	200
	Free T_4	15	Total T_3	2.0

The most likely explanation for these results is:

A pregnancy
B primary hyperthyroidism
C sick euthyroid syndrome
D subacute (de Quervain's) thyroiditis
E surreptitious treatment with thyroxine

6.6 Two thousand patients with multiple sclerosis were randomly allocated to treatment with interferon-β or placebo. At the end of 5 years 20 patients in the interferon-β group had severe relapse compared to 100 of the placebo group.

The absolute risk reduction in relapse due to interferon-β is:

A 0.02
B 0.08
C 0.10
D 0.12
E 0.80

6.7 A 49-year-old man with alcoholic liver disease was admitted with haematemesis. He had vomited 500 mL over the past 12 h. Four weeks ago, at another hospital, he had vomited blood and had had an endoscopy when some 'rubber bands' had been applied. He also complained of abdominal distension, much worse over the past 4 weeks. He had last drunk alcohol 24 h ago. He was not on any medication.

On examination he was apyrexial and jaundiced. He was verbally abusive and, although awake, was completely disorientated. His pulse was 72 regular and blood pressure 110/60. Respiratory examination was normal. He had spider naevi, 4 cm hepatomegaly and moderate ascites. Rectal examination revealed melaena.

Bloods	Hb	10.1	MCV	100.2
	WCC	9.4	Platelets	85
	INR	1.8	Na	125
	K	3.1	Urea	8.5
	Creatinine	96	Albumin	27
	Protein	54	Bilirubin	100
	ALT	68	ALP	125
	Amylase	77	Glucose	4.4
Urinalysis	Normal			
Chest X-ray	Normal			

The **NEXT** step in his **IMMEDIATE** management would be:

A give intravenous vitamin K
B give oral propranolol
C give oral spironolactone
D start intravenous cefotaxime and metronidazole
E start intravenous omeprazole infusion

6.8 A 23-year-old Afro-Caribbean man was referred with sudden abdominal pain, jaundice and haematuria. He was due to go to Egypt on holiday the following week and had been given malaria prophylaxis, which he had started to take 4 days ago. He had a normal appetite and no weight loss. He had no previous medical problems and was not on any other medication.

On examination he was jaundiced. His temperature was 37.0°C, pulse 100 regular and blood pressure 100/65. Cardiovascular and respiratory examination was normal. There was generalised abdominal tenderness but no organomegaly.

Bloods	Hb	8.2	MCV	99.5
	WCC	4.7	Platelets	300
	Reticulocytes	15%	INR	1.0
	Na	135	K	4.0
	Urea	3.3	Creatinine	70
	Protein	65	Albumin	37
	Bilirubin	80	ALT	25
	ALP	80		
Blood film	Heinz bodies			
Urinalysis	Urobilinogen 2+, no bilirubin, haemoglobin 2+, blood 1+			
Direct Coombs' test	Negative			

The most likely diagnosis is:

A autoimmune haemolytic anaemia
B Gilbert's syndrome
C glucose-6-phosphate dehydrogenase deficiency
D hereditary spherocytosis
E pyruvate kinase deficiency

6.9 A 31-year-old man with HIV was admitted with shortness of breath and cough productive of blood-streaked yellow sputum for the past 2 weeks. He had decreased appetite and loss of weight. He smoked 20 cigarettes a day but did not drink alcohol. He had no previous medical problems and was not on any medication.

On examination his temperature was 37.9°C, pulse 100 regular and blood pressure 110/62. His JVP was not elevated and heart sounds were normal. He had decreased breath sounds on the right side.

Chest X-ray Right hilar shadowing

Bronchoscopy was performed and washings were taken. (Figure 6.9, page, 396.)

The most likely diagnosis is:

A cytomegalovirus pneumonitis
B Kaposi's sarcoma
C lymphoma
D *Mycobacterium tuberculosis*
E *Pneumocystis jiroveci* (formerly *carinii*) pneumonia (PCP)

6.10 A 30-year-old HIV-positive woman was referred for treatment because she was 11 weeks pregnant. She was otherwise fit and well. She had no other medical problems and was not on any treatment.

No abnormalities were found on physical examination.

CD_4 500

Concerning this patient's management it is correct that:

A as she is asymptomatic she does not need to start anti-HIV treatment
B breast-feeding is safe in HIV-positive mothers
C normal vaginal delivery is not contraindicated
D the baby should be treated with AZT for the first 6 weeks of life
E vertical transmission of HIV is greatest during the first trimester

6.11 A 55-year-old woman presented with inability to walk but she had normal use of her arms. Her problem started 2 days ago and was getting worse. Bowels and micturition were normal. Two weeks ago she had a bout of gastroenteritis but made an uneventful recovery. There was no previous medical history and she was not on any medication. She smoked 20 cigarettes a day.

On examination she was not in pain. Her pulse was 90 regular and blood pressure 130/94. Her chest was clear. There was no palpable bladder and she had normal anal tone. She was unable to stand. There was no muscle wasting or fasciculation in her legs. Tone was decreased, power was 0/5 and reflexes were absent. Pinprick sensation was reduced up to the ankle. Upper limbs and cranial nerve examination were normal.

Bloods	Hb	13.5	WCC	5.6
	Platelets	198	ESR	30
	Glucose	4.5		
CSF	Glucose	3.0	Protein	1.2
	WCC	10		

The most likely diagnosis is:

A Guillain-Barré syndrome
B motor neurone disease
C multiple sclerosis
D poliomyelitis
E transverse myelitis

6.12 A 49-year-old woman was referred with deteriorating vision. Fundoscopy was performed. (Figure 6.12, page 397.)

The **TWO** abnormalities shown are:

A cholesterol embolus
B cotton wool spots
C flame-shaped retinal haemorrhage
D hard exudates
E microaneurysms
F optic atrophy
G papilloedema
H preretinal (subhyaloid) haemorrhage
I retinal detachment
J vitreous haemorrhage

6.13 A 45-year-old man with known squamous cell carcinoma of the lung was admitted because of progressive weakness. His condition was inoperable and he was being treated with chemotherapy. He complained of abdominal pain, nausea and loose stools but no bleeding anywhere.

On examination, he was not in pain but looked cachectic. He was apyrexial, pulse 100 regular and blood pressure 130/70. He had some crackles in the right mid-zone where the tumour was. Abdominal examination was normal. He had weakness but no wasting of the quadriceps and there was normal tone, reflexes and sensation.

Bloods	Hb	9.9	WCC	3.5
	Platelets	100	Na	138
	K	2.5	Urea	3.8
	Creatinine	69	Protein	62
	Albumin	34	Bilirubin	15
	ALT	30	ALP	120
	Glucose	7.5	Calcium	2.1
	Bicarbonate	34		
Chest X-ray	Solitary irregular lesion in right mid-zone			

The most likely cause of his deterioration is:

A carcinomatous neuropathy
B ectopic ACTH secretion
C hypocalcaemia
D hypomagnesaemia secondary to cisplatin
E metastatic disease

6.14 A 48-year-old woman was referred with progressive pain in her hands and wrists, worse in the morning, for about 6 months. She complained that her hands hurt a lot and that they changed colour when it got cold. She also described problems with chewing and swallowing her food. She had an underactive thyroid gland but apart from thyroxine was not on any other medication. She did not smoke or drink alcohol.

On examination her pulse was 74 regular and blood pressure 134/88. Respiratory examination was normal. Her wrists and metacarpophalangeal joints were swollen and tender but the other joints were normal.

Bloods	Hb	13.5	WCC	3.4
	Platelets	160	Na	139
	K	4.4	Urea	5.5
	Creatinine	88	Protein	80
	Albumin	38	Bilirubin	16
	ALT	19	ALP	78
	ESR	65	CRP	120
Rheumatoid factor	1 in 160			
Antinuclear antibody	1 in 80			
Anti-DS DNA	Negative			
Anticentromere antibody	Negative			
Anti-Ro antibody	1 in 80			
Anti-La antibody	1 in 40			
Anti-Jo1 antibody	Negative			

The most likely diagnosis is:

A mixed connective tissue disease
B Reiter's disease
C Sjögren's syndrome
D systemic lupus erythematosus
E systemic sclerosis

6.15 A 10-year-old girl was referred with temporary loss of vision. She had been deaf since birth. (Figure 6.15, page 397.)

The most likely congenital infection she has is:

A cytomegalovirus
B herpes simplex virus
C rubella
D syphilis
E toxoplasmosis

6.16 A 52-year-old man was referred because of progressive shortness of breath, chronic cough and weight loss. He had smoked 15 cigarettes a day for over 30 years. Until recently he was a coal miner.

A chest X-ray was performed.

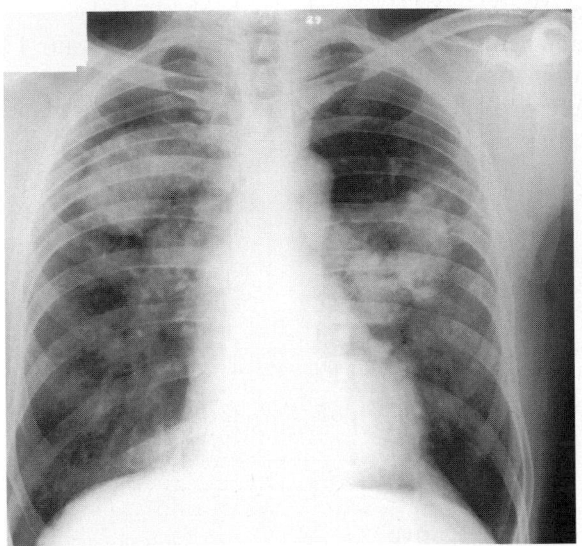

The likely interpretation of the radiological abnormality is:

- A Caplan's syndrome
- B cor pulmonale
- C cryptogenic fibrosing alveolitis
- D mesothelioma
- E metastatic thyroid carcinoma

6.17 A 14-year-old boy presented to Accident & Emergency very unwell. While riding his bike he fell and sustained a cut to his left thigh. He was able to walk and the bleeding was not heavy but his leg was now very swollen and tender.

On examination he was in a lot of pain. His temperature was 38.2°C, pulse 110 regular and blood pressure 90/55. He had decreased range of movements of his left lower limb due to pain, although sensation and peripheral pulses were normal.

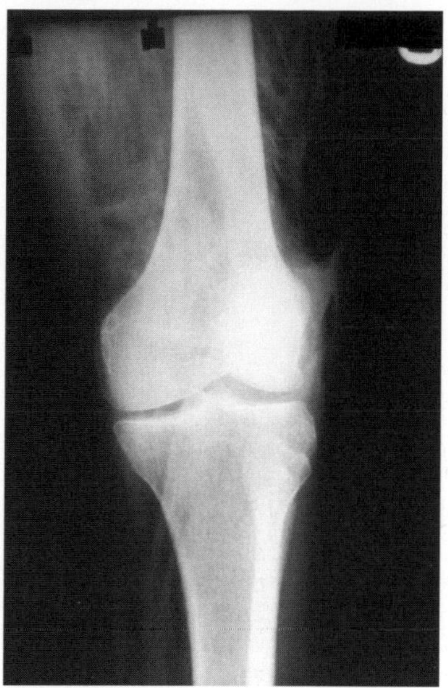

The most likely organism to have caused his symptoms is:

A *Clostridium botulinum*
B *Clostridium septicum*
C *Clostridium tetani*
D *Staphyloccus aureus*
E *Streptococcus pyogenes*

6.18 A 22-year-old man collapsed while playing squash. This was the third time he had had such an episode while playing sports. He had no chest pain or shortness of breath. He did not smoke or drink and was not on any medication. His father had died suddenly at the age of 35.

On examination he looked well. His pulse was 94 regular and blood pressure 122/88. The JVP was not elevated but there was a thrusting apex beat. There was an ejection systolic murmur that did not radiate to the carotids. Respiratory and central nervous system examinations were normal.

ECG Q waves in I, aVL, V_{5-6}
T wave inversion I, aVL, V_{5-6}
Voltage criteria for left ventricular hypertrophy present

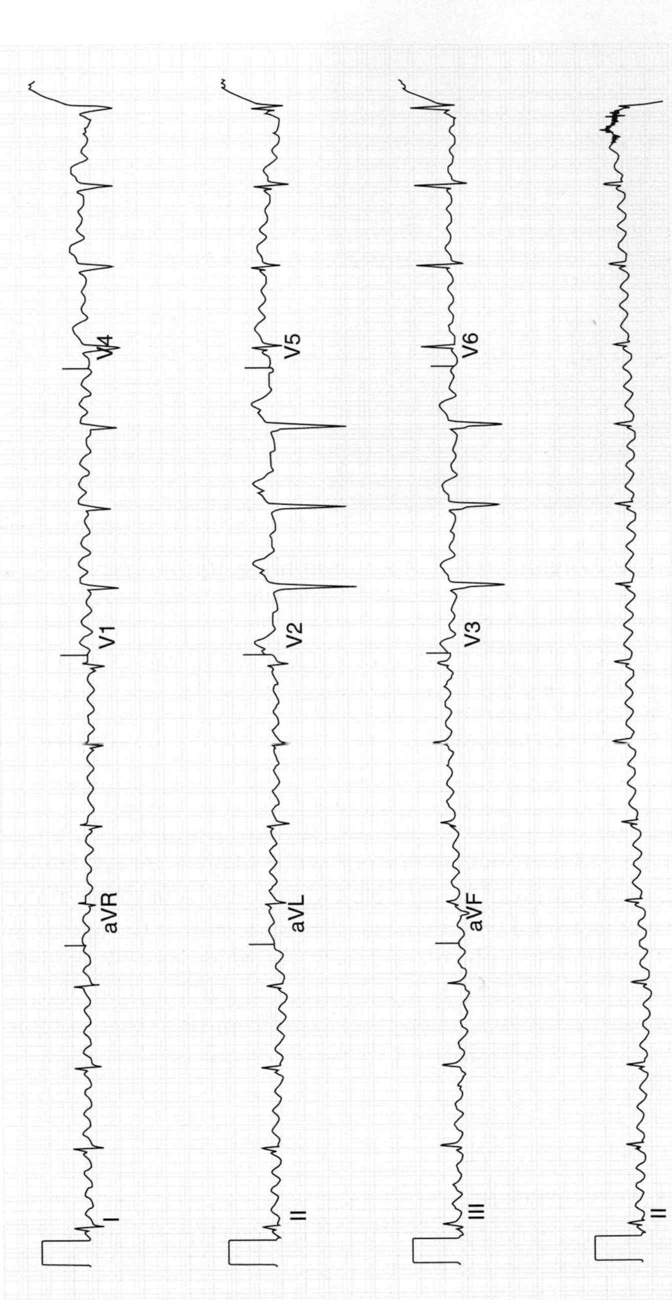
I
aVR
V1
V4
II
aVL
V2
V5
III
aVF
V3
V6
II

The drug treatment of choice for this patient is:

A atenolol
B digoxin
C enalapril
D furosemide
E isosorbide mononitrate

6.19 A 69-year-old man with a family history of ischaemic heart disease and strokes was admitted with progressive shortness of breath, but no chest pain. He did not smoke or drink alcohol. His only medication was aspirin.

On examination his temperature was 37.0°C, pulse 80 regular and blood pressure 120/79. His JVP was not elevated and heart sounds were normal. His chest was clear.

Bloods Normal. ECG: adjoining page

Concerning the management of this patient it is true that:

A adenosine often terminates this condition
B anticoagulation should be considered
C flecainide is contraindicated
D immediate DC cardioversion is the treatment of choice
E a permanent pacemaker should be inserted

6.20 A 35-year-old man was referred with a lesion on his right knee. He had similar lesions on his other knee and on both buttocks. (Figure 6.20, page 397.)

Concerning this patient it is **FALSE** that:

A he is likely to have a normal serum cholesterol and markedly raised serum triglycerides
B he is most likely to have type IIa hyperlipidaemia
C nephrotic syndrome is a recognised cause of this condition
D the serum is likely to be milky
E he is at risk of pancreatitis

6.21 A 12-year-old boy was referred because a screening test had shown hypercalcaemia. His father had a similar problem and had been operated on some years ago. He felt well in himself. He had no previous medical history and was not on any medication.

No abnormalities were found on examination.

Bloods	Calcium	2.92	Phosphate	0.8
	ALP	500	Albumin	40
	PTH	1.3		
Calcium/creatinine excretion	<0.01			

The most appropriate treatment for this patient is:

A calcitonin
B observation and follow-up
C parathyroidectomy
D prednisolone
E sodium pamidronate

6.22 Dipstick testing of urine for the presence of glucose was used as a screening test for diabetes mellitus; 800 patients were tested for glucosuria, of whom 200 who tested positive were later diagnosed as having diabetes mellitus, and there were 50 false positives.

The positive predictive value of this test is:

A 200/250
B 200/325
C 425/550
D 425/475
E 625/800

6.23 A 45-year-old man was referred with new onset diabetes and gynaecomastia. He also suffered with impotence over the past 3 months but was too embarrassed to tell anyone. He drank 8 units of alcohol a week and smoked 20 cigarettes a day. He was not on any medication. His only other symptom was longstanding painful knees.

On examination he had palmar erythema and gynaecomastia. His pulse was 72 regular and blood pressure 140/85. Chest and cardiovascular examinations were normal. He had 3 cm hepatomegaly but no abdominal distension or tenderness. Genital examination revealed small testes. Knee examination was normal.

Bloods	Hb	13.9	WCC	4.7
	Platelets	249	INR	1.1
	Bilirubin	20	Albumin	5
	Protein	67	ALT	45
	ALP	100	GGT	110
	Ferritin	1150	Calcium	2.20
	Phosphate	0.9	Glucose	12.1
Urinalysis	Glucose 1+, no protein			

Concerning the diagnosis and management of this patient it is true that:

A gene studies should be done to look for the YMDD mutation
B he is not at increased risk of developing hepatocellular carcinoma
C he should be venesected until his ferritin reaches 200
D his condition can be hereditary and his family should be screened
E diagnosis needs to be confirmed by performing a liver biopsy

6.24 A 5-year-old girl is seen recovering, having been treated successfully 1 day previously for the problem illustrated. She initially presented with irritability and inability to open her left eye. (Figure 6.24, page 398.)

The explanation for the findings is:

A bleeding disorder causing retro orbital haemorrhage
B ethmoid sinusitis causing orbital cellulitis
C fungal infection causing endophthalmitis
D lymphomatous infiltration of periorbital skin
E varicella zoster causing herpes zoster ophthalmicus

6.25 A 19-year-old man was referred because of progressive weakness in the lower limbs. His problems started a year ago when he found that he was walking like a 'drunkard' and noticed 'clawing' of his feet. Slurring of speech and tremor followed this. He was adopted and knew nothing about his family.

On examination he had a mild kyphosis and pes cavus. On shaking hands he was noted to have an intention tremor. He was fully orientated and mental test score was 10/10. He had difficulty pronouncing polysyllabic words. Cranial nerve examination revealed no abnormalities and his pupils were normal. Apart from his intention tremor his upper limbs were normal. There was weakness of both lower limbs with increased tone and reduced power; knee and ankle reflexes were absent but plantar responses were extensor. Pinprick sensation was intact but vibration sense and proprioception were reduced. He was unable to perform heel–shin movements and Romberg's sign was positive.

The most likely diagnosis is:

A Charcot–Marie–Tooth disease (HSMN)
B Friedreich's ataxia
C multiple sclerosis
D subacute combined degeneration of the cord
E tabes dorsalis

6.26 A 33-year-old farm worker was referred because of fatigue, progressive shortness of breath and productive cough over the past 6 months. His breathing was worse during the day but improved before going to sleep. He had normal appetite but had lost 3 kg over this time. His exercise tolerance was reduced to 200 m. There was no chest pain or palpitations. He had no previous medical history and was not on any medication. He did not smoke or drink alcohol.

On examination there was no clubbing, cyanosis, oedema or lymphadenopathy. His temperature was 37.3°C, pulse 100 regular and blood pressure 130/85. His JVP was not elevated and both heart sounds were normal. There were bilateral inspiratory crackles but no wheeze. Abdominal examination was normal.

Bloods	Hb	13.1	WCC	9.7
	Neutrophils	6.8	Lymphocytes	2.0
	Eosinophils	0.3	Platelets	239
	Na	140	K	4.7
	Urea	5.9	Creatinine	98
	Protein	65	Albumin	35
	Bilirubin	10	ALT	20
	ALP	78	Calcium	2.22
Chest X-ray	Bilateral patchy infiltrates			

The most likely diagnosis is:

A allergic bronchopulmonary aspergillosis
B bronchial asthma
C Churg–Strauss syndrome
D extrinsic allergic alveolitis
E Goodpasture's syndrome

6.27 A 61-year-old man known to suffer with Raynaud's phenomenon and rheumatoid arthritis was referred with rash on both legs, present for the past 2 months. He also complained of decreased sensation and pain in both his legs but no problems walking. Over the past week he had passed blood in his urine. His appetite had decreased and he had lost weight. Ten years ago he contracted hepatitis C through a blood transfusion abroad. He was not on any medication.

On examination he was apyrexial. His pulse was 88 regular and blood pressure 154/87. His JVP was not elevated and heart sounds were normal. His chest was clear. Abdominal examination revealed hepatomegaly. There was decreased sensation to light touch and pinprick up to the level of mid-shin. He had normal lower limb tone and power but absent ankle and plantar reflexes. The knee and ankle joints were tender but not inflamed. The rash on the legs was purpuric.

Bloods	Hb	11.9	MCV	92.4
	WCC	7.6	Platelets	459
	Na	138	K	4.8
	Urea	13.8	Creatinine	160
	Protein	74	Albumin	38
	Bilirubin	25	ALT	65
	ALP	100	ESR	65
	CRP	58	C_3	80
	C_4	8		
Rheumatoid factor	1 in 640			
Antinuclear antibody	Negative			
ANCA	Negative			
Hepatitis A, B serology	Negative			
Hepatitis C serology	Positive			
Urine dipstick	Blood 2+, protein 3+			
Chest X-ray	Normal			

The most likely diagnosis is:

A microscopic polyangiitis
B mixed cryoglobulinaemia
C polyarteritis nodosa
D systemic lupus erythematosus
E Wegener's granulomatosis

6.28 A 16-year-old girl was admitted with a 1-day history of headache, neck stiffness and photophobia.

She had a temperature of 38.5°C, pulse 110 regular and blood pressure 96/50. A lumbar puncture was undertaken and Gram stain analysis was performed on the CSF: (Figure 6.28, page 398.)

The most likely organism to have caused this is:

A *Escherichia coli*
B *Haemophilus influenza*
C *Mycobacterium tuberculosis*
D *Neisseria meningitidis*
E *Streptococcus pneumoniae*

6.29 An 83-year-old man complained of pain in his leg for 4 months.

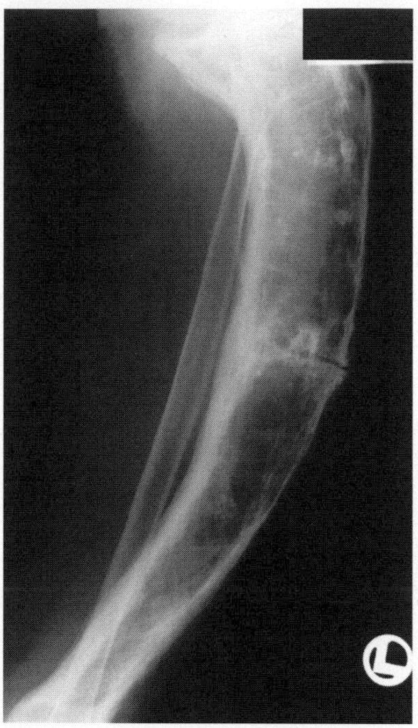

The X-ray is most consistent with:

A congenital syphilis
B hyperparathyroidism
C osteomalacia
D Paget's disease of bone
E sarcoidosis

6.30 A 57-year-old woman was referred because of severe pain in her hands.

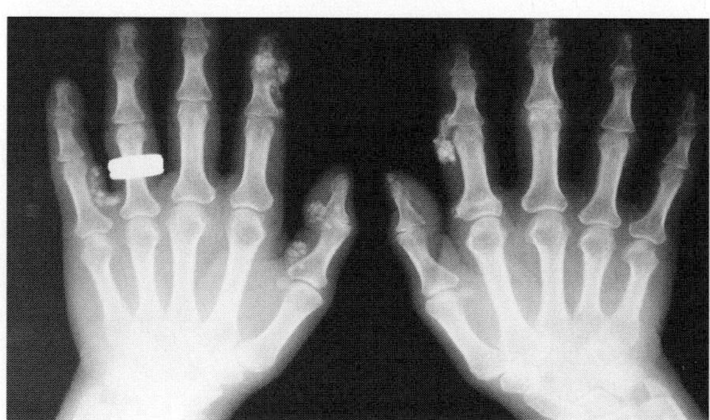

The X-ray findings would be most consistent with:

A gout
B hyperparathyroidism
C psoriatic arthropathy
D rheumatoid arthritis
E systemic sclerosis

6.31 A 14-year-old Nigerian girl was referred feeling lethargic and with pain and swelling in both knees for the past week. She had returned from visiting her family in Nigeria 2 weeks ago. While on holiday she had developed a sore throat. She had no previous medical history and was not on any medication.

On examination she had a temperature of 37.4°C. Her pulse was 66 regular and blood pressure 90/64. Her JVP was not elevated and she had an additional heart sound but no murmurs. Her chest was clear. Abdominal examination was normal. Both knees were hot, tender and swollen but there was no focal neurology.

Bloods	Hb	12.4	WCC	13.5
	Neutrophils	11.0	Platelets	330
	Na	136	K	4.5
	Urea	2.5	Creatinine	58
	Albumin	38	Protein	75
	Bilirubin	12	ALP	380
	ALT	24	Calcium	2.40
	Phosphate	0.98	ESR	120
	CRP	59	Urate	0.16
Rheumatoid factor	Negative			
Antinuclear antibody	Negative			
Hb electrophoresis	Normal			
Antistreptolysin O titre	1/160			
Hepatitis A, B, C serology	Negative			
Synovial fluid	WCC	350	50% polymorphs	
	No growth			
ECG	First-degree AV block			
Chest X-ray	Normal			

The most likely diagnosis is:

A infective endocarditis
B Kawasaki disease
C rheumatic fever
D Still's disease
E systemic lupus erythematosus

6.32 A 67-year-old man, admitted with an inferior myocardial infarction 2 days ago, developed palpitations and shortness of breath. As the doctor approached the patient he became pale, cold and clammy. The cardiac monitor showed the following trace.

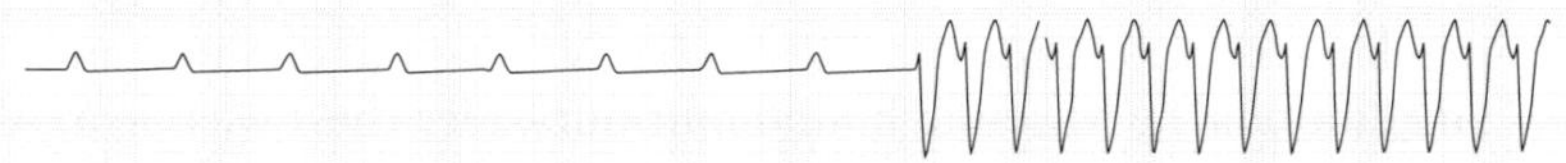

Assuming he improved after defibrillation, the next step in the immediate management of this patient would be:

A amiodarone infusion
B intravenous atropine
C lignocaine infusion
D magnesium infusion
E temporary pacing wire

6.33 A 70-year-old man was referred because of a 2-month history of a pruritic rash affecting the axillae, upper abdomen and neck. He had no previous medical problems and was not on any medication. (Figure 6.33, page 398.)

The most likely diagnosis is:

A bullous pemphigoid
B dermatitis herpetiformis
C epidermolysis bullosa
D pemphigus vulgaris
E scalded skin syndrome

6.34 A 45-year-old businessman was referred with progressive weight gain and lethargy. He smoked 20 cigarettes a day and drank 3 units of alcohol in the evening. He had a normal appetite. He found his job very stressful and was having some marital difficulties.

On examination he was plethoric and obese. There was some ankle oedema and bruising of his skin. His pulse was 98 and his blood pressure was 165/90. His chest was clear. Abdominal examination was normal.

	Urinary free cortisol (nmoL/24 h)	Cortisol (nmol/L) 9am	Cortisol (nmol/L) Midnight	ACTH (mg/L) 9am
Basal	400	900	150	50
0.5mg q.d.s. dexamethasone suppression test (48 h)		720		
2mg q.d.s. dexamethasone suppression test (48 h)		345		

The most likely diagnosis is:

A ACTH-secreting adrenal adenoma
B cortisol secreting adrenal adenoma
C ectopic ACTH secretion
D pituitary dependent adenoma
E pseudo-Cushing's due to alcohol

6.35 A 28-year-old woman was referred because she wanted to start a family. Her father suffered from haemophilia A but her mother had no clinical evidence of the disease. Her husband had also been tested and had a normal genotype.

Her risk of having a son with haemophilia A is:

A 0%
B 25%
C 50%
D 75%
E 100%

6.36 A 45-year-old publican was admitted with severe right-sided abdominal pain for the past 2 days, which radiated to the back and woke him from sleep. It came and went in severe spasms with no relieving factors. There was also some haematuria. He still drank 2 units of alcohol a day although he had cut down his intake. Over the past 4 months he had lost weight and had a decreased appetite. His stools were foul smelling and were difficult to flush away.

On examination he had a temperature of 37.4°C, pulse 88 regular and blood pressure 130/78. He was tender over the right loin but had no guarding. There was no organomegaly and bowel sounds were present. Rectal examination revealed steatorrhoea.

Bloods	Hb	13.5	WCC	12.3
	Neutrophils	10.0	Platelets	325
	Na	139	K	4.5
	Urea	5.6	Creatinine	100
	Albumin	35	Protein	67
	Calcium	2.01	Phosphate	0.80
	Amylase	100		
Urinalysis	Blood 2+			
Abdominal X-ray	Three small right renal calculi			

The likely composition of the renal calculi in this patient would be:

A cystine
B oxalate
C phosphate
D urate
E xanthine

6.37 A 77-year-old man was admitted with an acute facial and left limb weakness. He had no previous medical history. He smoked 30 cigarettes a day and drank 4 units of alcohol per night.

On examination he was unable to close his right eye and the angle of his mouth on the right was drooping down. He was able to raise his eyebrows. Ear examination was normal. There was left sided weakness of his upper and lower limbs. Tone was increased and power was reduced. His right plantar response was flexor and his left plantar was extensor. No sensory abnormalities could be detected.

The likely cause of the facial weakness is:

A Bell's palsy
B Foster Kennedy syndrome due to cerebral tumour
C middle cerebral artery occlusion
D pontine infarction
E posterior inferior cerebellar artery thrombosis

6.38 A 34-year-old man was admitted with severe shortness of breath and cough productive of yellow sputum. This was his third admission this year with chest problems. He was a heavy smoker. He took nebulised salbutamol and ipratropium bromide but did not have home oxygen therapy and had not required ventilation in the past. He had never been exposed to asbestos.

On examination he was breathless at rest. His temperature was 37.4°C, pulse 98 regular and blood pressure 135/86. His respiratory rate was 28 breaths/min and he had bilateral wheeze on chest auscultation. There was also 2 cm non-tender hepatomegaly.

The admitting doctor considered a possible diagnosis of α_1-antitrypsin deficiency.

Bloods	Hb	14.7	WCC	12.7
	Platelets	190	Na	145
	K	4.3	Urea	7.5
	Creatinine	110	Protein	58
	Albumin	38	Bilirubin	30
	ALT	34	ALP	76
Chest X-ray	Hyperinflated lung fields			
	Bulla at right base			
Arterial blood gases on air	pH	7.38	PCO_2	6.7
	PO_2	7.8	Bicarbonate	35.2
	Base excess	8.7		

Concerning this patient's condition it is correct that:

- A administration of influenza vaccination is contraindicated
- B he is likely to develop centrilobular emphysema
- C if a liver transplant for cirrhosis were performed, the condition would recur in the new donor organ
- D lung function tests are likely to show a decreased FEV_1/FVC ratio and increased residual volume
- E patients with a phenotype of PiMM are more likely to develop emphysema

6.39 A 53-year-old man was referred with a 12-month history of abdominal pain and bloating and loose stools. He had lost 4 kg, associated with decreased appetite. His stools were semi-liquid with some mucus but no blood. Recently he had become increasingly lethargic and short of breath on exertion. He had a previous medical history of arthritis that affected various joints for a few days before resolving: hips, knees, elbows and shoulders. He only took paracetamol. He did not drink alcohol or smoke. He had no recent travel abroad.

On examination he was thin and his skin was hyperpigmented but there was no rash. There was cervical lymphadenopathy. His temperature was 37.2°C, pulse 90 regular and blood pressure 120/78. His JVP was not elevated and heart sounds were normal. There was dullness to percussion at both lung bases. His abdomen was soft and mildly tender. There was no organomegaly and rectal examination was normal. Neurological examination was normal. The left knee joint was mildly swollen and inflamed but there was no effusion clinically.

Bloods	Hb	11.9	MCV	100.2
	WCC	4.6	Platelets	340
	Protein	64	Albumin	34
	Bilirubin	20	ALT	28
	ALP	120	Calcium	1.89
	Phosphate	0.71	ESR	35
	CRP	42	Amylase	40
Rheumatoid factor	Negative			
Chest X-ray	Bilateral pleural effusions			

The most likely diagnosis is:

A amyloidosis
B carcinoid syndrome
C coeliac disease
D Crohn's disease
E Whipple's disease

6.40 A 55-year-old man was referred for endoscopy because of intermittent dysphagia.

A fixed lesion was seen at endoscopy. (Figure 6.40, page 399.)

The endoscopic findings are consistent with:

A achalasia
B Barrett's oesophagus
C benign oesophageal stricture
D oesophageal carcinoma
E Schatzki ring

6.41 A 27-year-old man, known to suffer from HIV and a heavy drinker, was brought in confused and drowsy. He could not say whether he had suffered any trauma to his head.

On examination his GCS was 14/15. CT head was performed.

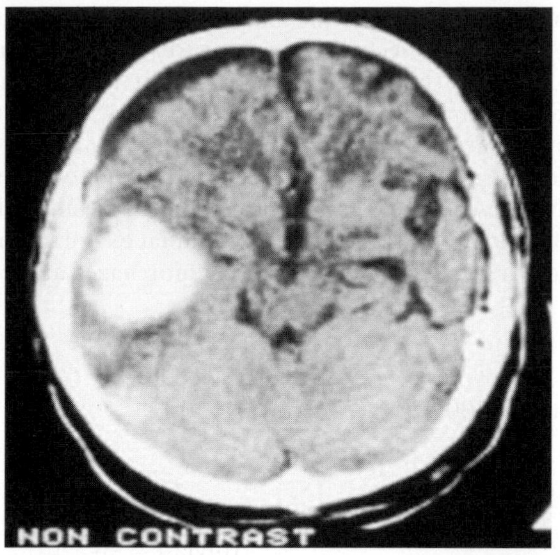

The **TWO** diagnoses that can be made from the scan are:

A acute cerebral infarct
B acute extradural haemorrhage
C acute intracerebral haemorrhage
D acute subdural haemorrhage
E cerebral abscess
F cerebral toxoplasmosis
G chronic cerebral infarct
H chronic extradural haemorrhage
I chronic intracerebral haemorrhage
J chronic subdural haemorrhage
K midline shift
L subarachnoid haemorrhage

6.42 A 50-year-old man known to suffer with muscle weakness and arthritis was referred with a rash on both hands. He also had had a rash on his face that involved the eyelids but not the eyes. (Figure 6.42, page 399.)

The most likely diagnosis is:

A dermatomyositis
B porphyria cutanea tarda
C rheumatoid arthritis
D systemic lupus erythematosus
E systemic sclerosis

6.43 A 25-year-old woman presented with a 3-month history of headaches, palpitations and sweating. She had been started on bendrofluazide because she was found to be hypertensive but that had not helped her symptoms. She had no previous medical history. She smoked 10 cigarettes a day but did not drink alcohol.

On examination her pulse was 100 regular and blood pressure 200/130. Her JVP was not elevated and heart sounds were normal. Her chest was clear. She had no neck swelling. Abdominal examination was normal. Fundoscopy revealed flame-shaped haemorrhages and cotton wool spots.

Bloods	Hb	15.6	WCC	6.7
	Platelets	400	Na	140
	K	4.0	Urea	5.0
	Creatinine	98	TSH	2.5
	Free T_4	20	Glucose	7.5
Chest X-ray	Enlarged heart			
ECG	Sinus tachycardia			
	Voltage criteria for left ventricular hypertrophy present			

The most likely diagnosis is:

A carcinoid syndrome
B Conn's syndrome
C Cushing's syndrome
D phaeochromocytoma
E T_3 thyrotoxicosis

6.44 A 20-year-old man presented with a 6-week history of abdominal pain and bloody diarrhoea. He was opening his bowels over eight times a day and his stools were liquid in consistency. He had a poor appetite and had lost >5 kg in weight over this time period. There was no previous medical history, he had not travelled abroad and he was not on any medication. He did not smoke or drink alcohol.

On examination his temperature was 37.5°C, pulse 110 regular and blood pressure 95/50. He had generalised abdominal tenderness. Rectal examination revealed fresh blood.

Bloods	Hb	10.5	WCC	12.5
	Neutrophils	10.2	Platelets	500
	Na	140	K	3.9
	Urea	5.9	Creatinine	100
	Albumin	28	Protein	56
	ALT	25	ALP	70
	Amylase	49	ESR	45
	CRP	200		
Chest X-ray	Normal			
Abdominal X-ray	Transverse colonic diameter 5.5 cm			

Regarding this patient's management it is true that:

A ciclosporin has no role in acute colitis
B he needs an urgent colonoscopy and then to start on intravenous steroids
C he should be treated initially with topical corticosteroids
D he should be treated with prophylactic subcutaneous heparin
E start intravenous antibiotics after stool cultures have been taken

6.45 A 48-year-old man was referred with sleep problems. He complained of excessive sleepiness and falling asleep at the wheel of his car. At night he had woken up and felt his whole body paralysed. On a number of occasions he had collapsed without warning but with no loss of consciousness and these attacks lasted a few minutes. There was no previous medical history. He did not smoke or drink alcohol. He had not been on any long-haul flights recently.

On examination he looked well. There were no clinical abnormalities to find on examination and his BMI was 25.

The most likely diagnosis is:

A bruxism
B complex partial epilepsy
C idiopathic insomnia
D narcolepsy
E obstructive sleep apnoea

6.46 A 64-year-old woman complained of headaches. She also had pain in her back and hips.

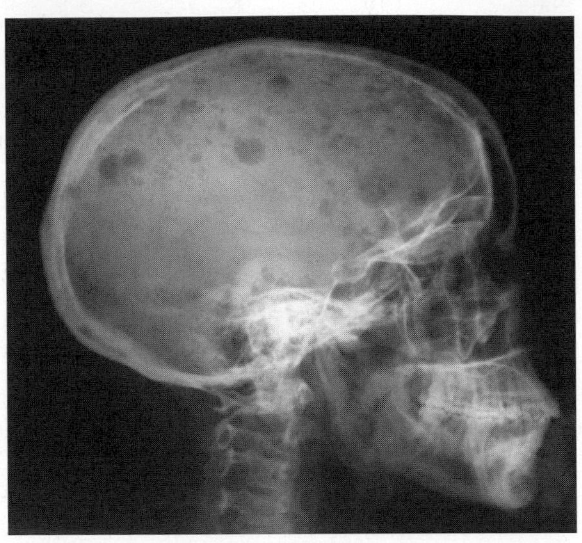

The most likely diagnosis is:

A hypoparathyroidism
B multiple myeloma
C osteoporosis
D Paget's disease of bone
E Sturge–Weber syndrome

6.47 A 12-year-old boy was referred to the dermatology clinic. (Figure 6.47, page 399.)

The dermatological sign elicited here is:

A cutis hyperelastica
B cutis laxa
C dermatographia
D Nikolsky's sign
E pathergy

6.48 A 30-year-old woman developed a non-tender swelling in her neck followed by tiredness, palpitations and sweating. She was 6 weeks post-partum. She had no previous medical history and had had no recent illnesses. She was not on any medication.

On examination, she had bilateral lid lag. Her skin was moist and she had palmar erythema. Her pulse was 110 regular and blood pressure 145/90. She had a smooth non-tender goitre.

Bloods	Hb	13.5	WCC	9.5
	Platelets	230	ESR	9
	TSH	0.01	Free T_4	35
24-h radioactive ^{131}I uptake scan	<1% uptake after 24 h			

The most likely diagnosis is:

A DeQuervain's thyroiditis
B Graves' disease
C postpartum thyroiditis
D sick euthyroid syndrome
E solitary toxic adenoma

6.49 A 45-year-old man with cirrhosis secondary to primary sclerosing cholangitis and hepatitis C was referred for orthotopic liver transplantation (OLT). He had now developed diuretic resistant ascites which required repeated drainage. He used to drink alcohol and inject drugs but not any more.

On examination he looked cachectic. No abnormalities were found apart from ascites. He was not encephalopathic and had never had spontaneous bacterial peritonitis.

OLT in this patient would be contraindicated if:

A Doppler ultrasound revealed portal vein thrombosis
B during assessment he was found to have developed cholangiocarcinoma
C he had a previous medical history of paracetamol overdose
D he was currently still taking methadone
E he was found to be co-infected with HIV

6.50 A 13-year-old boy was referred because of headaches and fits which had been occurring on and off for a number of years.

A CT head was performed.

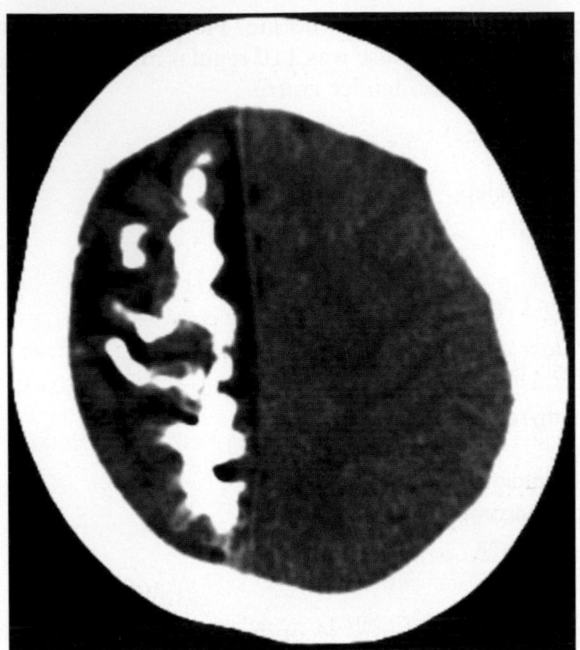

The CT findings are most consistent with:

A hypoparathyroidism
B Laurence–Moon–Biedl syndrome
C neurofibromatosis
D Sturge–Weber syndrome
E tuberous sclerosis

6.51 A 14-year-old boy presented with 'collapse'. He did not lose consciousness and did not fit. Prior to this he had been getting tingling in the hands for a number of years but had never received any treatment. He had no other medical problems and was not on any medication.

On examination he looked unwell. In his mouth there appeared to be some darkening of the buccal mucosa. His pulse was 100 regular and blood pressure 95/60. There were no other abnormalities on clinical examination.

Bloods	Hb	12.5	WCC	8.3
	Platelets	345	Na	130
	K	6.2	Urea	4.3
	Creatinine	50	Glucose	2.8
	Calcium	1.95	Albumin	40
	PTH	0.4		

The most likely diagnosis is:

A autoimmune polyglandular syndrome (APS) I
B APS 2
C multiple endocrine neoplasia (MEN) I syndrome
D MEN 2A syndrome
E MEN 2B syndrome

6.52 A 30-year-old woman was referred with a 6-month history of chronic diarrhoea. She had a normal appetite and no weight loss. There was no previous medical history or significant family history and she was not on any medication. A diagnosis of irritable bowel syndrome was suspected.

Of the following symptoms the one which is **NOT** typical of this condition is:

A feeling of incomplete evacuation
B passing loose, watery stools
C passing mucus in the stools
D severe bloating
E waking from sleep to open bowels

6.53 A 20-year-old man presented with a sore throat to his GP. He was diagnosed with tonsillitis and treated with amoxicillin. Three days later he re-presented to his GP complaining of haematuria. He reported no joint pain or rash. He had no other medical problems and was not on any other medication.

On examination he was apyrexial, had some cervical lymphadenopathy and red inflamed tonsils. The rest of the physical examination was normal.

Bloods	Hb	13.0	WCC	8.5
	Platelets	270	Na	138
	K	4.5	Urea	2.8
	Creatinine	68	Protein	0
	Albumin	40	CRP	25
Urinalysis	Protein 1+, red cells 1+, blood 1+, no white cells			
	Red cell casts and dysmorphic red cells			
Chest X-ray	Normal			

The most likely diagnosis is:

A acute interstitial nephritis secondary to amoxycillin
B Henoch-Schönlein purpura
C IgA nephropathy
D infectious mononucleosis
E poststreptococcal glomerulonephritis

6.54 A 45-year-old man presented to Accident & Emergency with pyrexia, malaise and abdominal pain. He had returned from Nigeria 10 days ago. (Figure 6.54, page 400.)

The organism seen in the film is:

A *Leishmania donovani*
B Loa loa
C *Plasmodium falciparum*
D *Schistosoma haematobium*
E *Trypanosoma brucei gambiense*

6.55 A 49-year-old man with advanced disease had a biopsy to assess prognosis. (Figure 6.55, page 400.)

Which one of the following prognostic scoring systems could be applied to this patient?

A Ann Arbor
B Rockall
C Childs–Pugh
D Dukes'
E Breslow

6.56 A 62-year-old man was referred feeling unwell. He had just finished a course of chemotherapy for lymphoma. He had no cough or urinary symptoms but reported malaise and decreased appetite for the past 2 days.

On examination his temperature was 38.5°C, pulse 100 and blood pressure 100/78. His chest was clear and abdominal examination was normal. There was no focal neurological defect and plantar responses were flexor. Examination of the oropharynx was also normal.

Bloods	Hb	12.1	WCC	1.8
	Neutrophils	0.9	Lymphocytes	0.5
	Platelets	130	INR	1.1
	Na	139	K	4.8
	Urea	10.6	Creatinine	139
	Protein	78	Albumin	31
	Bilirubin	12	ALT	22
	ALP	120	CRP	40
Chest X-ray	Normal			
Urinalysis	No WCC, no protein			

The most appropriate treatment for this patient is:

A ceftazidime and fluconazole
B cefuroxime and metronidazole
C rifampicin, isoniazid and pyrazinamide
D tazocin and gentamicin
E vancomycin and fusidic acid

6.57 A 63-year-old woman was referred because she had cervical lymphadenopathy and a palpable spleen.

A blood film was prepared. (Figure 6.57, page 400.)

The most likely diagnosis is:

A acute lymphoblastic leukaemia
B acute myeloid leukaemia
C chronic lymphocytic leukaemia
D chronic myeloid leukaemia
E infectious mononucleosis

6.58 A 54-year-old man was being assessed for a coronary artery bypass graft when he was noted to have cholesterol 8.2, urea 15 and creatinine 210. He had a previous history of intermittent claudication and hypertension but was not on any medication. He was a heavy smoker.

On examination his pulse was 90 regular and blood pressure 170/100. His JVP was not elevated and his chest and heart sounds were normal. Abdominal examination was normal but there were bilateral femoral bruits. Fundoscopy revealed flame-shaped haemorrhages and silver-wiring.

Renal ultrasound	Left kidney 9 cm, Right kidney 10.9 cm
	No hydronephrosis or extrarenal masses

The next most appropriate test to establish the cause of the renal findings would be:

- A DMSA scan
- B Doppler ultrasound
- C MAG 3 scan
- D magnetic resonance angiography
- E renal biopsy

6.59 A 43-year-old HIV-positive man was referred because of chronic watery diarrhoea that had been going on for 5 months. He also had associated abdominal pain, decreased appetite and weight loss of 6 kg in that time period. He had no other medical problems and was not on any medication.

He appeared cachectic but the rest of his physical examination was unremarkable.

Bloods	Hb	12.8	WCC 4.2
	Platelets	190	
CD_4	300		

The most likely cause of his symptoms is:

- A cryptosporidia
- B cytomegalovirus colitis
- C microsporidia
- D *Mycobacterium avium intracellulare*
- E non-Hodgkin's lymphoma

6.60 A 34-year-old Algerian refugee was referred because of malaise, ankle swelling and heavy proteinuria for the past month. In the past he had suffered from recurrent elbow and knee joint pain and intermittent abdominal pain. He had no surviving family members. He smoked 15 cigarettes a day but did not drink alcohol. He was not on any medication.

On examination he had bilateral pitting oedema up to the thighs. He was apyrexial, pulse 79 regular and blood pressure 125/84. His JVP was not elevated and heart sounds were normal. There was dullness at both lung bases. Abdominal and musculoskeletal examination was normal.

Bloods	Hb	10.6	MCV	93.4
	WCC	7.9	Platelets	346
	Na	140	K	4.8
	Urea	8.2	Creatinine	128
	Protein	50	Albumin	22
	ESR	40	CRP	26
	C_3	80	C_4	30
Urinalysis	Protein 4+, no blood, no red cells, no white cells			
24-h urinary protein collection	12.7 g/L			

The most helpful test to determine the diagnosis is:

- A antinuclear antibody
- B protein electrophoresis
- C rectal biopsy
- D renal biopsy
- E serum cryoglobulins

6.61 A 55-year-old man was referred to the clinic with chronic diarrhoea, lethargy and 5 kg weight loss. Three months ago he returned from southern India where he had been working as an engineer for the past 2 years. He opened his bowels up to four times per day and the motions were difficult to flush away but there was no blood. He had a normal appetite and was not vegetarian. He had no previous medical history or family history of note and was on no medication. He drank 5 units of alcohol a week but did not smoke.

On examination he was apyrexial. There was no jaundice but he was pale and had mild pitting oedema of both ankles. Abdominal and rectal examination was normal.

Bloods	Hb	9.4	MCV	103.7
	WCC	5.7	Platelets	220
	Folate	1.1	B12	135
	Iron	15	Ferritin	250
	Na	133	K	3.5
	Urea	3.5	Creatinine	66
	Albumin	33	Ca	2.05
	PO_4	0.60	ALP	135

Tissue transglutaminase	Negative
Upper GI endoscopy	Normal apart from some flattening
of duodenal folds	
Colonoscopy	Normal
Duodenal biopsies	Shortened, blunted villi with elongated crypts
Stool culture and microscopy	Negative

The **MOST** likely diagnosis is:

- A bacterial overgrowth
- B coeliac disease
- C Crohn's disease
- D giardiasis
- E tropical sprue

6.62 A 45-year-old man presented to Accident & Emergency feeling unwell and tired with muscle cramps and severe tremor. Four weeks previously he had had a liver transplant for hepatitis B cirrhosis. He had developed diabetes mellitus post transplant. He did not drink or smoke. He was taking his insulin and immunosuppressive medication as prescribed.

On examination he was apyrexial, pulse was 90 regular and blood pressure was 144/92. Examination of chest and abdomen was normal with no wound dehiscence. There was no evidence of encephalopathy but he had a marked tremor of his hands.

Bloods	Hb	10.1	WCC	4.4
	Platelets	200	PT	15
	Na	133	K	5.3
	Urea	10.5	Creatinine	160
	Bilirubin	20	Albumin	30
	ALT	35	ALP	120
	Calcium	2.30	Phosphate	0.73
	Magnesium	0.64	CRP	10
	Glucose	18.5	Cholesterol	4.5

Which one of the drugs he was taking is the **MOST** likely to have caused his symptoms?

A azathioprine
B insulin
C mycophenolate mofetil
D prednisolone
E tacrolimus

6.63 A 56-year-old man was admitted to the coronary care unit with non-ST elevation myocardial infarction (NSTEMI). He was treated with aspirin, atorvastatin, clopidogrel and atenolol. The next day he became acutely short of breath, cold and clammy but denied any chest pain.

On examination he was apyrexial. His pulse was 95 regular, blood pressure was 110/60, CVP +16 mmHg and heart sounds normal. Auscultation of his chest revealed bilateral crackles and respiratory rate of 24 breaths per minute. Abdominal examination was normal; he was oliguric. He was given intravenous furosemide and glyceryl trinitrate infusion but his symptoms did not improve.

Bloods	Na	128	K	2.9
	Urea	8.6	Creatinine	120
Chest X-ray	Bilateral pulmonary oedema			
Echo	Severely impaired left ventricular function			
	Ejection fraction 25%			

In view of his deteriorating condition it was felt that he should be started on inotropic support.

The following drugs should be given:

A adrenaline (epinephrine)
B dobutamine
C dopamine
D milrinone
E noradrenaline

6.64 A 48-year-old man was admitted to Accident & Emergency with a 5-week history of persistent cough, haemoptysis and weight loss. He was a heavy smoker. He had recently returned from Turkey but was well before he travelled there. He was also HIV-positive but not receiving any treatment.

On examination he had a temperature of 37.8°C, pulse of 78 and blood pressure of 120/82. He had bronchial breathing in the right upper zone. Abdominal and neurological examination was normal.

CD_4 count	200
Viral load	30000
Chest X-ray	Right upper lobe collapse and consolidation
Sputum	Acid fast bacilli seen with Ziehl–Nielson staining

The patient was suspected of having pulmonary tuberculosis

The correct statement regarding diagnosis and management is:

- A Mantoux test would give useful information about his possible TB status
- B he should be treated for TB before starting anti-HIV medication
- C anti-TB medication should be started with rifampicin, isoniazid and pyrazinamide for 6 months
- D detecting acid fast bacilli in the sputum confirms the diagnosis of *Mycobacterium tuberculosis*
- E radiological improvement is unlikely to occur for at least 4 months

6.65 A 16 year-old-boy was referred by his GP with a 3 month history of bloody diarrhoea and recurrent mouth ulcers. He opened his bowels up to four times per day. At age 10 he had developed *Staphylococcus* hepatic abscess and aged 13 he had contracted *Klebsiella* pneumonia.

On examination he looked thin and had bilateral cervical lymphadenopathy. He was apyrexial. Cardiovascular and chest examination was normal. Abdomen was soft with mild left sided tenderness, hepatosplenomegaly and perianal skin tags. He had a colonoscopy which revealed patchy ulceration and inflammation throughout his colon.

Bloods	Hb	9.8	MCV	96.5
	WCC	10.6	Platelets	340
	Neutrophils	8.5	Lymphocytes	1.5
	Na	134	K	4.2
	Urea	2.2	Creatinine	55
	Albumin	29	Bilirubin	12
	ALT	30	ALP	120
	CRP	25	ESR	60
	IgA	1.4	IgG	16.8
	IgM	2.0		
Colonic biopsies	Moderate inflammation with granulomas			

The most likely diagnosis is:

A Chediak-Higashi syndrome
B chronic granulomatous disease
C combined variable immunodeficiency
D severe combined immunodeficiency
E Wiskott-Aldrich syndrome

6.66 A 49-year-old man presented to Accident & Emergency with known alcoholic liver disease, and was admitted with ascites and variceal haemorrhage. He had had four previous admissions for variceal haemorrhage and had diuretic resistant ascites. He had never had encephalopathy.

He was treated successfully with medical therapy. When he was stable, transjugular intrahepatic portosystemic shunt (TIPSS) was inserted to prevent recurrence of these complications.

	Pre-TIPSS (mmHg)	Post-TIPSS (mmHg)
Wedged hepatic vein pressure	17	9
Free hepatic vein pressure	3	4

The new portal pressure gradient is:

A −1
B 5
C 8
D 9
E 14

6.67 A 24-year-old man was admitted to Accident & Emergency with severe head injuries following a car crash. CT head revealed traumatic brain injury with intracerebral bleeding not amenable to neurosurgery. His GCS was 3/15. He was intubated and ventilated and transferred to intensive care. After 2 days he showed no signs of regaining consciousness.

Prior to this accident he had expressed a wish to donate his organs after his death. Before harvesting of organs can occur the patient has to be declared brain stem dead.

The **TWO** following criteria are correct for diagnosing brainstem death:

A absent corneal reflex but pupils can react to light
B absent gag reflex
C absent spinal reflexes
D assessment can be done by transplant team
E assessment has to be done by three consultants
F haemoglobin concentration needs to be > 8 mg/dl
G no evidence of sepsis
H no motor responses in cranial nerve distribution after sedation and relaxants have been stopped
I no spontaneous respiration when disconnected from ventilator and PO_2 <6.7 kPa
J no testing until at least 24 h after the development of coma

6.68 A 20-year-old man was referred by his GP. The patient had noticed when in the shower that his left testicle was larger than his right. There was no history of trauma or urinary tract infection. He had no previous medical history.

On examination his left testicle was tender and 3 cm larger than the right. Abdominal examination was normal.

Regarding his diagnosis it is correct that:

A choriocarcinoma is the least aggressive of the germ cell tumours
B development of pulmonary metastases still carries a good prognosis
C diagnosis should be confirmed histologically by transscrotal biopsy
D elevated carcinoembryonic antigen (CEA) is associated with a worse prognosis in testicular cancer
F seminoma is the most common testicular tumour in this age group

6.69 A 35-year-old Caucasian man was referred by his GP with a 4-week history of rash on his trunk, palms and soles. He had also noticed patchy hair loss. He was homosexual and had multiple sexual partners. He did not complain of any dysuria or rash on his penis or groin. He was not on any medication. He was HIV-negative. He had no recent foreign travel.

On examination he had a scaling maculopapular rash on his trunk, palms and plantar surfaces of his feet. He had bilateral cervical lymphadenopathy and patchy alopecia. He was also noted to have warty lesions in the perianal region. The rest of his physical examination was normal.

Treponemal enzyme immunoassay (EIA)	IgG positive
Treponema pallidum **particle agglutination (TPPA) assay**	Positive
Rapid plasma reagin/ Venereal Disease Research Laboratory (VDRL)	1:128

This patient's diagnosis is:

A early latent syphilis
B gummatous syphilis
C late latent syphilis
D primary syphilis
E secondary syphilis

6.70 A 33-year-old woman was admitted with a ruptured cerebral aneurysm that required surgical intervention for drainage of haematoma. Following surgery she remained intubated and ventilated and was transferred to ITU. Seventy-two hours after admission her GCS was 6/15; she developed a fever of 38.9°C and became hypoxic despite high inspired oxygen concentration. She had no previous medical history and was not on any medication prior to this admission.

On examination her pulse was 110 regular and blood pressure was 120/70. She was on synchronised intermittent mandatory ventilation (SIMV) with an inspired oxygen concentration of 60%. She had decreased breath sounds at both lung bases.

Chest X-ray	Bilateral pulmonary infiltrates

Regarding this patient's condition it is correct that:

A gastric acid suppression with histamine receptor antagonists (H2RA) increases the risk of developing chest infections
B she should be treated with vancomycin
C the likelihood of her developing infections is decreased by a tracheostomy
D the most likely infective organism is *Streptococcus pneumoniae*
E tracheal aspiration is the best method of culturing an organism

6.71 A 15-year-old boy was admitted with a painful, swollen left knee following a game of football. He was known to suffer from moderate haemophilia A. He was not on any medication and could not remember how he was treated in the past.

On examination he was apyrexial but in some pain. His pulse was 90 regular and blood pressure 108/74. He had an obvious tender, bruised, swollen left knee but no external bleeding. There was pain on movement and weight bearing, with a decreased range of movements.

Bloods	Hb	13.0	WCC	9.6
	Platelets	200	PT	12
	APTT	75	Fibrinogen	2.0
	APTT with 50:50 mix of normal plasma 42			

The **MOST** appropriate treatment is:

A cryoprecipitate
B fresh frozen plasma
C recombinant factor IX
D recombinant factor VIII
E tranexamic acid

6.72 A 73-year-old man was referred by his GP with terminal dribbling and dysuria. Examination was normal apart from a large, firm, craggy prostate on rectal examination.

His PSA was raised at 25 (normal < 4.1 ng/mL).

Concerning the patient's management and prognosis it is correct that:

A spread direct to the rectum is common in prostate cancer
B metastatic disease can be controlled by bilateral orchidectomy
C post surgery he should be treated with a luteinising hormone releasing hormone antagonist depot injection
D post surgery PSA cannot be used to screen for disease recurrence
E radiotherapy has not been shown to be effective in treating prostate cancer

6.73 A 58-year-old man with COPD and Type 1 diabetes was admitted to ITU with respiratory failure. He was slow to wean off mechanical ventilation. At the time of his intubation he had a nasogastric (NG) tube inserted for feeding. After 5 days he still had not opened his bowels and was having large aspirates from his NG tube. The rate of NG feed was reduced to 20 ml/h and he was given metoclopramide and erythromycin (for its prokinetic effect) but still continued to have large aspirates despite normal plasma electrolytes.

The **NEXT** step in his nutritional management is to:

A insert a nasojejunal feeding tube
B insert a percutaneous endoscopic gastrostomy (PEG)
C leave him on intravenous fluids only
D reduce the NG feed rate to 10 ml/h
E start total parenteral nutrition (TPN)

6.74 A 65 year old man presented to Accident & Emergency with a headache and vomiting for the past 2 days. There was no history of trauma. His GCS was 13/15.

A CT head was performed.

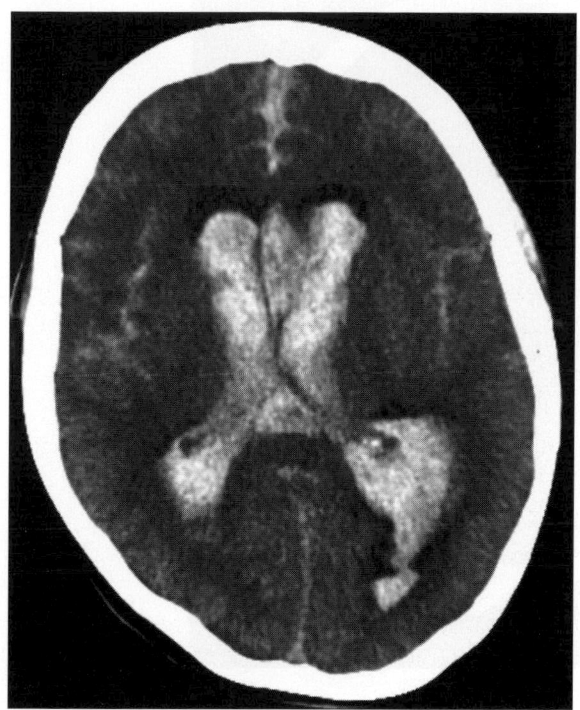

The **THREE** diagnoses that can be made from the CT head are:

A acute cerebral infarct
B acute extradural haemorrhage
C acute intracerebral haemorrhage
D acute subdural haemorrhage
E cerebral abscess
F cerebral metastases
G cerebral toxoplasmosis
H chronic cerebral infarct
I chronic extradural haemorrhage
J chronic subdural haemorrhage
K hydrocephalus
L interventricular haemorrhage
M midline shift
N skull fracture
O subarachnoid haemorrhage

6.75 A 72-year-old man was referred to Accident & Emergency with collapse and unsteadiness.

Physical examination was normal. A CT head was performed.

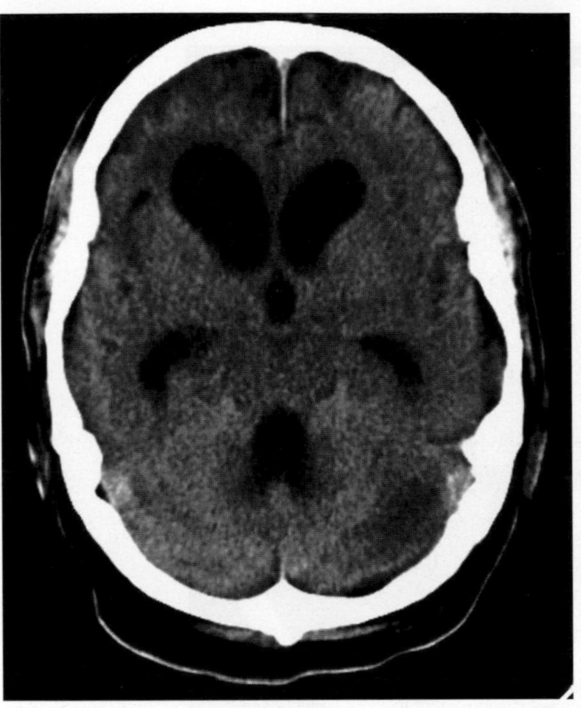

His CT scan shows:

A anterior falx haemorrhage
B communicating hydrocephalus
C non-communicating hydrocephalus
D normal CT showing age-related changes
E previous cerebrovascular accident

Paper 6

Answers

6.1 **C*** Patients with inferior or inferoposterior myocardial infarction are at risk of infarcting the right ventricle. The clinical presentation is of a patient who becomes acutely unwell, hypotensive, with an elevated JVP and clear lung fields. An ECG will usually show ST elevation in the inferior leads (II, III and aVF) and ST elevation in V_4R–V_6R. The correct management of these patients is to fluid resuscitate with possible inotropic support to ensure high filling pressures. Rupture of the interventricular septum to produce acute ventricular septal defect, and rupture of the papillary muscles to produce acute mitral regurgitation may also cause hypotension and elevated JVP. However, a murmur would be expected, and the development of acute pulmonary oedema. Cardiac tamponade is very difficult to diagnose but should be suspected if heart sounds are difficult to hear, and there is an elevated JVP, pulsus paradoxus and a globular heart on chest X-ray.

6.2 **E**** The ECG shows ST elevation in leads II, III and aVF with ST depression in V_{1-3} consistent with an inferoposterior MI.

6.3 **B*** This young girl may well have taken amphetamines, 'ecstasy' or MDMA (methylenedioxymetamphetamine) while in the nightclub, which could account for her malignant hyperpyrexia, acute renal failure, imminent DIC and decreased conscious level. If her creatinine kinase were measured, it would be very raised consistent with rhabdomyolyis in which myoglobin is released; hence, urine dipstick and microscopy will reveal blood but no red cells. The mainstay of treatment is rehydration and alkalinization of urine. Furosemide acidifies urine and may enhance myoglobin tubular damage. With rhabdomyolysis there is a risk of compartment syndrome and so fasciotomy may be necessary.

6.4 **C**** This patient has acanthosis nigricans, which is a rare darkly pigmented velvety thickening of flexural skin. It can be associated with insulin resistance, obesity and various endocrinopathies, such as insulin dependent diabetes, Cushing's syndrome, polycystic ovary disease and thyroid disease. In the absence of these, malignant disease should be excluded. Intra-abdominal adenocarcinoma should be suspected: stomach, colon, pancreas, gallbladder and oesophagus. Renal cell carcinoma is not an association.

6.5 **A**** During pregnancy women may develop goitre. There is an increase in total thyroxine but normal levels of free T_4 and free T_3. Virus-induced subacute thyroiditis may cause transient thyrotoxicosis but is usually associated with thyroid tenderness and, unlike other forms of hyperthyroidism, reduced radioactive iodine uptake.

6.6 **B**** The absolute risk reduction (ARR) is the absolute amount by which interferon-β reduces the risk of relapse at the end of 5 years. As patients are randomly assigned, there are 1000 patients in each group.

Relative risk of relapse in interferon-β group = 20/1000 = 0.02

Relative risk of relapse in placebo group = 100/1000 = 0.1

ARR = 0.1–0.02 = 08

6.7 **D*** This patient is most likely to have had a further variceal haemorrhage; the fact that he has had banding of his varices in the past suggests that he has oesophageal varices rather than gastric varices, which are usually treated with histoacryl glue injections. Proton pump inhibitors like omeprazole should be given to patients who present with an upper gastrointestinal haemorrhage where the cause is unclear (see **1.25**). The bleeding is due to portal hypertension and in the long term management, non-selective β-blockers, like propranolol, are the best drugs for secondary prophylaxis against further variceal haemorrhage to lower the portal pressure; they should not be given when there is an acute haemorrhage, especially when patients may be shocked and unable to tolerate them. This patient should have his circulating volume corrected with blood. Care must be taken to prevent hypokalaemia and hyponatraemia. In this case dextrose, even with potassium supplementation, will worsen the low sodium; normal saline may make the ascites worse but this can be therapeutically drained in due course. Spironolactone may make the hyponatraemia worse. Glypressin, a vasopressin analogue, is a powerful vasoconstrictor which reduces blood flow to the splanchnic organs, resulting in decreased portal blood flow and portal pressure and, unlike octreotide, which is a somatostatin analogue, is the only drug proven to improve mortality in variceal haemorrhage. Patients with variceal haemorrhage are at high risk of hepatic decompensation, resulting in encephalopathy, developing infections and fluid retention. Even though this patient shows no signs of infection there is good evidence that prophylactic treatment with third-generation cephalosporins reduces the risk of bacterial translocation from the gut. Other measures in this patient's acute management include administration of clotting factors (i.e. fresh frozen plasma) and platelets, early endoscopy and avoiding sedation.

6.8 C** Glucose-6-phosphate dehydrogenase (G6PD) is an essential enzyme, which prevents denaturation of haemoglobin and the cell membrane during periods of oxidative stress. Deficiency results in the production of Heinz bodies and reticulocytosis. Type A G6PD deficiency disease is associated with acute haemolysis after the ingestion of certain drugs like antimalarials, sulphonamides and phenacetin. Type B G6PD deficiency disease tends to affect individuals of Mediterranean origin and results in severe intravascular haemo-lysis with exposure to fava beans. Pyruvate kinase deficiency is associated with extravascular haemolysis, splenomegaly and prickle cells on blood film. The Coombs' test detects autoimmune haemolytic anaemia.

6.9 D** This slide is stained with Ziehl–Nielson stain and shows clumped red–purple bacilli on a green background. This is characteristic of *Mycobacterium tuberculosis. Pneumocystis jiroveci* (formerly *carinii*) pneumonia (PCP) would stain with silver stain.

6.10 D** Pregnant mothers with HIV should be given anti-HIV treatment during pregnancy even if they are asymptomatic; the choice of drugs will depend on the viral load as the higher this is the more drugs will be given. Risk of vertical transmission is greatest during the intrapartum period and so elective Caesarian section should be planned. Breast-feeding can transmit the virus and so should be avoided. The baby should be given AZT for the first 4–6 weeks of life to reduce the risk of vertical transmission.

6.11 A*** The diagnosis is Guillain–Barré syndrome or postinfective polyneuropathy with progressive ascending peripheral neuropathy following a viral infection. The CSF protein is very high and this would not be found with the other conditions.

6.12 D, H* This patient is diabetic and has a ring of hard exudates close to the macula. There is also a boat-shaped lesion characteristic of preretinal haemorrhage/subhyaloid haemorrhage, which is due to bleeding into the small space between the retina and posterior vitreous.

6.13 D* The most obvious abnormalities on his blood picture are pancytopaenia and hypokalaemia. The patient is on chemotherapy, which could include platinum compounds like cisplatin. Side effects of cisplatin include hypomagnesaemia, myelosuppression, gastrointestinal disturbances, nephrotoxicity and ototoxicity. Ectopic ACTH secretion occurs with small cell bronchial carcinomas, not squamous cell, and gives rise to hypokalaemic alkalosis.

6.14 C** This patient is likely to have Sjögren's syndrome, as suggested by dry mouth, Raynaud's phenomenon, the presence of other autoimmune disease and confirmatory blood tests. The positive serological tests associated with Sjögren's syndrome are rheumatoid factor (80–95%), positive antinuclear antibodies (90%), raised anti-Ro and anti-La antibodies (50–90%). Classically patients also present with dry eyes and bilateral parotid gland swelling. The autoimmune profile is not consistent with systemic sclerosis and polymyositis. Mixed connective tissue disease is an overlap syndrome of rheumatoid arthritis, systemic lupus erythematosus, scleroderma and myositis; such patients lack other autoantibodies like anti-Ro, anti-La and anti-ds DNA.

6.15 D** This picture shows Hutchinson's teeth, which appear as barrel-shaped upper incisors. Normal incisors narrow towards the base; Hutchinson's incisors are broad at the base and narrow towards the cutting surface. 'Hutchinson's triad' consists of Hutchinson's teeth, inner ear deafness and interstitial keratitis, which could account for the temporary loss of vision. This triad and saddle-shaped nose are reliable signs of congenital syphilis.

6.16 E** There are bilateral confluent shadows. Caplan's syndrome is coal worker's pneumoconiosis associated with rheumatoid arthritis; there is no mention of the latter. There is no pleural thickening to suggest mesothelioma. The apparent absence of a goitre does not exclude a thyroid carcinoma that has metastasised to the lung. Teratoma and renal cell carcinoma metastases could also give this X-ray picture.

6.17 B** The X-ray shows gas gangrene in the young boy's thigh. The most likely organism is *C. septicum. C. perfringens* can also cause gas gangrene.

6.18 A** This patient has hypertrophic (obstructive) cardiomyopathy (HOCM). This is a primary heart muscle disorder characterised by inappropriate myocardial hypertrophy of a non-dilated left ventricle and often associated with a degree of outflow tract obstruction. Syncope is usually exertional and is due to a combination of ischaemia, arrhythmias, outflow tract obstruction and poor diastolic ventricular filling. Drugs such as diuretics, nitrates and ACE inhibitors reduce preload and decrease chamber size, making the condition worse. They may increase the outflow tract gradient and, along with inotropic agents like digoxin, can induce arrhythmias that can worsen diastolic function. β-Blockers and verapamil slow the heart rate, increase the diastolic filling period and reduce outflow obstruction.

6.19 B** This patient's ECG shows atrial flutter with 4:1 block. It is unusual to develop idiopathic atrial flutter, but it may be caused by any of the causes of atrial fibrillation. Drugs like sotalol, flecainide, propafenone and disopyramide are effective in terminating flutter; adenosine can often slow the heart rate down to reveal flutter as the underlying rhythm but does not usually terminate it. This patient is not haemodynamically compromised so DC cardioversion is not indicated. As there is the risk of thromboembolic event like stroke, he should be anticoagulated, especially if cardioversion is going to be attempted. A pacemaker is not indicated.

6.20 **B*** This patient has eruptive xanthoma. These are small papules or nodules, which have a predilection for the gluteal regions and extensor surfaces. They are indicative of hypertriglyceridaemia and such patients are likely to have raised chylomycrons and very low-density lipoproteins. The serum cholesterol may be normal or slightly elevated. Acute pancreatitis is a very serious risk. Eruptive xanthomas are associated with types I, IV and V hyperlipidaemia where triglycerides are raised. Nephrotic syndrome, diabetes, gout and hypothyroidism are all associated with hypertriglyceridaemia. Type IIa hyperlipidaemia is associated with raised cholesterol only.

6.21 **B*** This patient has familial autosomal dominant hypercalcaemic hypocalciuria. It is a rare but benign condition that can be confused with primary hyperparathyroidism, leading to inappropriate surgery, as may have happened to his father. Patients have a normal PTH level and the calcium/creatinine excretion <0.01. The seemingly high ALP is normal for a boy of his age.

6.22 **A**** The positive predictive value is the probability that a patient who tests positive really does have the condition.

	Diabetes +	**Diabetes -**	
Glucosuria +	200 (a)	50 (b)	250

Positive predictive value = a/a + b = 200/250 = 0.80

6.23 **D*** This patient most likely has haemochromatosis, which can be primary/idiopathic, or secondary to iron overload conditions like alcoholic liver disease. Both conditions may present in a number of ways due to iron overload: 'bronze' diabetes, congestive cardiac failure (due to cardiomyopathy), hypo gonadism and arthropathy (due to pseudogout, which primarily affects the metacarpals, wrists, hips and knees). He does not have a history suggestive of alcoholic liver disease. Idiopathic haemochromatosis can be inherited in an autosomal recessive pattern and has an increased incidence in Caucasians of Celtic origin. Ninety per cent of patients with hereditary haemochromatosis are positive for the C282Y mutation on the HFE gene on chromosome 6; a less common mutation is associated with H63D mutation on the same gene. Patients who have a ferritin >1000 and are homozygous for the C282Y gene do not need a liver biopsy to confirm the diagnosis. A liver biopsy is useful to determine cirrhosis and to estimate the hepatic iron index. Hereditary haemochromatosis does not usually present with deranged liver function tests but can still progress to cirrhosis; 30% of cirrhotics develop hepatocellular carcinoma. The mainstay of treatment is regular venesection to reduce the excess iron. A standard venesection removes 450 ml of blood which contains about 250 mg of iron. Regular (often weekly) venesection is performed to reduce the ferritin to 50. The YMDD mutation is associated with the development of lamivudine resistance in patients with hepatitis B.

6.24 **B**** Especially in children, the walls of the ethmoid sinuses are very thin and infection can spread into the adjacent orbit very easily. A Penrose drain can be seen entering into the ethmoid sinus to drain pus from a subperiosteal abscess. Prompt treatment with systemic antibiotics can lead to a rapid recovery. Endophthalmitis is a severe infection within the globe itself, usually following trauma or surgery; it presents with a hot painful eye and a hypopyon. There is no clear involvement of the ophthalmic division of the trigeminal nerve to support a diagnosis of herpes zoster ophthalmicus. The skin has features of marked cellulitic change as opposed to an infiltration with lymphoma or the dusky red swelling associated with bleeding.

6.25 **B**** Friedreich's ataxia is an autosomal recessive (or very rarely X-linked recessive) disorder affecting the cerebellum, spinal cord and peripheral nerves. There is pyramidal weakness in the legs. Ankle and knee reflexes may be lost due to peripheral neuropathy. The sensory deficits are due to involvement of the dorsal columns and maybe the lateral spinothalamic tract. Other features include cardiomyopathy, optic atrophy, diabetes and dementia. Multiple sclerosis can also produce cerebellar, pyramidal and dorsal column signs but is not associated with pes cavus and absent reflexes. Tabes dorsalis can produce absent reflexes and positive Romberg's sign but only taboparesis is associated with extensor plantars. Tabes dorsalis would also be associated with Argyll Robertson pupils: small, irregular and responding to accommodation but not light.

6.26 **D*** Extrinsic allergic alveolitis is a type of hypersensitivity syndrome that results in a diffuse interstitial granulomatous lung disease caused by an allergic response to inhaled organic dust or chemicals; here fungal spores are probably causing farmer's lung. This patient has progressive dyspnoea with cough, which is worse during the day, presumably when he is at work and exposed to the allergen. When he is removed from the allergen his symptoms improve. With chronic exposure, irreversible lung damage may occur. Lung function tests would show a restrictive pattern (FEV_1:FVC ratio 92%); normal eosinophil count and lack of wheeze excludes asthma and allergic bronchopulmonary aspergillosis. Churg–Strauss syndrome is unlikely in a patient with a lack of renal involvement; it would also be associated with a positive ANCA. With Goodpasture's syndrome there would be a history of pulmonary haemorrhage.

6.27 B** Peripheral neuropathy, vasculitic rash, arthritis, haematuria and renal impairment suggestive of a glomerulonephritis, history of hepatitis C infection, a raised globulin, low C_4 and positive rheumatoid factor are all features consistent with mixed cryoglobulinaemia. There are a number of causes of cryoglobulinaemia, including other autoimmune conditions like systemic lupus erythematosus and Wegener's granulomatosis, but negative ANA and ANCA fail to support these diagnoses. Fifty per cent of patients with cryoglobulinaemia have antibodies to hepatitis C. Renal complications are common and are associated with a poorer prognosis.

6.28 E** This Gram stain shows purple Gram-positive diplococci. Gram-negative organisms would stain pink. All the other organisms are Gram negative (except *Mycobacterium tuberculosis*).

6.29 D*** This is a 'sabre tibia' where the tibia is grossly bowed with sparing of the fibula. Although characteristic of Paget's disease, the term was originally applied to the osteitis of congenital syphilis; however, this is hardly likely to present at this age!

6.30 D** The X-ray shows terminal phalangeal resorption and soft tissue calcification. With gout, there is no calcification of tophi. Psoriatic arthropathy has a 'pencil-in-cup' deformity. There are no features of rheumatoid arthritis such as ulnar deviation. Compare this X-ray with that of hyperparathyroidism (see **4.30**)

6.31 C** This young girl presents with low-grade pyrexia, arthritis, first-degree heart block, a possible pericardial rub, a raised ESR and antistreptolysin O (ASO) titre, and a history of a sore throat. There is no single pathognomic test for rheumatic fever but she has enough of the Jones criteria to meet this diagnosis. To diagnose rheumatic fever there needs to be evidence of streptococcal infection (history of sore throat and raised ASO titre) and two major criteria (carditis, polyarthritis, chorea, erythema marginatum and subcutaneous nodules); or one major criteria and two minor criteria (arthralgia, fever, raised ESR or CRP, and prolonged PR interval). Still's disease is a form of juvenile rheumatoid arthritis, which would have high spiking fevers, splenomegaly, lymphadenopathy and serositis. Kawasaki disease/syndrome is a severe childhood illness that causes inflammation of blood vessels, especially coronary vessels, associated with fever, swollen hands and feet, swollen lips and tongue and lymphadenopathy. It rarely affects children aged over 8 years.

6.32 E* The cardiac monitor shows ventricular standstill followed by ventricular tachycardia. Assuming defibrillation works, he will need a temporary pacing wire as his problem is most likely due to bradycardia leading to ventricular fibrillation as an escape rhythm.

6.33 A** This man has symmetrical tense blisters affecting the upper part of his body, which are characteristic of bullous pemphigoid. There are linear deposits of IgG and C3 complement within the basement membrane. The condition is lethal in up to 50% of cases if left untreated but does respond to steroids. Dermatitis herpetiformis is a bullous disease associated with coeliac disease that tends to affect shoulder girdle, gluteal region, scalp and extensor surfaces of the limbs. While it can cause burning pain and pruritus it is not life-threatening. Pemphigus is discussed in **1.47**.

6.34 D** This patient has a form of Cushing's syndrome as shown by the raised 24-h urinary free cortisol and failure of the serum cortisol to normalise with a low dose dexamethasone suppression test (0.5 mg q.d.s). The next step is to determine whether his condition is ACTH-dependent or -independent. The serum cortisol is partly suppressed when the patient is given high dose dexamethasone (2 mg q.d.s.) and is consistent with pituitary-dependent adenoma.

6.35 C** Haemophilia A is an X-linked recessive disease. The patient's father must have been carrying the haemophilia gene to develop the gene. With X-linked recessive disorders all the daughters (including the patient in this case) will be obligate carriers and all the sons will be clear of the disease. If the patient has a child with an unaffected person, then, as she is heterozygous for the gene, half of her sons will be unaffected and half will develop haemophilia A. Antenatal diagnosis can be undertaken in a female fetus who has a high chance of being a carrier, as well as in the male fetus, by chorionic villus sampling.

6.36 B** This patient has chronic pancreatitis. Patients with steatorrhea have high concentrations of long chain fatty acids in their colon. These can bind to calcium salts so that there is less calcium available to bind dietary oxalate. The possible consequence of this is that more unbound oxalate can be absorbed and so lead to formation of oxalate stones.

6.37 D** He appears to have had a stroke (cerebrovascular accident) causing a left hemiplegia and, simultaneously, also causing a right lower motor neurone facial palsy with no other localising features. As it is most likely that there is a single rather than multiple lesions responsible, this localises such a lesion to the right side of the pons. There is close proximity of VII and VI but the latter has been spared. A VI nerve palsy can sometimes be a false localising sign caused by raised intracranial pressure in the Foster Kennedy syndrome.

6.38 D* A young man who has signs and symptoms of bullous emphysema and hepatomegaly should raise the suspicion of α_1-antitrypsin deficiency. α_1-Antitrypsin is a glycoprotein produced by the liver, that prevents the lung being attacked by proteolytic enzymes. Patients have three main phenotypes depending on their level of α_1-antitrypsin: PiMM (normal homozygous), PiMZ (heterozygous deficient) and PiZZ (homozygous deficient). Of PiZZ patients, 60% will develop panacinar-type emphysema and 12% will develop liver cirrhosis, for which the only curative treatment is liver transplantation. Fortunately the recipient's phenotype changes to that of the donor liver so that this produces normal α_1-antitrypsin. The patient is likely to have an 'obstructive' lung function pattern. All respiratory infections should be treated promptly, so influenza vaccination is prudent.

6.39 E** A history of a malabsorption syndrome associated with polyarthritis, lymphadenopathy, pleural effusions and hyperpigmented skin suggests Whipple's disease. It is a systemic disorder caused by the Gram-positive bacterium *Tropheryma whippelii.* The disease may also affect the heart, central nervous system, causing dementia and nerve lesions, and kidney, resulting in interstitial nephritis. Amyloidosis would be unusual without a history of myeloma or rheumatoid arthritis. Carcinoid is associated with flushing and diarrhoea and not arthritis. There is nothing to suggest inflammatory bowel disease.

6.40 E* Schatzki ring is a benign mucosal ring that occurs at the squamocolumnar junction. Its exact aetiology is unknown but patients typically present with intermittent dysphagia for solid foods, made worse by anxiety or hurrying down a meal. As it is a fixed lesion this would differentiate it from problems with peristalsis and oesophageal motility.

6.41 C, J* The scan shows a right chronic subdural haematoma in the frontal lobe. In the right temporal lobe is a high density lesion consistent with an acute intracerebral haemorrhage. There is no midline shift.

6.42 A*** This photograph shows characteristic red–blue plaques over the knuckles and metacarpophalangeal joints, as well as ragged cuticles and dilated nailfold capillaries. Dermatomyositis is also associated with a heliotrope, erythematous rash that also involves the eyelids but not the eye. Systemic lupus erythematosus is associated with a 'butterfly' rash on the face but this typically spares the eyelids, and on the hands often spares the knuckles.

6.43 D** A young woman presents with headaches, severe hypertension, palpitations and sweating. This could be caused by thyrotoxicosis but the thyroid function tests are normal and she is clinically euthyroid. Hypertension that is resistant to antihypertensives should always raise the possibility of a phaeochromocytoma. Ninety per cent of phaeochromocytomas arise as tumours of the adrenal medulla and secrete amines and peptides, including catecholamines like adrenaline (epinephrine), noradrenaline (norepinephrine) and dopamine. The diagnostic tests of choice would be 24-h urinary catecholamines and imaging with CT, MRI or MIBG to localize the tumour.

6.44 **D**** The history is highly suggestive of severe colitis, most likely ulcerative colitis. In the acute setting he will require intravenous hydrocortisone, not oral or topical steroids. In time, full colonoscopy will be necessary to establish the extent of the disease, but there is a higher risk of perforation if it is attempted while the patient is in this state. It would be much safer to do a flexible sigmoidoscopy and gather diagnostic biopsies but treatment should not be delayed. A transverse colonic diameter >5.5 cm or caecum >9 cm is indicative of toxic megacolon and requires urgent surgical referral. This patient will require daily abdominal X-rays and monitoring of CRP and stool frequency to assess progress; a CRP >45 and stool frequency >8 on day 3 post-admission is associated with an 85% chance of the patient requiring a colectomy. Ciclosporin has been shown to be very useful in the management of acute ulcerative colitis but its introduction should not delay surgery. There is an increased risk of neurotoxicity with ciclosporin in patients with hypomagnesaemia and low cholesterol. Patients with colitis are at increased risk of thromboembolism and should be given venous thromboembolism prophylaxis. There is no indication for antibiotics except preoperatively or if there is evidence of perforation.

6.45 **D**** This patient complains of abnormal daytime somnolence, cataplexy (episodes of muscular weakness) and paralysis (inability to move during sleep). All these are consistent with narcolepsy. Also associated with narcolepsy are hypnagogic hallucinations, which are hallucinations that typically occur during the sleep–wake transition. Bruxism is forcible teeth grinding that usually occurs at night.

6.46 **B***** The X-ray shows a skull with multiple lytic lesions consistent with multiple myeloma. Compare and contrast this image with that of Paget's disease of bone (see **2.44**).

6.47 **A***** This patient has Ehlers–Danlos syndrome. The skin has unusual elasticity in that it can be lifted up from its supporting tissues and springs back again on release. Cutis laxa is where the skin lacks elasticity and hangs in loose folds. Dermatographia is where touching or slightly scratching the skin causes raised reddish marks. Nicolsky's sign (see **1.47**) and pathergy (see **3.42**) are discussed elsewhere.

6.48 **C*** This patient develops symptoms and signs of hyperthyroidism post-partum. She has a painless smooth goitre and she is biochemically hyperthyroid. She has no recent illnesses and her ESR is normal, thereby making deQuervain's thyroiditis unlikely. In Graves' disease and toxic solitary adenoma there is increased uptake in the radioactive iodine scan. Postpartum thyroiditis can be a form of autoimmune thyroiditis. During pregnancy there is partial suppression of the immune system. After delivery there can be a dramatic increase in thyroid hormones. The clinical picture may follow a hyperthyroid phase, then a hypothyroid phase, followed by a euthyroid state.

6.49 B* A patient who is requiring repeated drainage of ascites should be considered for liver transplantation. Contra-indications to liver transplantation include: extrahepatic malignancy; extrahepatic sepsis; total porto-mesenteric system thrombosis; and severe pulmonary hypertension. Patients with HIV/HCV co-infection can be considered for OLT but their CD_4 count should be >200 with absence of viraemia and no AIDS-defining illness after immune reconstitution. Active intravenous drug misuse and alcohol abuse are absolute contraindications to OLT assessment.

O'Grady JG, Taylor C (2005) BHIVA guidelines for liver transplantation in patients with HIV. www.bhiva.org

6.50 D* The patient has a history of headaches and epilepsy. The CT reveals obvious intracranial calcification throughout the right side of the brain consistent with Sturge–Weber syndrome.

6.51 A* This patient has Addison's disease, as evidenced by his collapse, low blood pressure, hypoglycaemia, hyponatraemia and hyperkalaemia. He also has buccal mucosa pigmentation. The low calcium and PTH along with the symptoms of tetany are due to hypoparathyroidism. The APS type I is a disorder that usually manifests in childhood. It requires the combination of two of the following: hypoparathyroidism, adrenal insufficiency and chronic mucocutaneous candidiasis. Other endocrine diseases can also be associated with this syndrome, such as gonadal failure, thyroid disease and type I diabetes.

6.52 E** The history is suggestive of irritable bowel syndrome (IBS). The Rome II criteria for the diagnosis of IBS consider all the answers. Most patients with IBS do not wake up from sleep to open their bowels; their symptoms are typically worse in the morning when they may open their bowels a number of times. Other symptoms that would be unusual include the passage of blood, weight loss, anaemia and change in bowel habit.

Rome II: A Multinational Consensus Document on Functional Gastrointestinal Disorders. *Gut* 1999: **45** (Suppl II).

6.53 C** Patients with IgA nephropathy tend to present with synpharyngetic haematuria, in that the renal problem occurs at about the same time as the streptococcal infection. There is no evidence of systemic vasculitis, so this cannot be Henoch–Schönlein purpura (HSP) because IgA nephropathy is a limited version of HSP. Acute interstitial nephritis tends to present with fever, arthralgia, skin rash, decreased renal function and eosinophilia; urinalysis would show blood and protein. Epstein–Barr virus infection does not cause haematuria.

6.54 C*** The blood film shows the characteristic intracellular ring trophozites. Of all the options, this is the only one that shows intracellular organisms.

6.55 C** This biopsy is of the liver and shows cirrhosis. There are nodules, which stain deep pink, and surrounding fibrosis, which stains blue. The Childs–Pugh scoring system is used to determine prognosis with cirrhosis.

Score	**1**	**2**	**3**
Albumin	>35	28–35	<28
Ascites	None	Mild	Moderate
Bilirubin	<35	35–50	>50
Encephalopathy	None	Grade I–II	Grade III–IV
Prothrombin time (above control/s)	1–4	4–6	>6

Childs A = 5–6; B = 7–9; C = 10–15: operative mortality: A = 10%; B = 30%; C = 75%

Ann Arbor is associated with Hodgkin's lymphoma staging; Rockall's criteria is associated with severity of upper gastrointestinal bleeding; Dukes' classification is concerned with colorectal carcinoma staging; and Breslow's thickness is associated with depth of invasion of malignant melanoma.

6.56 D* This patient has a neutropaenic sepsis, most likely following his chemotherapy. The normal neutrophil count is 1.5–7 x 10^9/L. He is most at risk of sepsis from *Pseudomonas* spp, staphylococci, *Escherichia coli* and *Klebsiella* spp. Management of such patients includes isolation in a side room and avoidance of contact with individuals with infections; scrupulous hand washing should be undertaken and gloves and aprons put on before entering the room. First-line antibiotic treatment should be aimed at treating the above organisms and tazocin and an aminoglycoside like gentamicin would be the best options. Persistent pyrexia may be due to fungal infection but fluconazole should not be started first line in a patient with no evidence of candidiasis.

6.57 C** The blood film shows purple 'smear' or 'smudge' lymphocytes characteristic of chronic lymphocytic leukaemia. Acute lymphoblastic leukaemia is associated with large, round lymphocytes with very little cytoplasm. Lymphocytes in acute myeloid leukaemia are larger but are not always round, and have granular cytoplasm which may contain Auer rods. Chronic myeloid leukaemia is often characterised by seeing a number of different cells in varying degrees of maturation: basophils, myelocytes, metamyelocytes and blasts. Infectious mononucleosis is characterised by 'atypical' lymphocytes that have a cytoplasm which is pushed out towards the rim and has a tendency to 'stream' around adjacent red cells.

6.58 D* This patient most probably has renal artery stenosis, as suggested by unilateral small kidney on ultrasound, bilateral femoral bruits, hypercholesterolaemia, hypertension and renal impairment. The gold standard test for diagnosing this is renal angiography but magnetic resonance angiography could diagnose the condition. Doppler ultrasound would help identify whether the blood vessels were patent. DMSA scans look for renal scarring. MAG 3 scans are used to see if there is divided function between left and right kidney.

6.59 E* All the pathogens may cause diarrhoeal disease in HIV-positive patients but at this CD_4 count only non-Hodgkin's lymphoma would be a possibility. All the others are unlikely to present until the patient has a CD_4 count <100.

6.60 D* This patient has familial Mediterranean fever, as characterised by intermittent abdominal and joint pains in a patient of Mediterranean extraction. In general this is a fairly benign condition but it may lead to amyloidosis and this is the cause of his nephritic syndrome. Renal biopsy would be the definitive test to establish the cause of his nephrotic syndrome.

6.61 E*** This patient, who has worked in the Tropics and has a B_{12} and folate deficiency, chronic diarrhoea with probable steatorrhoea, hypoalbuminaemia and partial villous atrophy on duodenal biopsy but negative tissue transglutaminase most probably has tropical sprue. It is a chronic condition which possibly follows intestinal infection, which can lead to mucosal injury and malabsorption of nutrients and folate and B_{12} deficiency. Many patients have overgrowth of *Escherichia coli* and *Enterobacter* in their ileum and symptoms improve after trials with antibiotics. Bacterial overgrowth is usually associated with small intestinal stasis either due to anatomical abnormalities such as the development of a blind loop or to decreased small bowel motility. With bacterial overgrowth, the bacteria tend to generate folate and so folate levels are usually increased rather than low. Giardiasis can cause very similar symptoms and must always be excluded in patients with chronic diarrhoea even if there is no history of foreign travel. Duodenal biopsies may show the organisms lying above the crypts (see **3.9**). Stool culture and microscopy will detect either the trophozoites or cysts in >70% of cases.

6.62 E* This patient presents feeling unwell, and with tremor, worsening diabetes, renal impairment, hyperkalaemia, hypomagnesaemia and hypophosphataemia. These features are all consistent with tacrolimus toxicity. Other side effects that can occur with tacrolimus include confusion, psychosis, depression, paraesthesia and hypertension. All of these are usually reversible with dose reduction. Similar side effects occur with ciclosporin. Methylprednisolone is given to patients who have evidence of cellular rejection and can cause hyperglycaemia but not the other symptoms. Mycophenolate mofetil is often started in patients who develop renal impairment due to tacrolimus and its main side effects are bone marrow suppression and diarrhoea. Sirolimus can be used instead of tacrolimus for liver and renal transplants and is associated with pancytopaenia, diarrhoea, hyperlipidaemia and renal impairment when given with ciclosporin. Azathioprine is still used in some immunosuppressive regimens but not without ciclosporin or tacrolimus, and it is not used first line for renal or liver transplants; it is associated with bone marrow suppression. Insulin does not cause these side effects.

6.63 **B**** This patient has developed acute left ventricular failure post acute coronary syndrome. He is hyponatraemic and hypokalaemic and so cannot continue with furosemide. He has oliguria but giving intravenous fluids will make his pulmonary oedema worse. Dobutamine is a β_1-agonist and improves left ventricular function by being a positive inotrope and reducing systemic vascular resistance, which leads to decreased afterload. Dopamine also has β_1-agonist activity but its α_1-actions can cause tachycardia and arrhythmias, along with vasoconstriction and increased systemic vascular resistance. It would be of more benefit in a hypotensive patient. Milrinone is a phosphodiesterase inhibitor with inotropic and vasodilatory actions. Although not a first-line inotrope, it could be useful in the treatment of acute heart failure, especially if there was evidence of pulmonary hypertension.

6.64 **B***** Identifying acid-fast bacilli in sputum is diagnostic of *Mycobacterium* spp, but this could include *M. kansasii*, *M. avium intracellulare* or any other non-tuberculous mycobacteria. He should still be treated for pulmonary tuberculosis (TB) pending culture results, starting with quadruple therapy using rifampicin, isoniazid, pyrazinamide and ethambutol; the latter two for at least 2 months and rifampicin and isoniazid for 6 months. The gold standard diagnostic test is microscopy followed by culture (of the sputum in this case), which will also determine the species and sensitivities. Given the risk of drug interactions, drug toxicity and effects on immune reconstitution inflammatory syndrome, current expert opinion is that, if possible, anti-HIV treatment should be delayed until the completion of anti-TB treatment, especially if the CD_4 count is >100–200. Treatment is assessed by monitoring the patient's weight, reduction in symptoms, possible seroconversion of sputum to smear negative if positive initially, and sputum culture at 2 months. There should be radiological evidence of improvement after 2 months of therapy; if the chest X-ray was severe initially, this may take a long time to change and CT chest is then better for monitoring changes. A Mantoux test can be used to detect patients with latent TB but it is not very sensitive or specific in patients with HIV, especially those who have had BCG vaccinations, in whom false-negatives can occur; hence the need for new diagnostic tests such as interferon-γ assays.

6.65 **B*** Chronic granulomatous disease (CGD) is a rare inherited disorder of phagocytes, which is characterised by recurrent infections, hepatosplenomegaly, lymphadenopathy and hypergammaglobulinaemia. A defect in the enzyme NADPH oxidase prevents the generation of reactive oxygen-free radicals. Bacteria normally produce hydrogen peroxide which is converted to H_2O by the enzyme catalase; some bacteria like *Streptococcus pyogenes* and *Haemophilus influenzae* cannot produce catalase and so the H_2O_2 produced is utilised by host phagocytes to generate free radicals and neutralise these organisms, even in CGD patients. It is the bacteria that are catalase-positive, like *Staphylococcus aureus, Klebsiella* spp and *Escherichia coli*, along with fungi such as *Candida* spp and *Aspergillus*, that CGD patients cannot deal with. Such patients are prone to pneumonia, abscesses, enteritis, osteomyelitis and skin infections. WCC counts may be normal but are increased during acute infections. Anaemia is due to chronic disease. Treatment is with prophylactic septrin, interferon-γ infusions and ultimately haemopoietic stem cell transplantation. Unlike the other types of immunodeficiency, in which there are decreased levels of immunoglobulin, as in combined variable immunodeficiency and severe combined immunodeficiency, CGD patients have raised levels of IgG but normal levels of IgA and IgM. Chediak–Higashi syndrome is characterised by recurrent infections, especially of skin and respiratory tract, partial oculocutaneous albinism and neurological defects, such as seizures, nystagmus and peripheral neuropathy.

6.66 **B*** Portal hypertension depends on flow in the portal vein and resistance to flow, which in turn depends on the radius of the blood vessels (Poisseuille's law). Patients with portal hypertension can develop ascites and portosystemic varices. The aim of TIPSS is to dilate the portal vein and insert a shunt so as to reduce flow and resistance. The pressure in the (free) hepatic vein is the same as in the systemic circulation (i.e. inferior vena cava), and in a normal patient this would be 4 mmHg. The pressure in the portal venules is the same as in the portal system and normally this would be 7 mmHg. If a catheter were inserted into a small hepatic vein and wedged there to prevent blood flow (wedged hepatic vein pressure [WHVP]), this would give an indication of the pressure in the portal vein. The portal pressure gradient in a normal patient would be 3 mmHg (7–4). Variceal haemorrhage tends not to occur in patients whose portal pressure gradient is <12 mmHg. In this case the TIPSS has been successful, with the portal pressure gradient dropping from 14 (17–3) to 5 (9–4). The causes of portal hypertension can be classified as prehepatic, hepatic and posthepatic. A high WHVP suggests an hepatic cause with obstruction of flow between the portal venule to above and the hepatic vein. Ideally the pressure between the suprahepatic inferior vena cava and the hepatic vein should be measured to make sure there is no gradient, as is seen with hepatic webs.

Boyer TD, Haskal ZJ (2005) AASLD Practice Guideline: The role of transjugular intrahepatic portosystemic shunt on the management of portal hypertension. Hepatology 41: 386-400

6.67 H*** Brainstem death can be diagnosed if certain preconditions and exclusions are fulfilled and there is no evidence of brainstem function. Assessment must be done by two senior doctors, neither of whom should be part of the transplant team. Patients must be in a coma, not breathing independently and being ventilated. There must be conclusive evidence that there is no chance of regaining brainstem function. Before testing can be undertaken the patient must be free of the effects of drugs such as alcohol, sedatives and muscle relaxants. The diagnosis cannot be made in a patient with hypothermia or electrolyte abnormalities, and so these have to be corrected because they can alter neurological function; this does not apply to anaemia. Tests of brainstem function are: (1) absence of pupillary reaction to light, (2) absence of corneal reflex, (3) absence of the vestibulo-ocular reflex with caloric testing, (4) no motor responses in cranial nerve distribution, (5) absent gag reflex, (6) no spontaneous respiration when the patient is disconnected from ventilator and a $PCO_2 \geq 6.7$ kPa; a high PCO_2 would normally be expected to stimulate central chemoreceptors and so prompt breathing. The patient should be given oxygen to prevent hypoxia before disconnection of the ventilator; spinal reflexes do not need a functioning brainstem to still be elicited.

6.68 B** A man with a solid, firm testicular mass must be assumed to have a testicular cancer until proven otherwise. Scrotal ultrasound can show a solid mass and blood tests like α-fetoprotein (AFP), β-HCG and LDH are all increased with testicular tumours, but these cannot diagnose the condition. The scrotum has a different lymphatic drainage to the testicle and so a trans scrotal biopsy could contaminate the scrotum with malignant cells. The patient needs radical inguinal exploration with ligation of the spermatic cord and orchidectomy. Ninety-five per cent of testicular tumours are germ cell tumours and these can be differentiated into seminomas and non-seminomas: embryonal carcinomas, teratomas, teratocarcinomas, choriocarcinomas and yolk sac tumours. Non-seminoma germ cell tumours are more common in young men but seminomas are more prevalent in men aged over 35 years. Choriocarcinoma is the most aggressive of the testicular carcinomas. According to the international germ cell cancer consensus group (IGCCG) 1997 prognostic factors, poor prognosis is associated with: elevated AFP, β-HCG or LDH, non-seminomas, non-pulmonary visceral metastases and a mediastinal primary.

6.69 E* The blood results suggest that this patient has active treponemal disease. His symptoms could occur with HIV but this has been excluded; although potentially it could be HIV seroconversion. EIA is a specific test for *Treponema pallidum* and is used as a screening test. Confirmation of treponemal disease is with TPPA or TPHA. RPR and VDRL are non-specific for anti-treponemal antibodies. They are used to measure disease activity and assess response to treatment. Infectious syphilis refers to primary, secondary and early latent syphilis and occurs within 2 years of contracting the disease. Late latent, gummatous syphilis, cardiovascular syphilis and neurosyphilis are all types of non-infectious syphilis and usually occur in patients who have had the disease for more than 2 years. Primary syphilis is characterised by a painless papule which ulcerates to produce a primary chancre. Secondary syphilis is characterised by systemic infection of the trepenomal bacteria beyond the primary chancre, resulting in constitutional symptoms, patchy alopecia, skin rashes which can affect the palms and soles, lymphadenopathy and wart-like lesions in moist areas (condylomata lata). Early latent syphilis refers to asymptomatic patients with positive serology; late latent syphilis is the same as early latent syphilis but occurs in a patient who has had the disease for >2 years. Gummata are large, granulomatous lesions in the skin, soft tissues and internal organs.

6.70 A** This patient has ventilator assisted pneumonia (VAP). It can be diagnosed in patients who have been ventilated for >48 h and who develop a fever, leucocytosis and new pulmonary infiltrates on chest X-ray. The most likely organisms to cause this condition are *Pseudomonas aeruginosa*, coliforms and MRSA. Antibiotic therapy should include anti-*Pseudomonas* cover, such as tazobactam and piperacillin or imipenem. Tracheostomy does not decrease the risk of developing VAP. Other conditions which predispose to VAP include: age >70 years, chest surgery, nasogastric tube insertion, chronic lung disease, depressed conscious level and aspiration. Stomach acid acts as a natural antimicrobial barrier and increasing the pH with H_2 antagonists increases the risk of pneumonia. Tracheal aspirations are often non-specific for the diagnosis of VAP as tracheobronchial colonisation is common in critically ill patients; better yield is achieved by bronchoscopic alveolar lavage and non-bronchoscopic deep pulmonary aspiration.

6.71 D*** Bleeding is a common complication in patients with haemophilia. The best treatment to give this patient is factor VIII to prevent further haemorrhage. Factor IX is given to patients with haemophilia B. The aim of treatment is to correct the factor VIII activity to 100% of normal in a major haemorrhage and 30–50% of normal for minor haemorrhages. The amount to give depends on the patient's weight and the difference between the desired factor VIII level and the patient's native factor VIII activity level. Other drugs that can be given as an adjunct are DDAVP (desmopressin), which can increase factor VIII levels, and tranexamic acid and aprotonin, which inhibit fibrinolysis and promote clot stability.

6.72 B** Prostate cancer can spread by direct extension to the seminal vesicles and pelvic lymph nodes. It can also metastasize via the haematogenous route to the bones. Bone pain often responds well to external beam radiation. Spread to the rectum is rare because of Denonvillier's fascia which prevents extension from the gland to the rectum. Reducing testosterone levels has been shown to curb metastatic disease. This can be achieved by surgical removal of the testicles. Another method is using LHRH agonists such as goserelin (Zoladex); these affect the hypothalamo–pituitary–testes axis by having a negative feedback effect on the testes, causing decreased release of testosterone. No chemotherapeutic agent or combination of agents has been shown to improve survival in patients with prostate cancer.

6.73 A** Malnutrition is common in hospitalized patients and there is good evidence that if nutritional support is started early, especially in patients with critical illness, it can reduce hospitalization and mortality. This patient is clearly not absorbing his NG feeds. In many cases this is due to an ileus, which may be precipitated by electrolyte abnormalities such as hypokalaemia. With a history of diabetes this patient may also have a gastroparesis. Reducing the rate of his NG feed and intravenous fluids is not going to give him the calories he needs. PEG insertion involves a feeding tube being inserted into the stomach, either endoscopically or radiologically, and is used in patients with an unsafe swallow or who cannot tolerate long-term NG feeding; in this case the feed will still accumulate in his stomach. NJ feeding should be used in those patients who are at risk of aspiration pneumonia, recurrent vomiting and large gastric aspirates, and those with dysmotility syndromes. TPN could be used but there are the complications of line insertion (arterial puncture, bleeding, pneumothorax, misplacement and sepsis), volume overload, and increased hepatic steatosis.

6.74 K, L, O* The CT shows a subarachnoid haemorrhage with blood in the Sylvian fissure and in the lateral ventricles. There is some developing hydrocephalus in the anterior horns of both lateral ventricles, which suggests this is not a hyperacute bleed. There is no bleeding into the cerebrum and no midline shift.

6.75 B*** The CT shows dilatation of the lateral ventricles, third and fourth ventricles and the temporal horns, which would be consistent with a communicating hydrocephalus. In communicating hydrocephalus the CSF pathways are competent from the ventricles to the basal cisterns, just below the third ventricle. In non-communicating, obstructive hydrocephalus there is a blockage to the flow of CSF, usually between the third and fourth ventricles at the level of the Sylvian aqueduct.

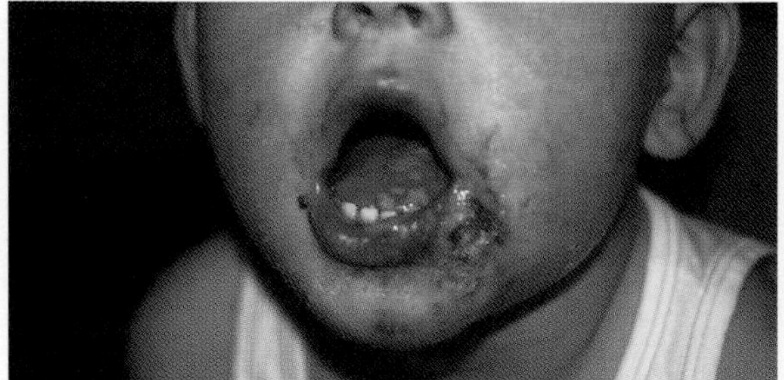

Plate 1.4

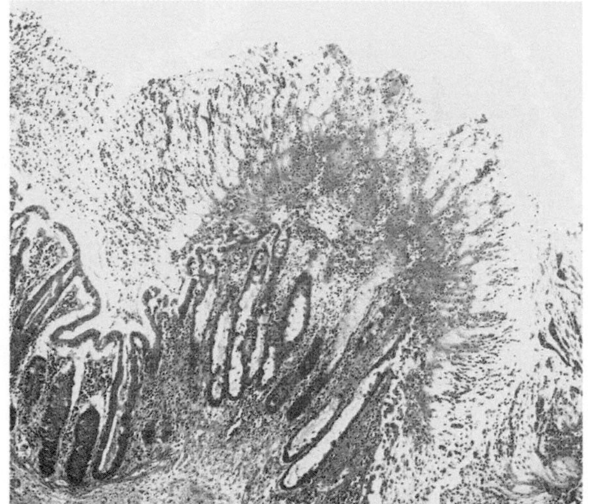

Plate 1.10

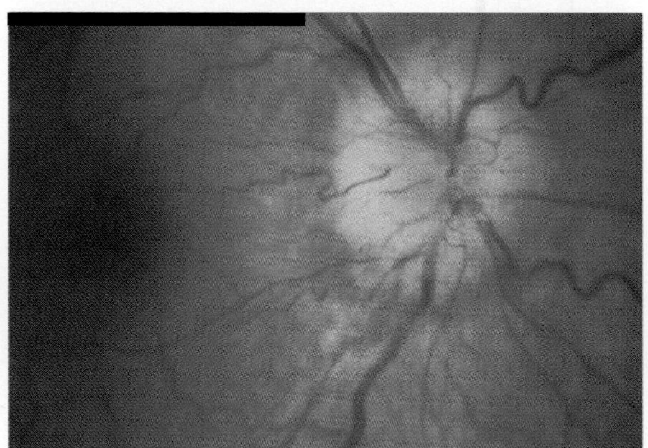

Plate 1.12

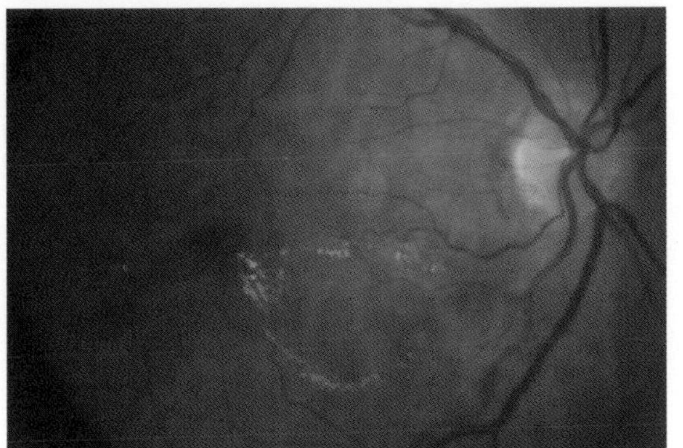

Plate 1.13

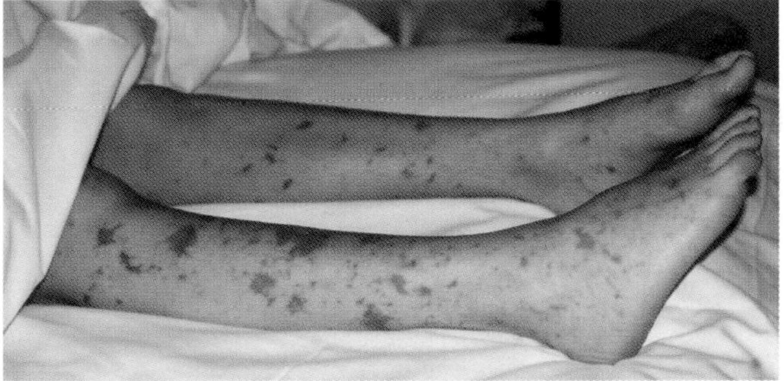

Plate 1.16

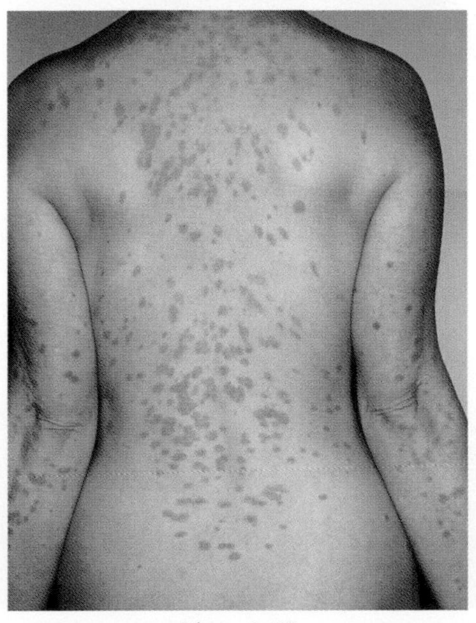

Plate 1.22

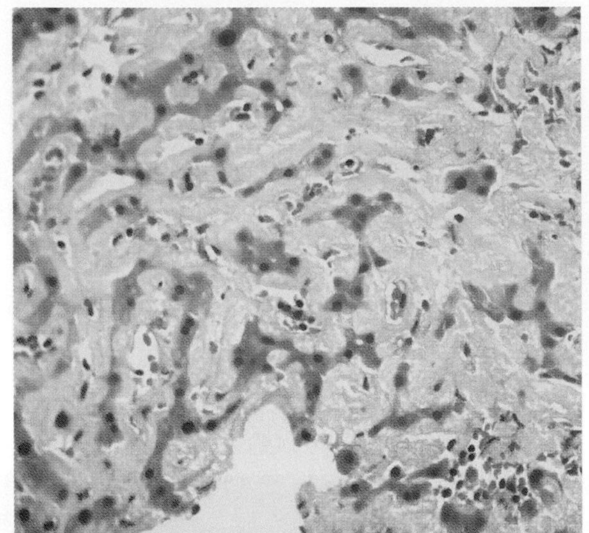

Plate 1.27

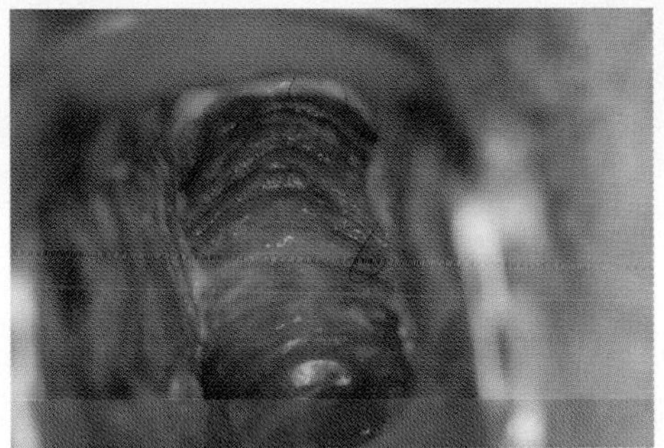

Plate 1.32

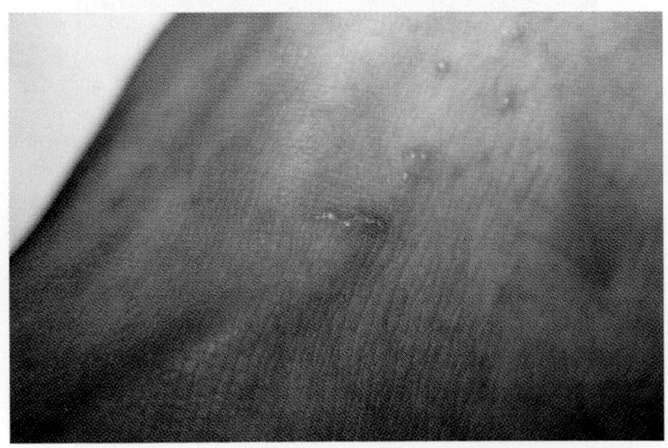

Plate 1.37

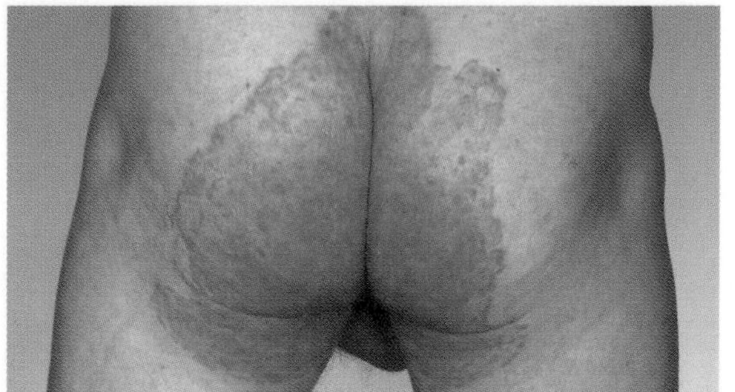

Plate 1.44

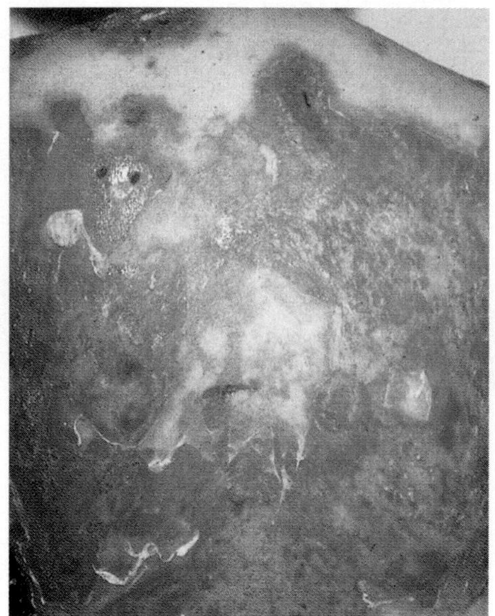

Plate 1.47

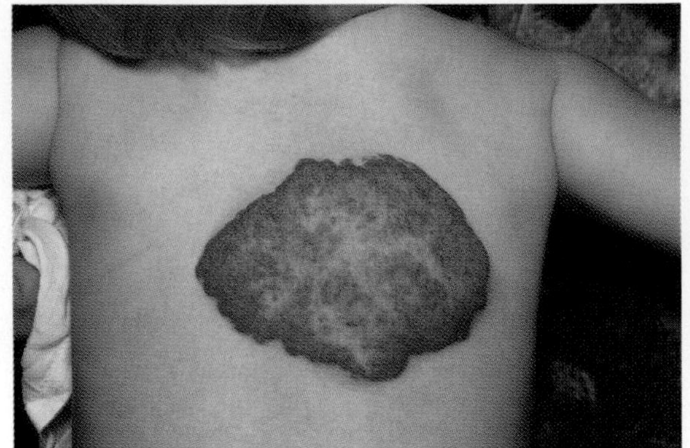

Plate 1.52

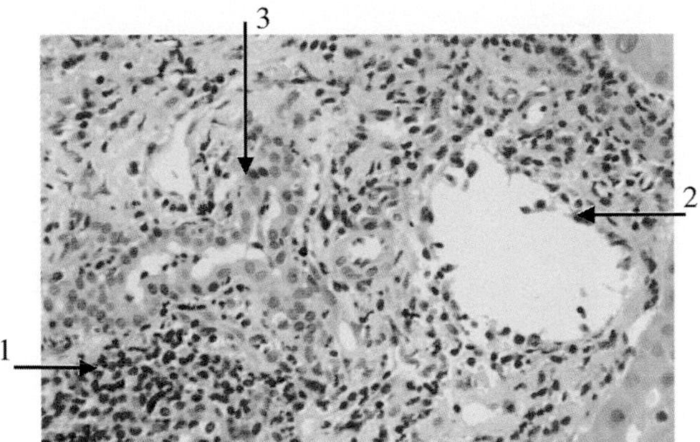

Plate 1.62

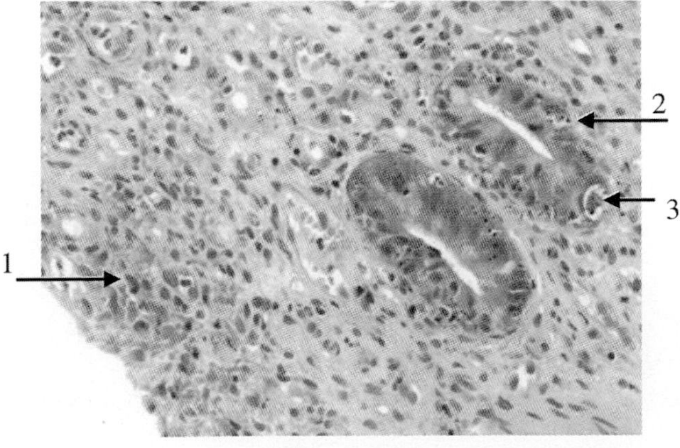

Plate 1.71

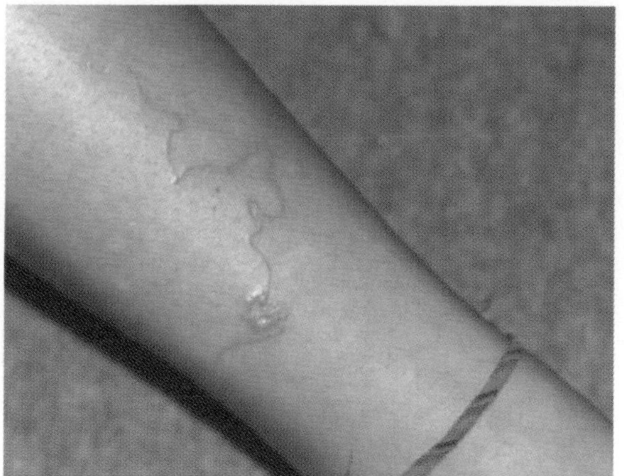

Plate 2.4

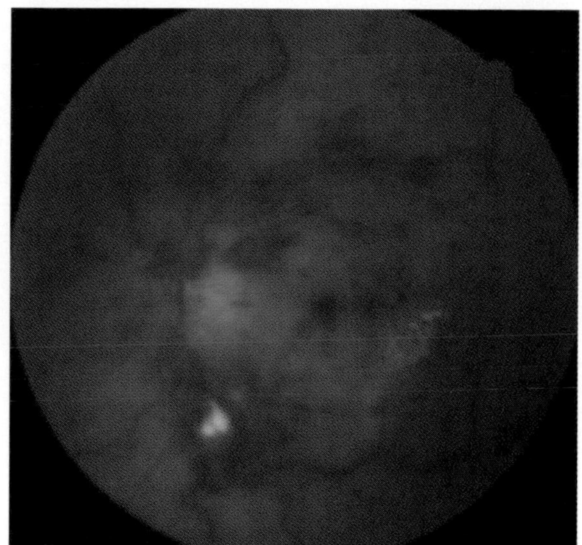

Plate 2.8

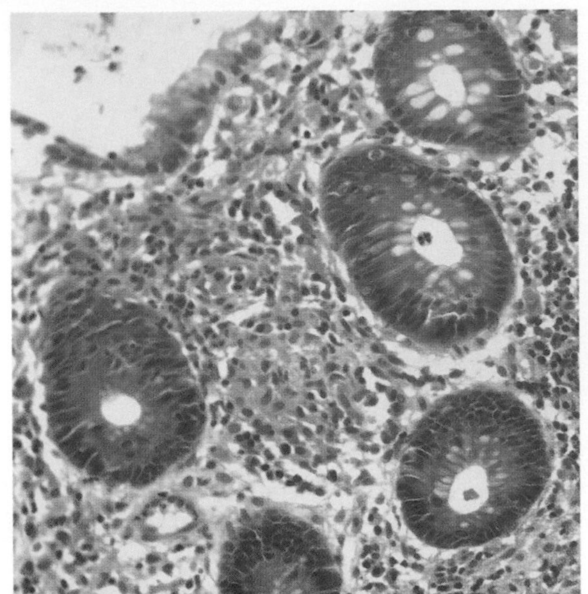

Plate 2.10

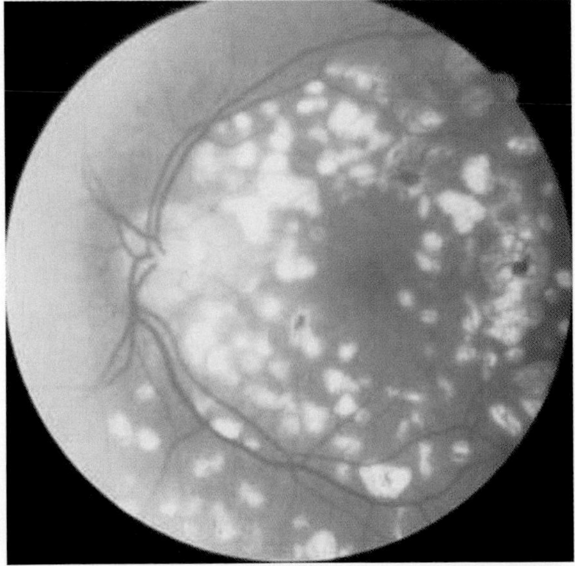

Plate 2.13

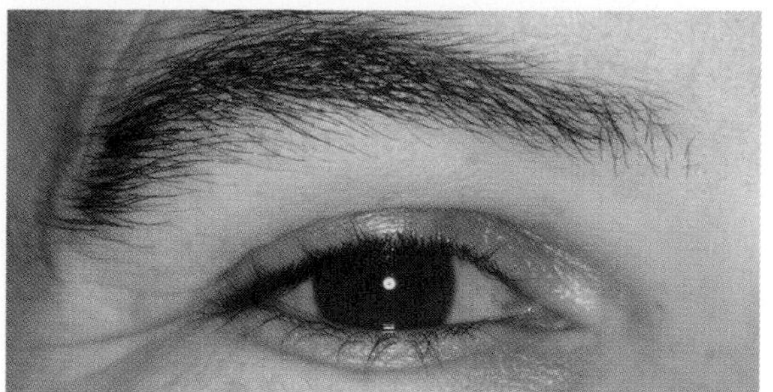

Plate 2.16

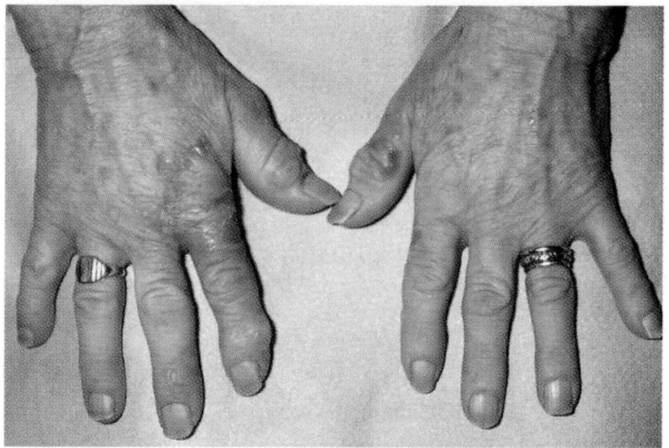

Plate 2.22

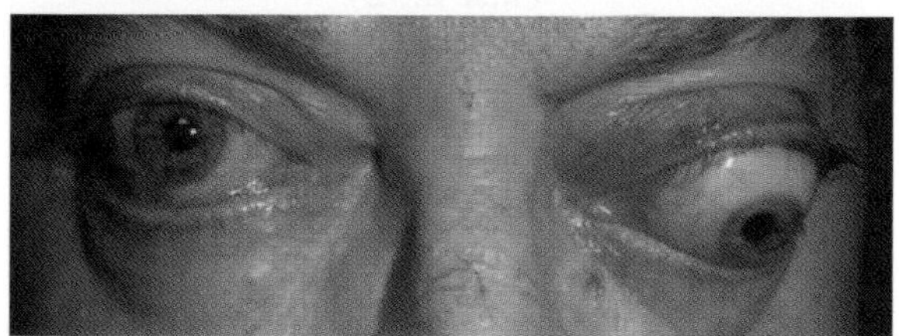

Plate 2.26
(with kind permission from Dr Shamira Perera)

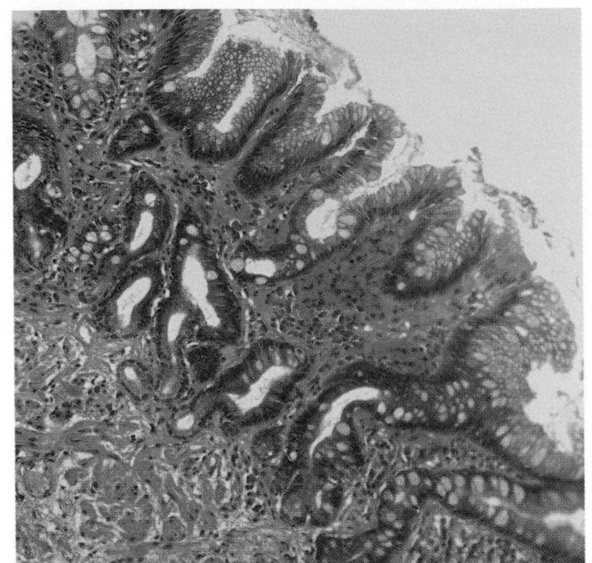

Plate 2.27

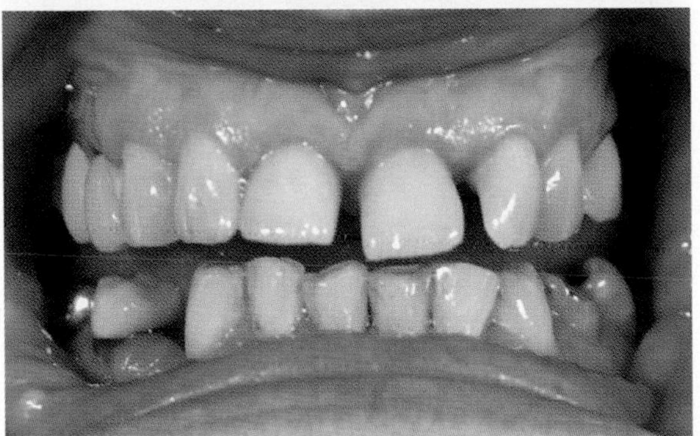

Plate 2.32

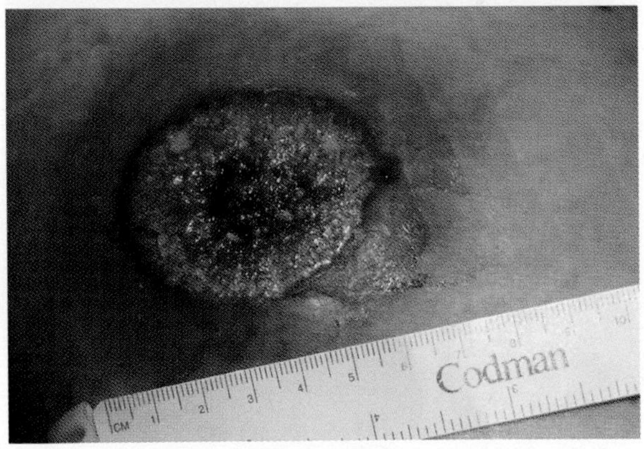

Plate 2.37

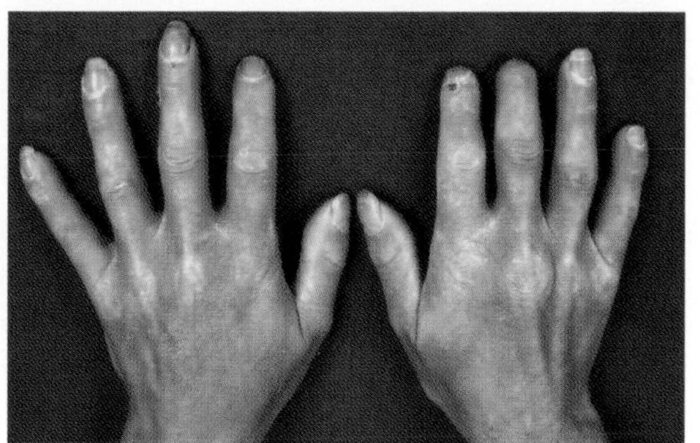

Plate 2.45

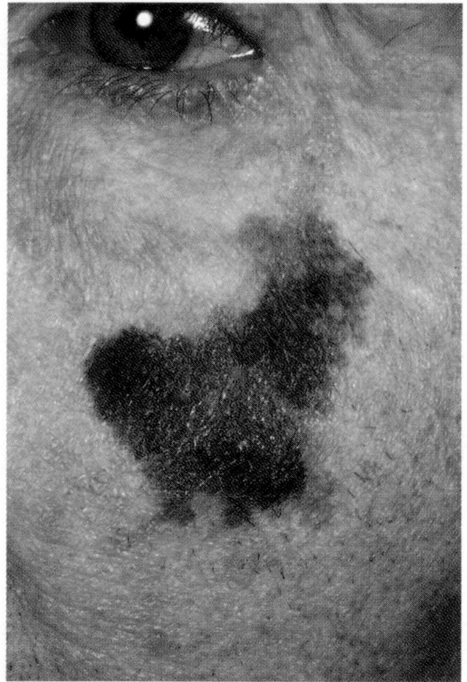

Plate 2.52

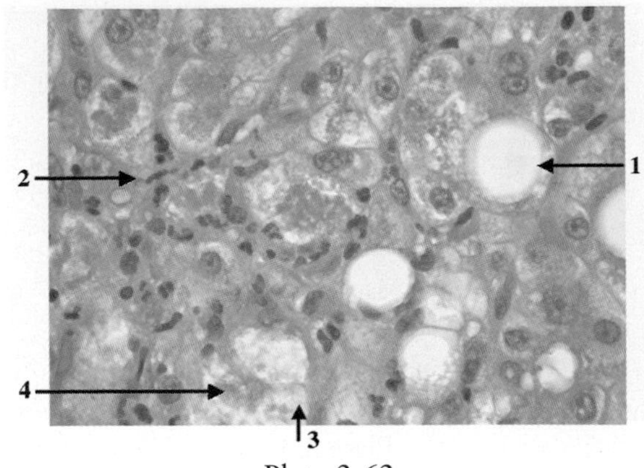

Plate 2.62

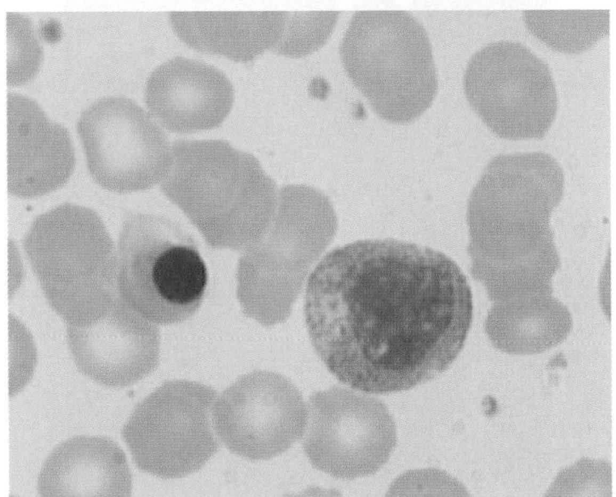

Plate 2.71

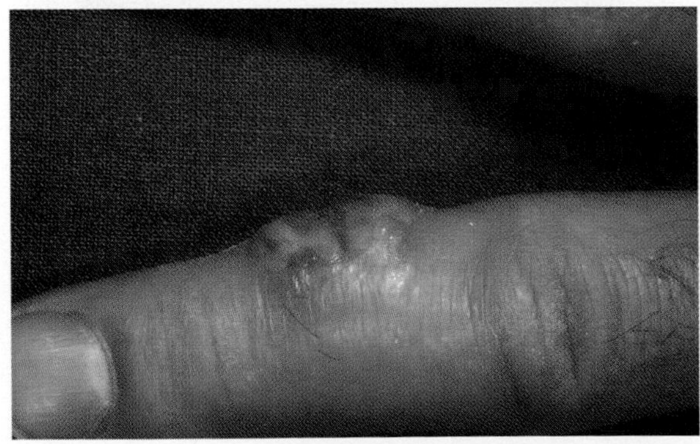

Plate 3.4

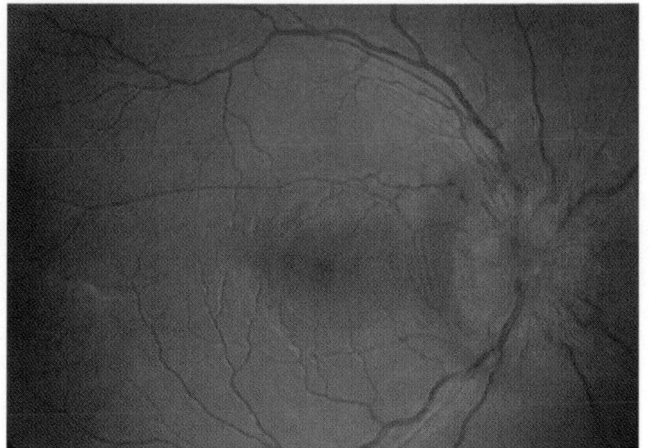

Plate 3.7

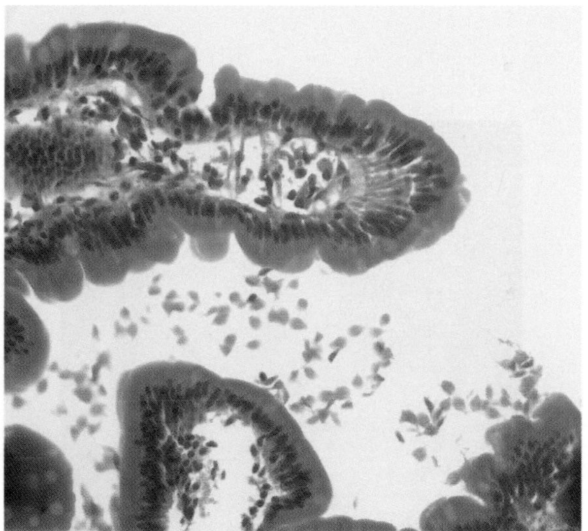

Plate 3.9

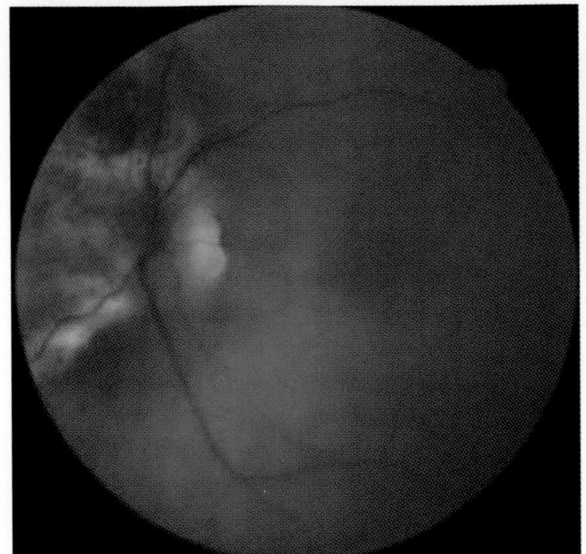

Plate 3.12

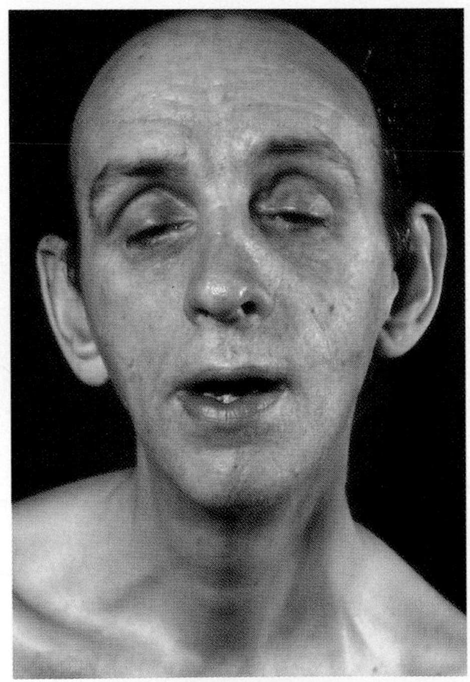

Plate 3.15
(with kind permission from Dr Stuart Coltart)

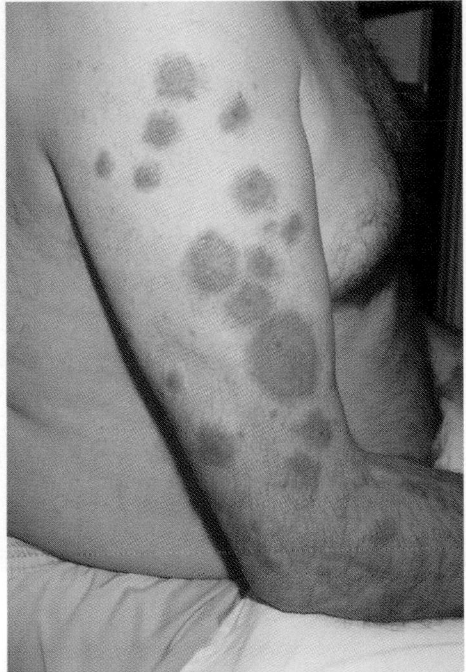

Plate 3.21

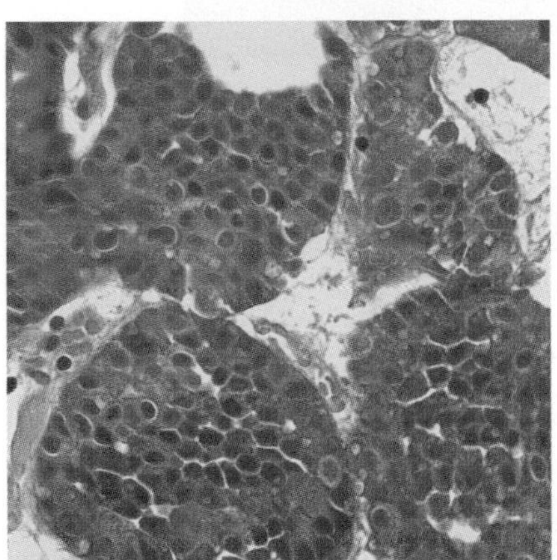

Plate 3.26A

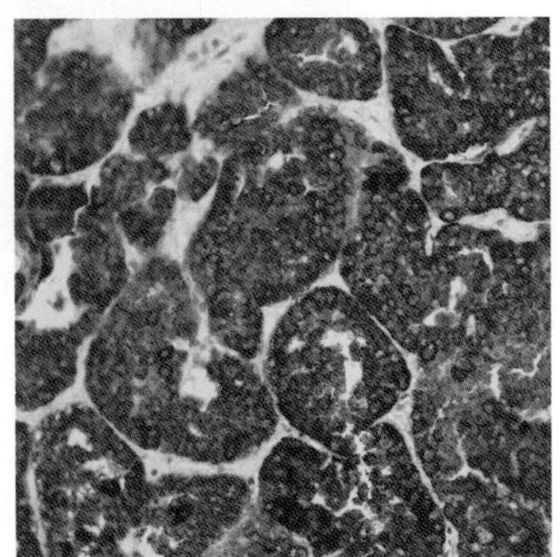

Plate 3.26B

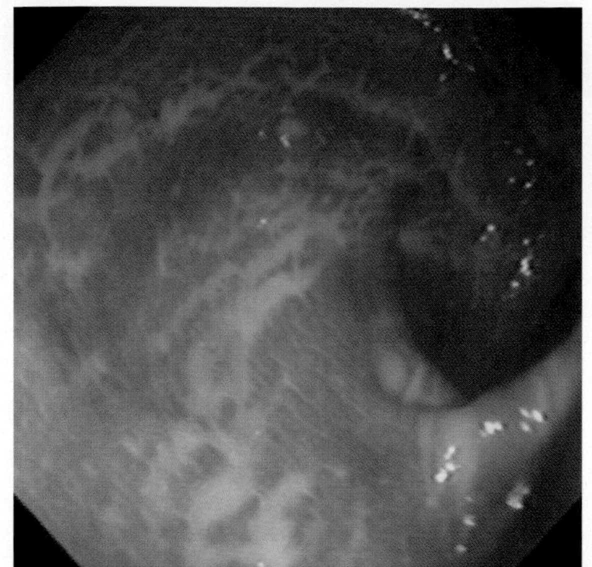

Plate 3.31

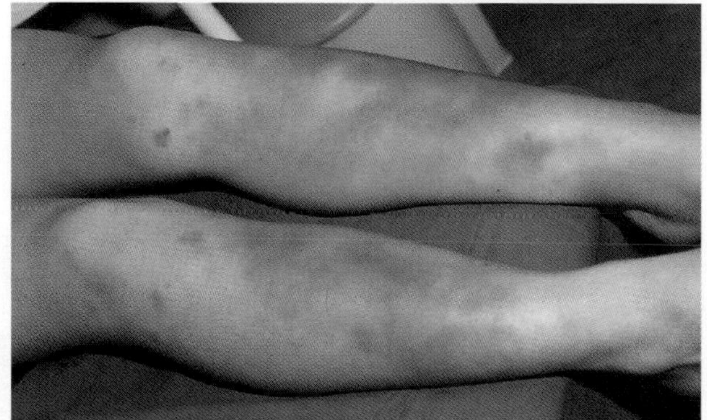

Plate 3.36

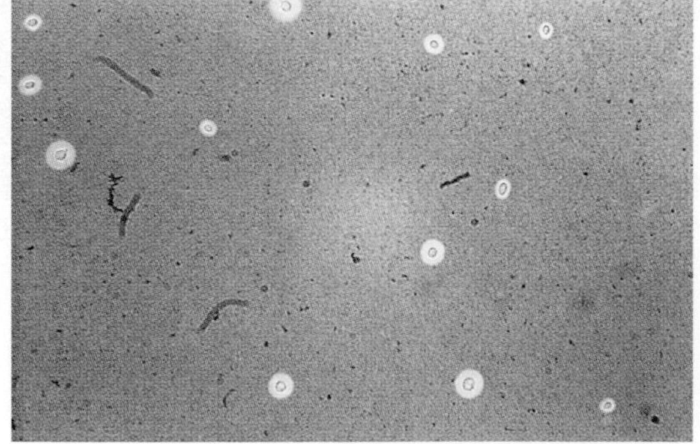

Plate 3.43

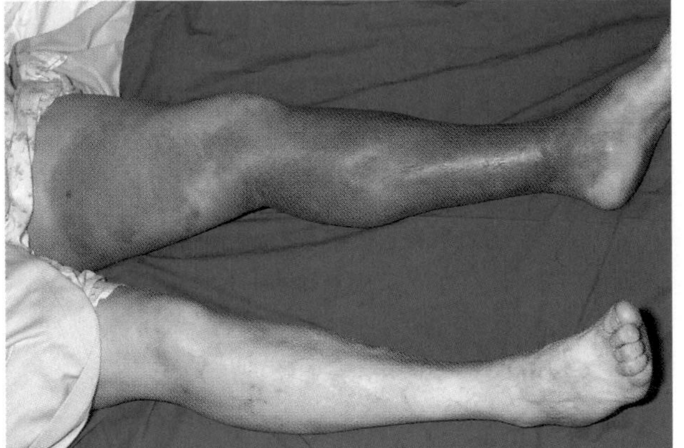

Plate 3.45

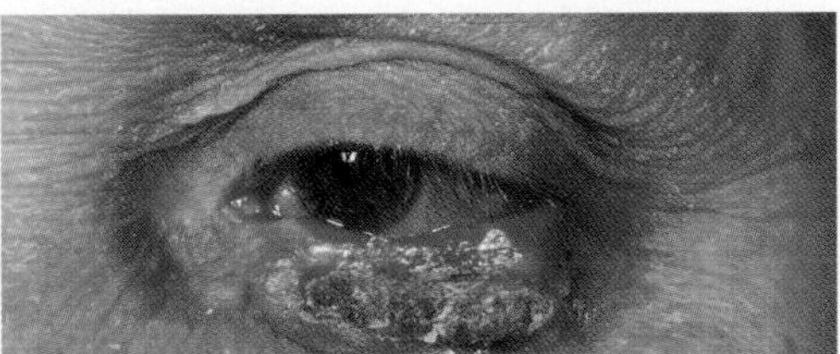

Plate 3.52

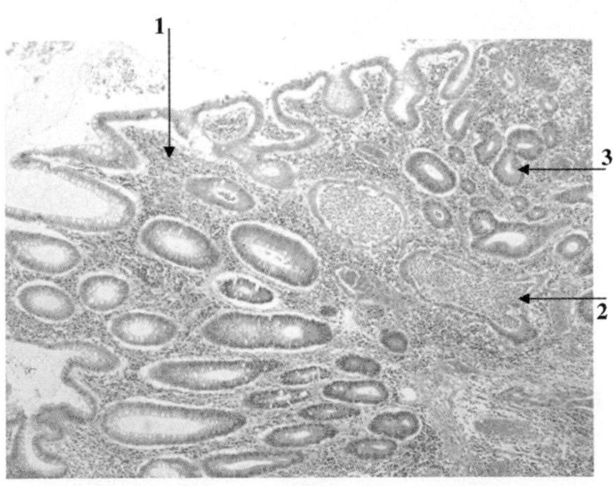

Plate 3.61

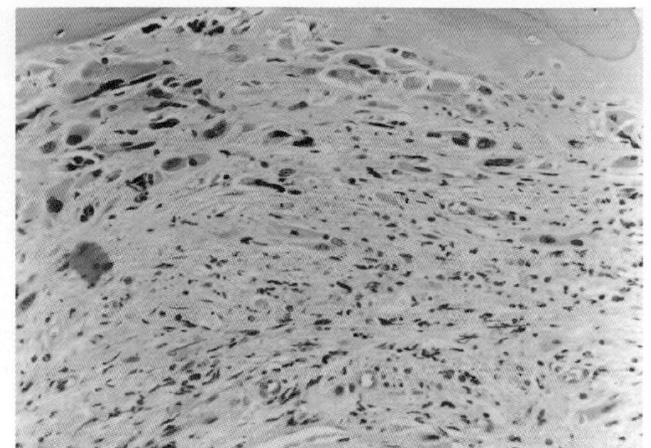

Plate 3.71

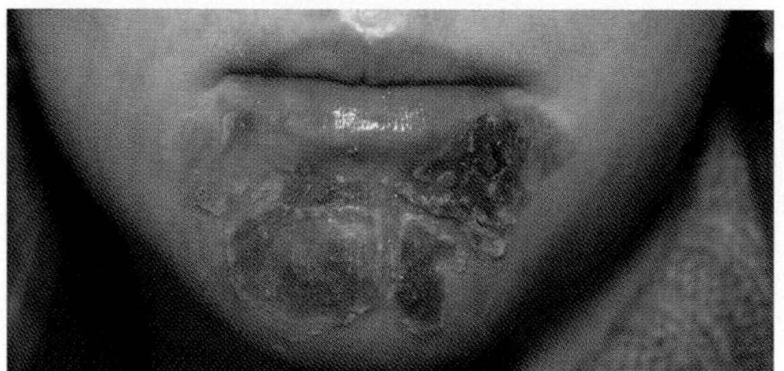

Plate 4.4

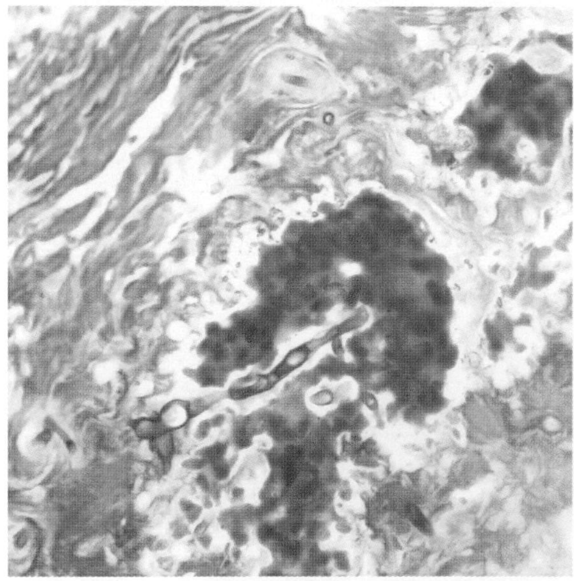

Plate 4.9B

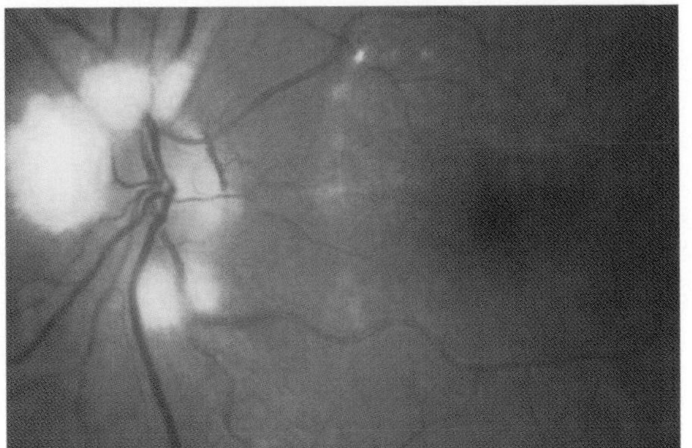

Plate 4.12

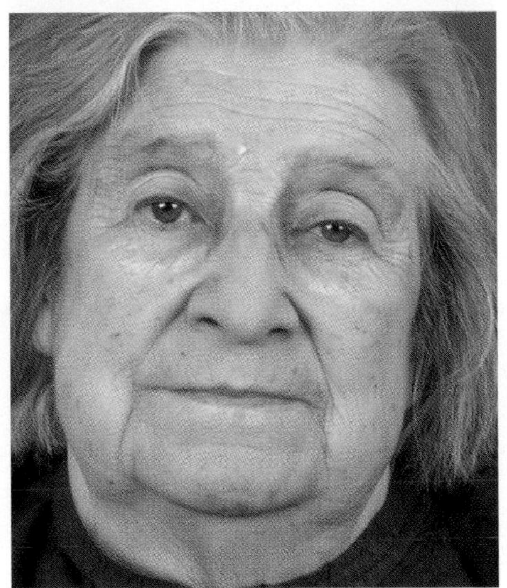

Plate 4.15
(with kind permission from Dr Stuart Coltart)

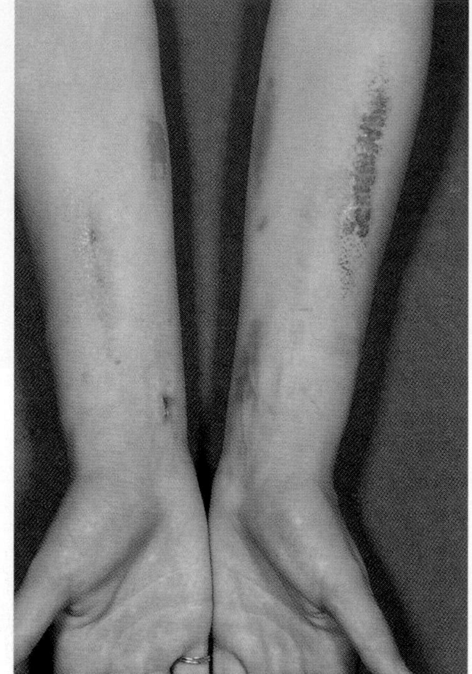

Plate 4.21

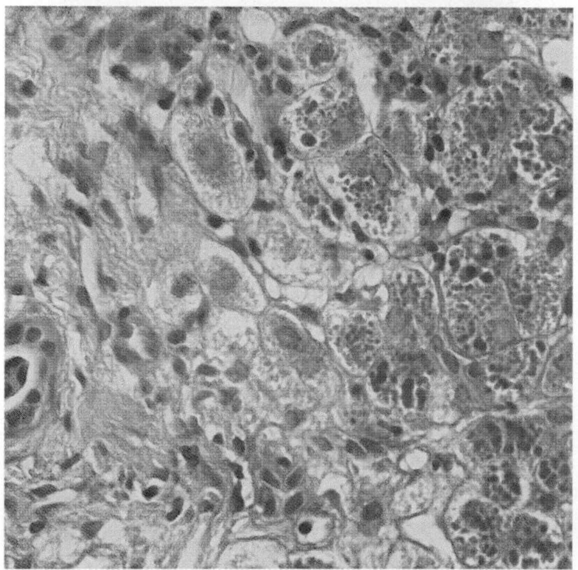

Plate 4.25

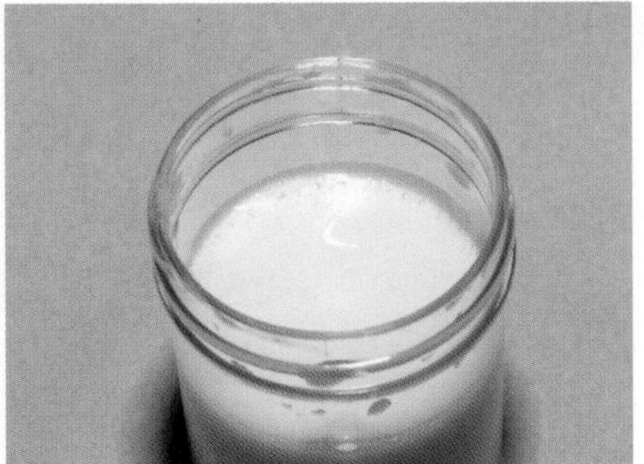

Plate 4.29

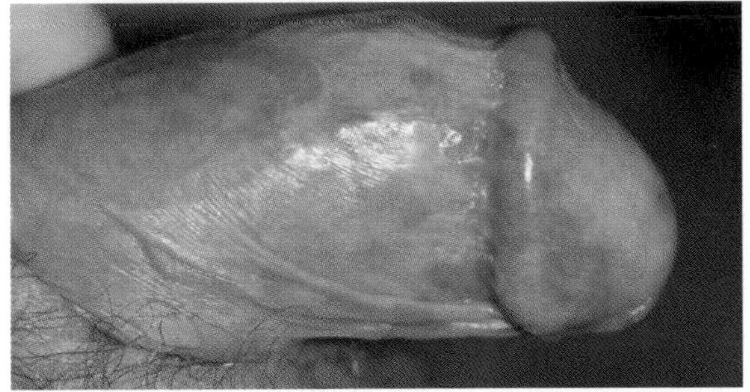

Plate 4.34

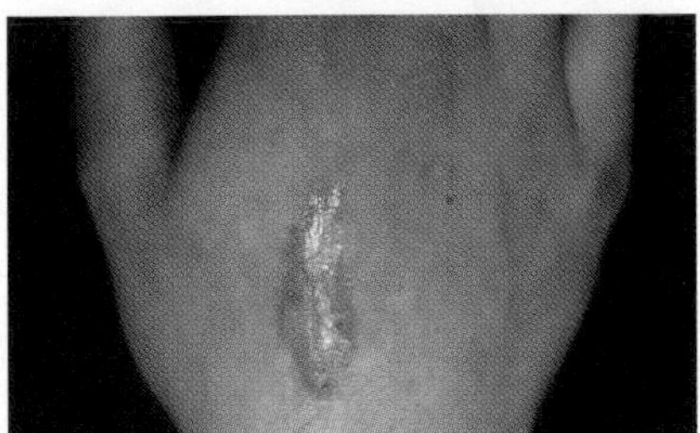

Plate 4.43

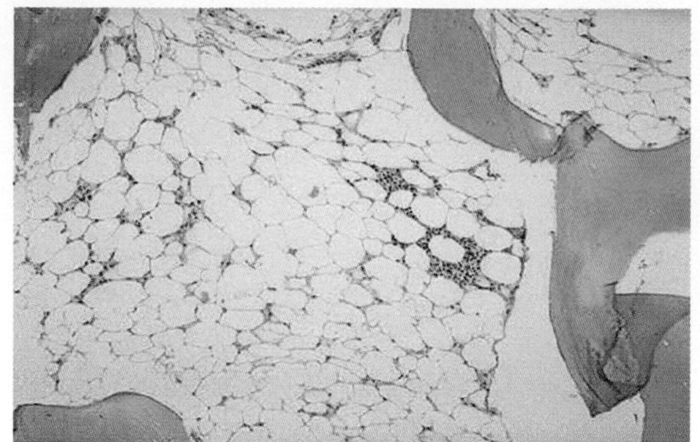

Plate 4.44

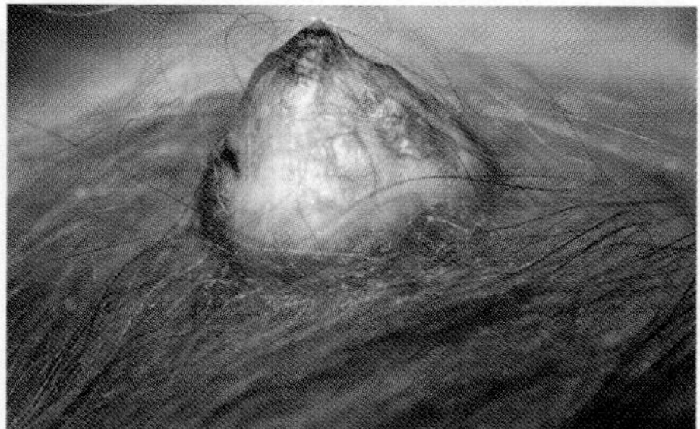

Plate 4.50

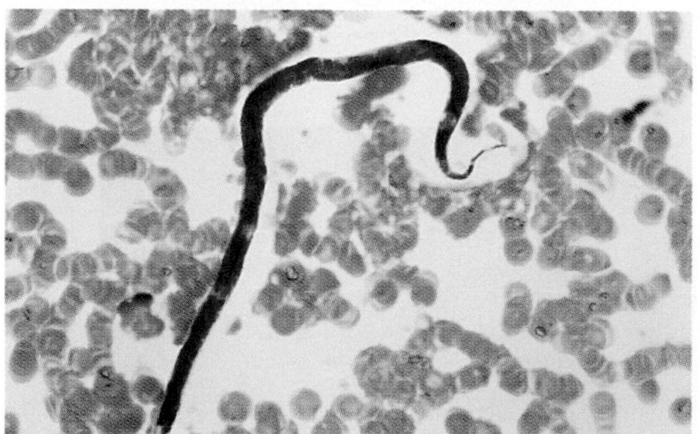

Plate 4.57

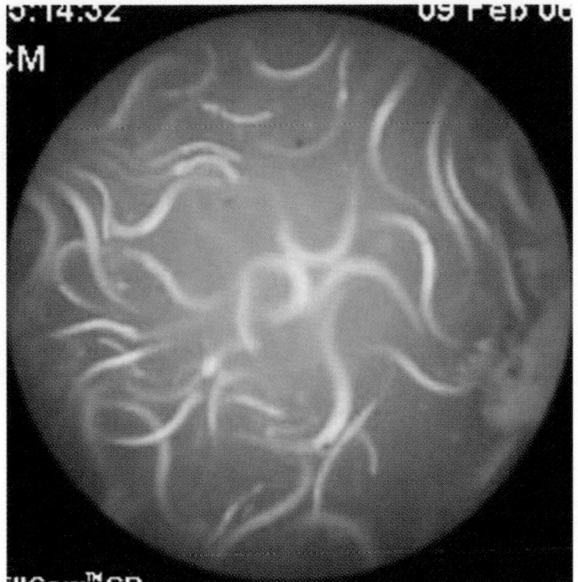

Plate 4.61

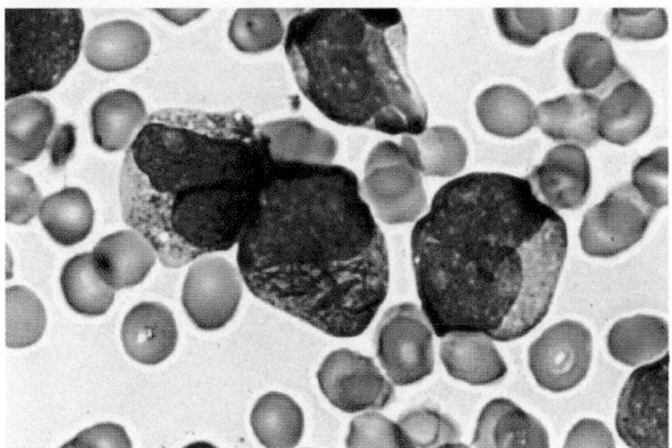

Plate 4.71

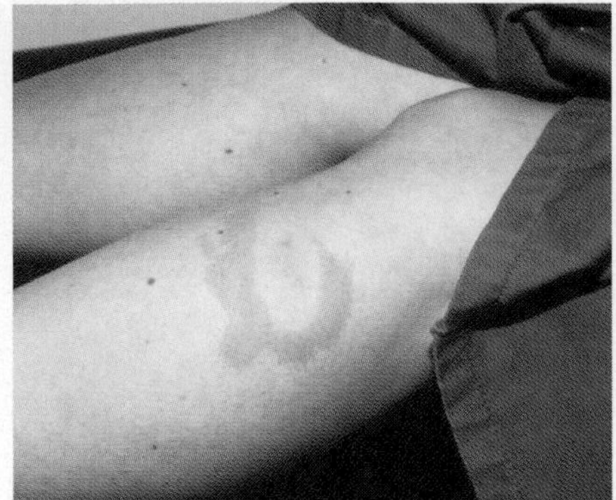

Plate 5.4

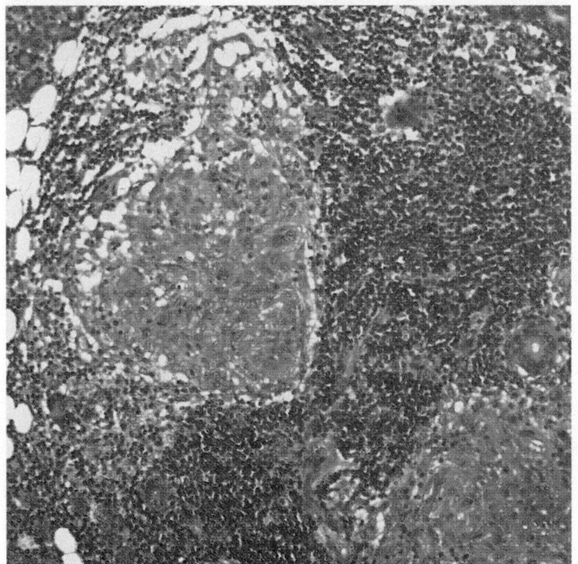

Plate 5.9

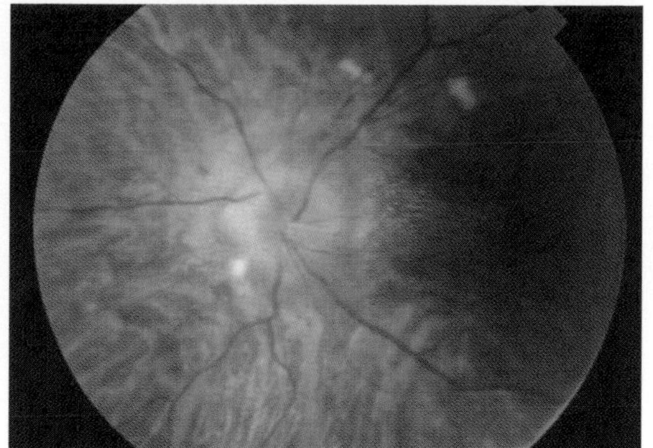

Plate 5.12

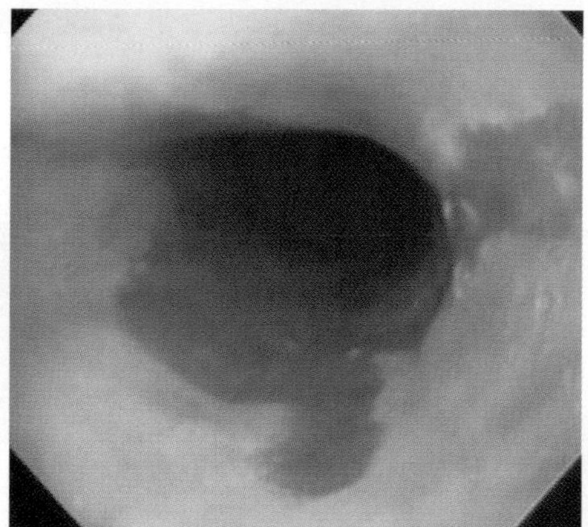

Plate 5.15

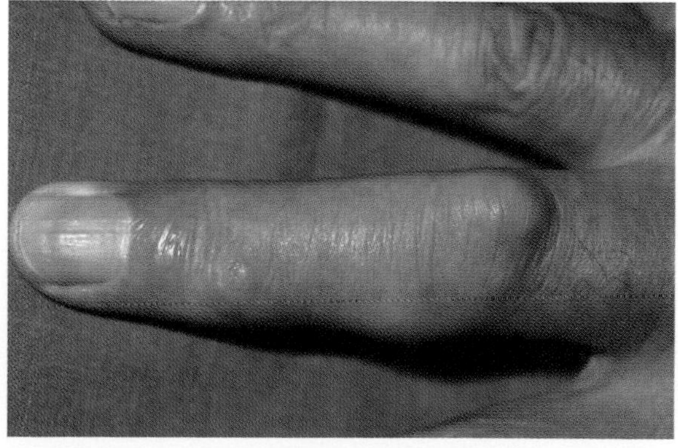

Plate 5.20

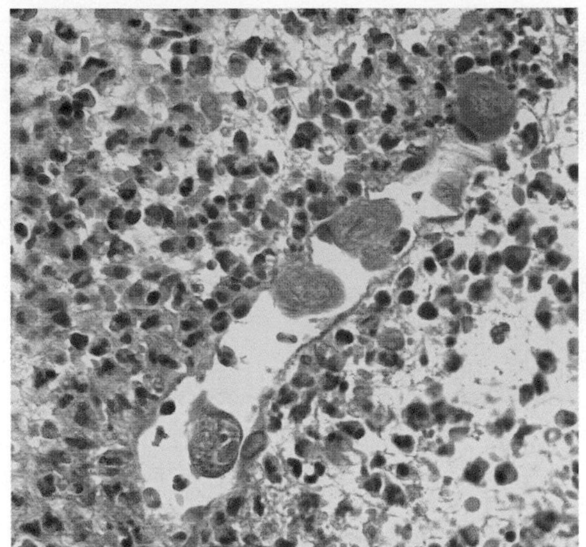

Plate 5.26

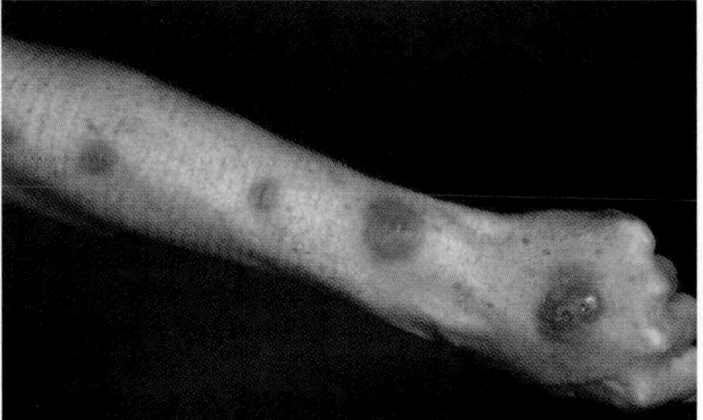

Plate 5.30

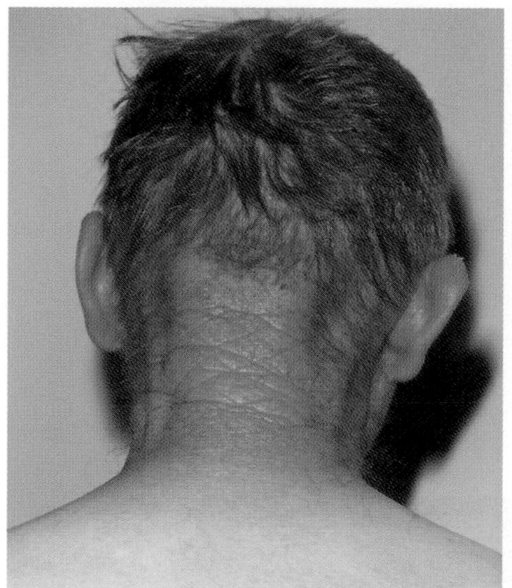

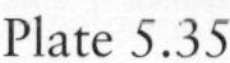

Plate 5.35

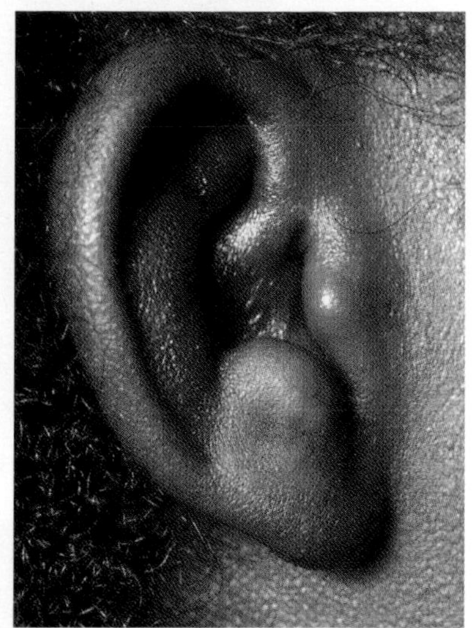

Plate 5.42

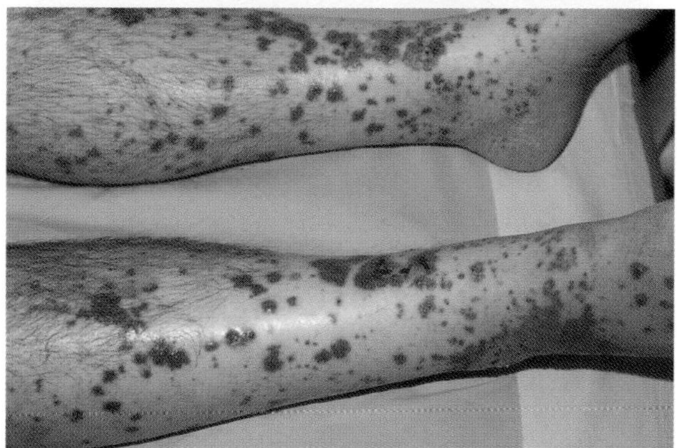

Plate 5.44

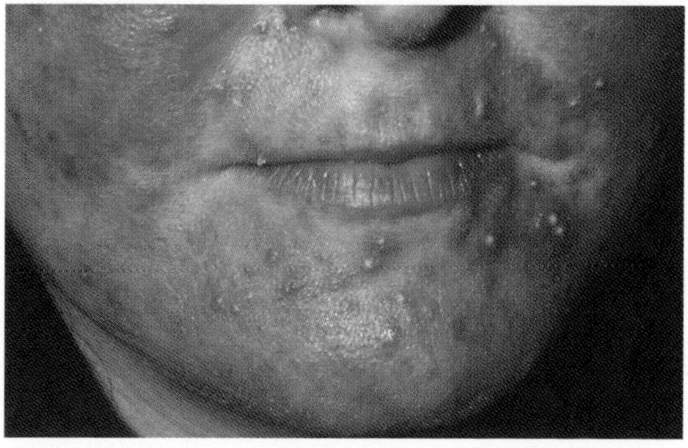

Plate 5.50

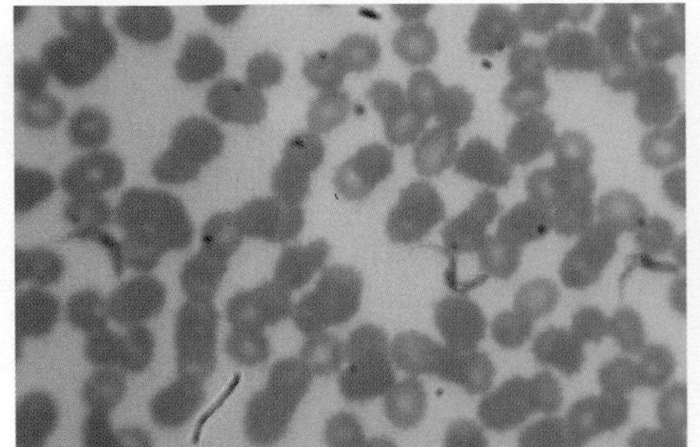

Plate 5.57

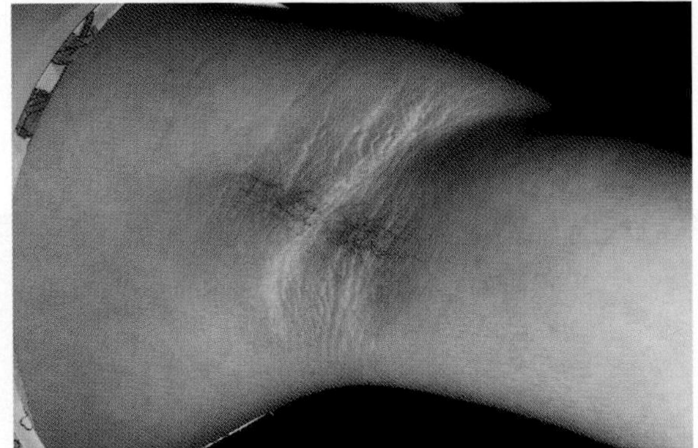

Plate 6.4

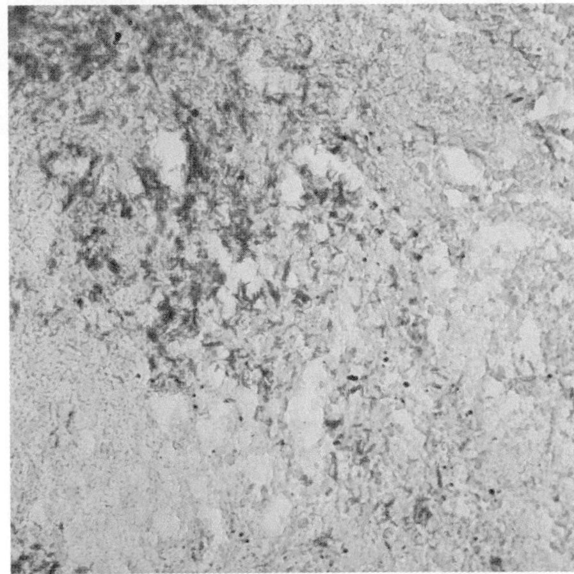

Plate 6.9

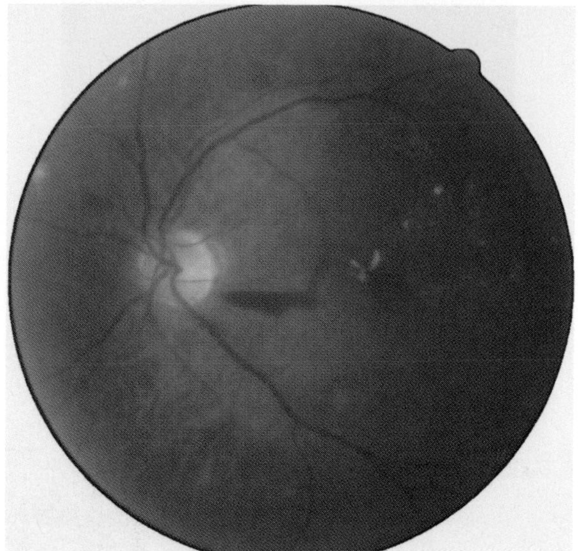

Plate 6.12

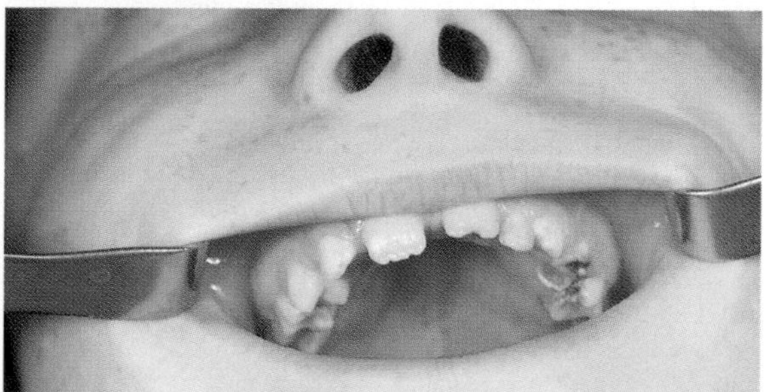

Plate 6.15

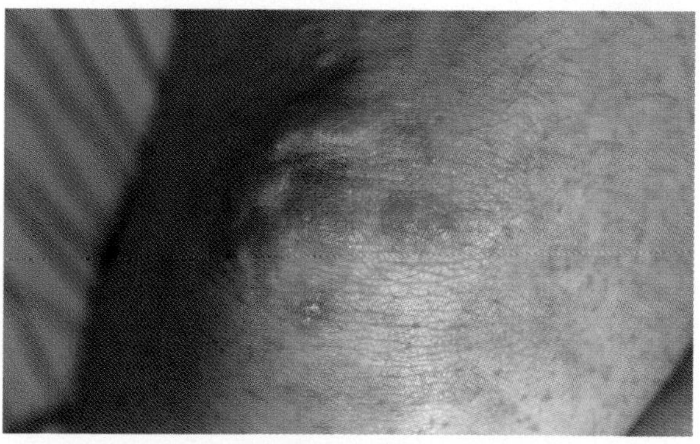

Plate 6.20

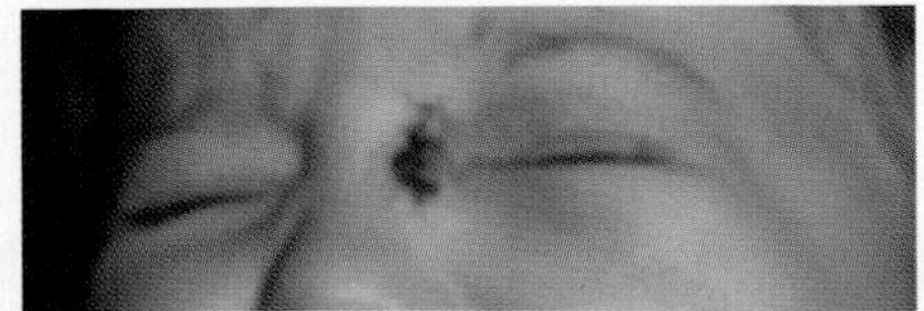

Plate 6.24
(with kind permission from Dr Shamira Perera)

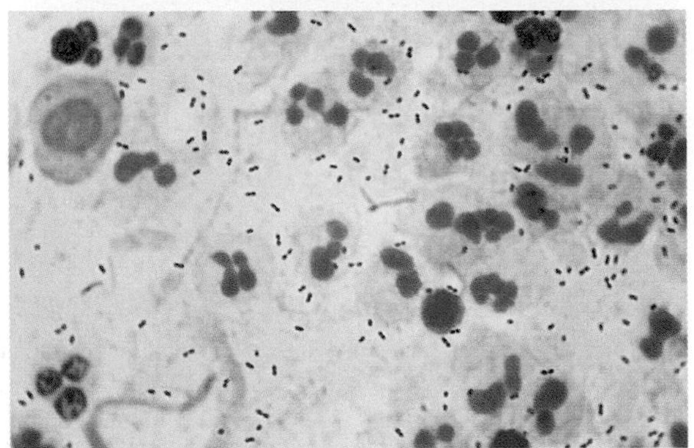

Plate 6.28

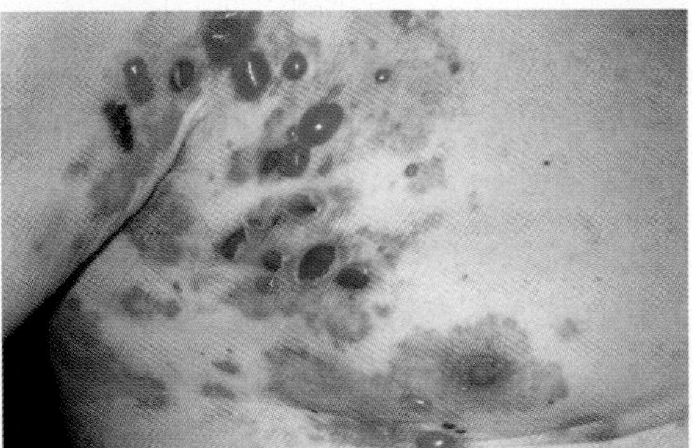

Plate 6.33

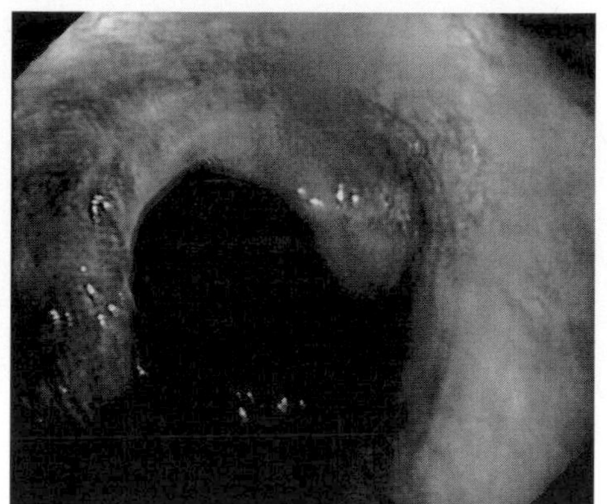

Plate 6.40

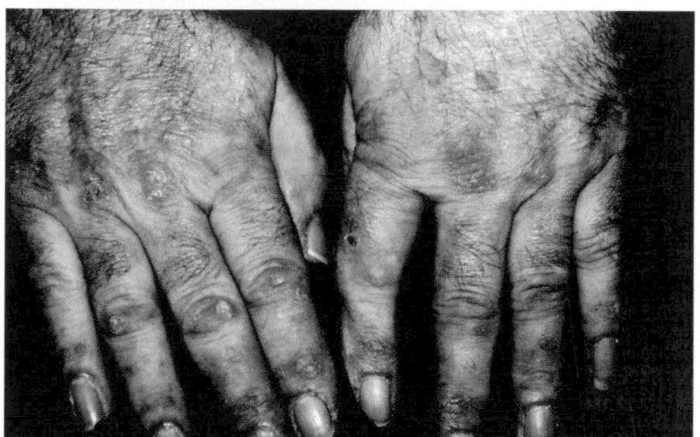

Plate 6.42

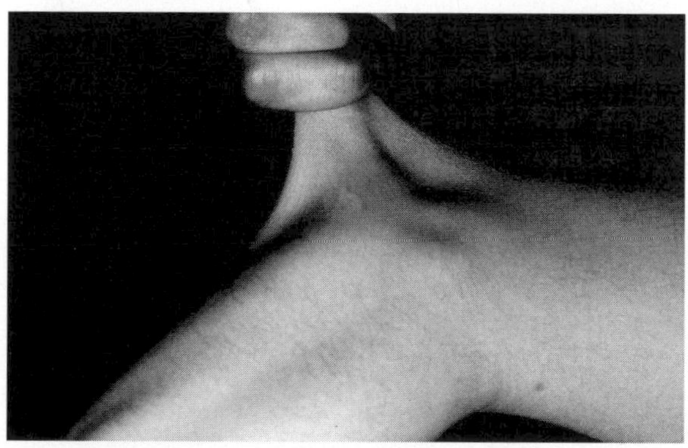

Plate 6.47

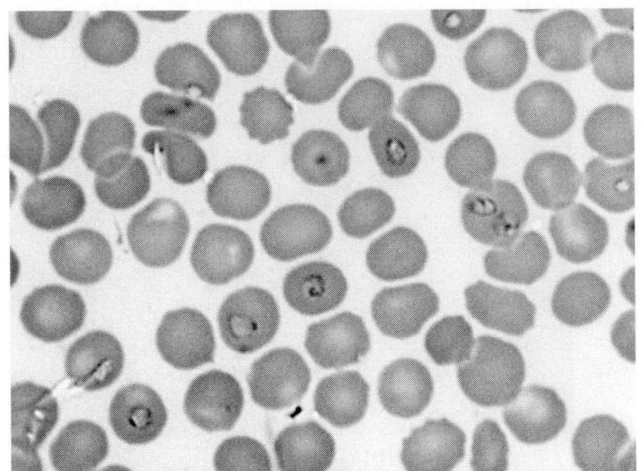

Plate 6.54

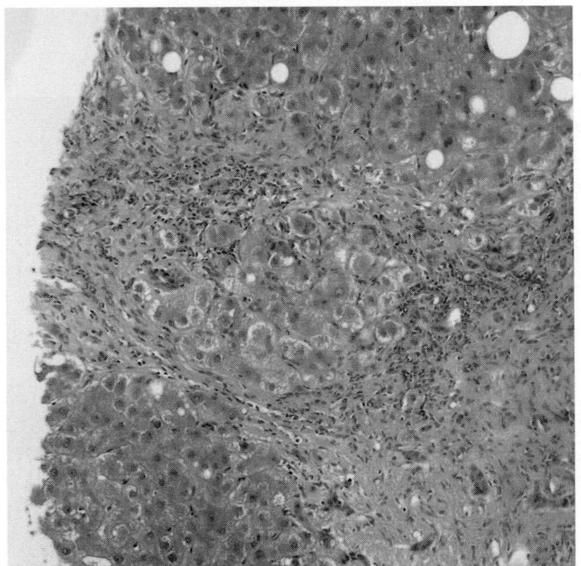

Plate 6.55

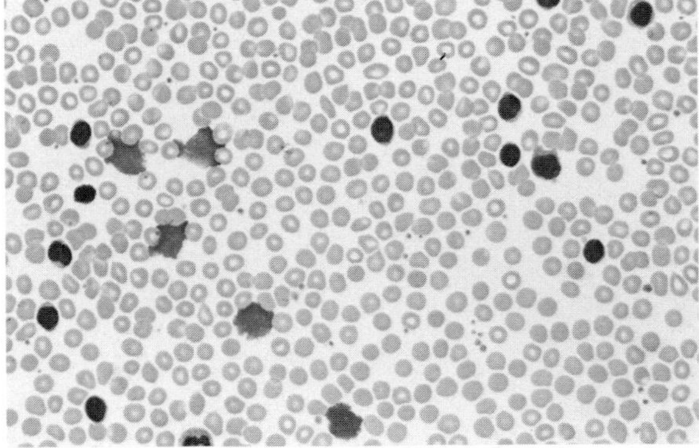

Plate 6.57

Index

α_1-antitrypsin deficiency 4.25, 6.38
Absence seizures 5.58
Absolute risk reduction 6.6
Acanthosis Nigricans 6.4
Achalasia 1.18, 3.59
Acromegaly 2.32
Acute cellular rejection 1.62
Acute colitis 5.46
Acute coronary syndrome 5.1
Acute liver failure 5.52
Acute Myeloid Leukaemia 4.71
Acute Pancreatitis 5.38
Addisons disease 4.5
Adult respiratory distress syndrome (ARDS) 3.41
Alcoholic cirrhosis 6.7
Alcoholic hepatitis 2.62
Alcoholic neuropathy 1.67
Alkaptonuria 4.48
Allergic bronchopulmonary aspergillosis (ABPA) 1.42
Alport's Syndrome 4.60
Alzheimer's disease 4.67
Amoebic liver abscess 2.11
Amyoidosis 1.27, 2.31
Androgen insensitivity 2.53
Ankylosing Spondylitis 2.18
Aortic stenosis 4.18, 4.32
Aplastic Anaemia 4.44
Arterial blood gases 1.30, 2.14, 2.30, 3.29, 4.27
Asbestos plaque 1.74
Ascending cholangitis 4.7, 2.56
Ascites 1.40, 4.29, 5.54
Aspergillosis 4.9
Asthma–acute 5.13
Asthma–chronic 1.64
Asthma–ventilation 1.73
Asystole 4.33
Atrial fibrillation–Rx 4.1
Atrial flutter 6.19
Atrial septal defect 5.18
Autoimmune hepatitis 3.24
Autoimmune polyglandular syndrome 1 6.51
Autoimmune polyglandular syndrome 2 1.57
Avian influenza 1.68

Bacterial gastroenteritis 2.68
Back pain 5.48
Bacterial vaginosis 1.32
Barrett's Oesophagus 2.27 5.15
B-blockers 4.3
Basal cell carcinoma 3.52
Behçet's syndrome 2.16
Benign intracranial hypertension 1.12
Bile acid malabsorption 1.54
Biliary colic 1.56
Botulism 3.68
Brain tumour 3.74
Brainstem death 6.67
Brittle diabetes 5.55
Bronchiectasis 4.49
Brucellosis 3.27
Budd Chiari Syndrome 4.37

Capsule endoscopy 4.61
Carbon monoxide poisoning 1.21
Carcinoid 1.49, 3.26
Carcinoma of Colon 1.14, 2.54, 3.16
Carcinoma of Oesophagus 4.17
Carcinoma of Stomach 1.34
Carcinoma of Unknown Origin 1.72
Cardiac Arrest 2.2 4.33 5.34
Cardiogenic shock 1.63
Case control study 3.6
Cellulitis 3.45
Central diabetes insipidus 1.48
Central Retinal Vein Occlusion 2.8
Cerebellarpontine angle lesion 3.67
Cerebral haemorrhage 6.41
Cerebral infarct 4.16
Cerebral oedema 2.73
Cerebrovascular accident 2.12
Charcot Marie Tooth Disease 2.29
Cholesterol embolus 5.60
Choroidal melanoma 3.12
Chronic granulomatous disease 6.65
Chronic lymphocytic leukaemia 5.71, 6.57

Chronic obstructive pulmonary disease (COPD) 5.28
Chronic Pancreatitis 2.7
Chronic renal failure 2.66
Churg Strauss 1.70
Circinate balanitis 4.34
Cirrhosis 6.55
CMV colitis 5.26
Coeliac disease 2.40
Cohort study 1.6
Common bile duct stone 3.51
Complete heart block 3.2
Congenital syphilis 6.15
Conn's Syndrome 1.35, 3.58, 5.45
Consent to feeding 3.38
Consent to treatment 4.36
Constitutional growth delay 3.53
Continuous ambulatory peritoneal dialysis (CAPD) Peritonitis 1.66
CREST 5.14
Crohn's diseasel 2.61, 4.45
Cross sectional study 2.6
Cryoglobulinaemia 6.27
Cryprotococcal meningitis 3.43
Cushing's Syndrome 6.34
Cutaneous larva migrans 2.4
cutis hyperelastica 6.47
Cystic fibrosis 4.49

Decompensated liver disease–Ix 2.25, 6.7
Dengue Fever 3.10
Dermatitis Artefacta 4.21
Dermatomyositis 6.42
DEXA scan 1.7, 2.50, 5.21
Diabetic maculopathy 1.13
Discitis 1.75
Dissecting thoracic aortic aneurysm 2.63
Diverticular D 4.54
Dressler's syndrome 2.35
Drug induced cholestasis 4.24
Dystrophia myotonica 2.46 3.15

ECG 1.2, 1.20, 2.2, 2.20, 2.36, 2.41, 3.2, 3.19, 3.35, 3.60, 4.2, 4.19, 4.33, 5.2, 5.34, 6.2 6.19, 6.32
Ecstasy overdose 6.3
EEG 5.58
Ehlers–Danlos Syndrome 4.43, 6.47
Emphysema 4.47 5.40
Empyema 2.64
Erythema multiforme 3.21 3.42
Erythema nodosum 3.36
Exercise testing 3.1
Exophthalmos 2.26
Extradural haematoma 1.17
Extrinsic allergic alveolitis 6.26

Fallot's tetralogy 5.33
Familial Hypocalcaemic Hypercalcuria 6.21
Familial Mediterranean Fever 6.60
Fibromyalgia 2.15
Flow volume loop 5.40
Focal Segmental Glomerulosclerosis 5.56
Food intolerance 1.61
Friedreich's Ataxia 6.25

Gas gangrene 6.17
Gastrinoma 2.57
Giardia 3.9
Gilbert's Syndrome 3.39
Glucose-6-phosphate deficiency 6.8
Gonococcal arthritis 4.40
Goodpasture's Syndrome 2.42
Gout 5.20
Graft versus Host disease 1.71
Guillain Barre Syndrome–prognosis 1.29, 6.11
Guttate psoriasis 1.22

Haematuria 3.56
Haemochromatosis 6.23
Haemodialysis indications 1.3
Haemolytic uraemic syndrome 3.66
Haemophilia 6.35, 6.71
Henoch Schonlein Purpura 5.44
Hepatitis B 5.10
Hepatitis C 4.10, 5.62
Hepatocellular carcinoma 2.72
Hereditary Angioedema 1.9
Hereditary non-polyposis colon cancer (HNPCC) 4.52
Hereditary spherocytosis 3.8
Herpes simplex genitalis 1.69
Hiatus hernia 2.74
HIV–diarrhoea 6.59
HIV–HBV coinfection 4.69
HIV–needlestick 3.69
HIV–oppurtunistic infections 2.9 6.59

HIV–TB coinfection 6.64
HIV–treatment 1.28
HIV–vaccinations 2.69
HIV & Pregnancy 6.10
Hodgkin's lymphoma 3.72
Homocystinuria 3.50
Hydrocephalus 6.75
Hypercalcaemia of malignancy 1.38
Hyperkalaemia–ECG 2.20
Hypertriglyceridaemia 5.5
Hyperosmolar non-ketotic state (HONK) 2.5, 4.55
Hyperparathyroidism 4.30
Hypertension in pregnancy 3.63
Hypertensive retinopathy 5.12
Hypertrophic obstructive cardiomyopathy 2.59, 6.18
Hypoglycaemia 3.65
Hypogonadotrophic hypogonadism 1.55
Hyponatraemia 1.65
Hypopituitarism 2.65
Hypothyroidism 3.22, 4.15
Hypovolaemic shock 3.73

Idiopathic thrombocytopaenic purpura 1.8
IgA Nephropathy 6.53
Impetigo contagiosa 4.4
Implantable cardioverter defibrillators 4.63
Infectious Mononucleosis 5.25
Infective Endocarditis 1.36, 3.34
Infero posterior MI 6.2
Inhaled foreign body 4.41
Inotropic support 6.63
Insecticide poisoning 3.3
Insulin dependent diabetes 5.55
Intraventricular bleed 6.74
Irritable bowel syndrome 6.52
Ischaemic hepatitis 5.66

Jehovah's Witness 2.39

Kallman's syndrome 1.55
Klinefelter's syndrome 4.51

Lateral medullary syndrome 5.19
Left ventricular failure 1.1
Legionnaire's Disease 3.33
Leptospirosis 4.58
Lithium toxicity 2.21
Liver transplantation 1.62, 6.49, 6.62
Loa Loa 4.57
Long term oxygen therapy 2.49
Lung Cancer 4.39, 6.13
Lung function test 3.13 4.47
Lyme Disease 5.4
Lymphogranuloma venereum 5.69
Lymphoma 4.22
Leucoerythroblastic reaction 2.71

Malaria 6.54
Melanoma 2.52
Melanosis coli 3.31
MEN 2A syndromes 5.53
MEN I syndrome 4.53
Meningitis–Meningococcal 1.16
Meningitis–Pneumococcal 6.28
Menopause 5.51
Mesenteric angiogram 3.47
Mesenteric ischaemia 3.57
Metabolic acidosis 1.30
Methanol poisoning 3.20
Mixed metabolic & respiratory acidosis 4.27
Mobitz type 1 AV block–ECG 5.2
Mobitz type 2 AV block–ECG 4.2
Motor neurone disease 4.26
Multiple sclerosis 2.51
Myasthenia gravis 4.11, 5.11
Mycobacterium marinuum 5.30
Myelinated Fibres 4.12
Myelofibrosis 3.71

Narcolepsy 6.45
Non-alcoholic steatohepatitis (NASH) 4.62
Nasojejunal feeding 6.73
Nephrotic syndrome 5.56, 6.60
Neuroblastoma 4.72
Neutropaenic sepsis 6.56
Nodular goitre–Ix 5.36
Non-invasive positive pressure ventilation (NIPPV) 5.73
Number needed to treat 1.24

Obstructive sleep apnoea 3.64
Oculogyric crisis 5.3
Odds ratio 2.24
Oesophageal candidiasis 2.33
Oesophageal Carcinoma Rx 5.72

Oesophageal Variceal haemorrhage 6.7
Optic neuritis 2.67, 3.7
Orbital Cellulitis 6.24
Osteoarthritis 1.50
Osteomalacia 3.44
Osteonecrosis 2.50
Osteopaenia 1.7
Orf 3.4

Pacemaker–permanent 1.20
Pacemaker–temporary 3.60
Paget's disease 2.44, 3.5, 6.29
Pancreatic carcinoma 3.17, 4.74
Pancreatic pseudocyst 5.74
Papilloedema 1.12
Paracetamol overdose 4.20, 5.52
Paraspinal abscess 2.75
Parkinson's disease 2.48
Paroxysmal nocturnal haemoglobinuria (PNH) 1.26
Patent ductus arteriosus 2.19
PEG feeding 5.7
Pemphigoid 6.33
Pemphigus 1.47
Pericardial effusion–Echo 1.59
Periodic paralysis 5.67
Phaeochromocytoma 1.53, 6.43
Photocoagulation scars 2.13
Photosensitivity 5.35
Pinworm infection 4.61
Pituitary tumour 3.37
Pleural Effusion 4.64
Pneumonia 4.13
Pneumothorax 1.33
Polyarteritis nodosa 5.29
Polycystic ovarian syndrome (PCOS) 4.65
Polycythaemia rubra vera 4.8
Polymyalgia Rheumatica 1.31
Polymyositis 3.11
Pontine infarction 6.37
Porphyria cutanea tarda 2.22
Portal vein thrombosis 5.54
Post MI–Diabetic control 2.1
Post MI–Rx 1.19
Post parathyroidectomy hypercalcaemia 5.65
Post partum thyroiditis 6.48
Predictive Value–Negative 1.39
Predictive Value–Positive 6.22
Pregnancy & TFTs 6.5
Pre-proliferative Retinopathy 6.12
Preretinal Haemorrhage 6.12
Primary biliary cirrhosis 5.24
Primary polydipsia 3.28
Primary pulmonary hypertension 5.63
Progressive supranuclear palsy 3.48
Prolactinoma 4.35
Prostate Carcinoma 6.72
Pseudobulbar Palsy 5.39
Pseudohypoparathyroidism 2.38
Pseudomembranous colitis 1.10
Psoriatic Arthritis 2.70
Pulmonary embolus 3.29, 3.49, 5.75
Pulseless electrical activity 5.34
Pyoderma gangrenosum 2.37

Radiculopathy 3.40 4.38
Randonmised control trial 4.6
Refeeding Syndrome 2.47
Reiter's Disease 4.34 5.41
Relapsing polychondritis 5.42
Relative risk 3.23
Renal artery stenosis 6.58
Renal carcinoma 1.38
Renal stones 3.55 6.36
Renal transplant 4.66
Renal tubular acidosis type 1 4.56
Respiratory acidosis 2.14
Respiratory alkalosis 2.30 3.29
Retrosternal goitre 4.42
Rhabdomyolysis 6.3
Rheumatic Fever 6.31
Rheumatoid Arthritis 3.14, 3.70
Right middle lobe collapse 1.45
Right ventricular infarction 6.1
Ringworm 1.44
Rosacea 5.50

Salicylate overdose 1.3
Sarcoidosis 1.51, 2.17, 3.54, 5.9
Scabies 1.37
Schatzki ring 6.40
Schistosomiasis 2.28
Screening 5.37
Scurvy 1.58
Selection bias 5.6
Sensitivity 4.23
Sepsis 4.73
Short bowel syndrome 5.61

Sick euthyroid syndrome 2.23
Sickle cell disease 5.8
Simple partial seizures 4.46
Sjogren's Syndrome 6.14
Specificity 5.23
Spinal cord compression 3.75
Squamous cell carcinoma of skin (SCC) 4.50
Staghorn calculi 3.55
Status epilepticus 5.47
Stokes–Adams syncope 1.46
Strawberry Naevus 1.52
Sturge–Weber syndrome–Brain 6.50
Subacute degeneration of cord 1.41
Subarachnoid Haemorrhage 5.43
Subcapsular haematoma 5.70
Subdural haematoma 5.16 6.41
Superior vena cava obstruction 5.68
Supraventricular tachycardia 2.36
Syndrome of inappropriate antidiuretic hormone secretion (SIADH) 3.46
Syphilis–congenital 6.15
Syphilis–secondary 6.69
Syringomyelia 4.75, 5.27
Systemic sclerosis 2.45, 6.30

Tacrolimus toxicity 6.62
Takayasu's arteritis 4.28
Temporal arteritis 3.30
Temporal lobe encephalitis 2.34
Testicular Carcinoma 6.68
Thromboangitis obliterans 1.43
Thrombotic thrombocytopaenic purpura 5.22
Thyroid cancer 6.16
Thyroid nodule 5.36
Thyrotoxicosis 1.23
Torsades de Pointes 3.19
Toxic megacolon 5.46
Toxic Shock Syndrome 4.68
Toxoplasmosis 5.17
Transfusion reaction 3.25
Transjugular intrahepatic portosystemic shunt (TIPSS) 6.66
Tricyclic overdose 2.3
Trifascicular block 1.2
Tropical Sprue 6.61
Trypanosomiasis 5.57
Tuberculosis (TB) 2.10, 3.32, 4.31, 5.64, 6.9
Tumour lysis syndrome 1.60
Turner's syndrome 2.55
Typhoid 1.11

Ulcerative Colitis 3.61, 6.44
Upper GI haemorrhage 1.25
Uraemic pericarditis 2.60

Variceal haemorrhage 6.7
Varicella zoster 1.4
Ventilator associated pneumonia 6.70
Ventricular fibrillation (VF) 2.2
Ventricular septal defect 3.18
Ventricular tachycardia (VT) 3.35
Ventricular tachycardia with cardiacstandstill 6.32
Vitamin B6 deficiency 2.58
Vitamin C deficiency 1.58
Volvulus 5.32

Waldenstrom's Macroglobulinaemia 2.8
Wegener's Granulomatosis 2.43
Whipple's disease 6.39
Wilson's Disease 3.62
Wolff–Parkinson–White syndrome 2.41, 4.19

Xanthomata 6.20
X-linked recessive disease 6.35

Zollinger–Ellison syndrome 2.57